DEVELOPING AN EVIDENCE-BASED CLASSIFICATION OF EATING DISORDERS

Scientific Findings for DSM-5

DEVELOPING AN EVIDENCE-BASED CLASSIFICATION OF EATING DISORDERS

Scientific Findings for DSM-5

Edited by

Ruth H. Striegel-Moore, Ph.D.
Stephen A. Wonderlich, Ph.D.
B. Timothy Walsh, M.D.
James E. Mitchell, M.D.

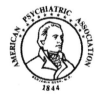

Published by the
American Psychiatric Association
Arlington, Virginia

Copyright © 2011 American Psychiatric Association
ALL RIGHTS RESERVED

Manufactured in the United States of America on acid-free paper
15 14 13 12 11   5 4 3 2 1
First Edition

Typeset in Adobe's Frutiger and AGaramond.

American Psychiatric Publishing, Inc.
1000 Wilson Boulevard
Arlington, VA 22209-3901
www.appi.org

Library of Congress Cataloging-in-Publication Data
Developing an evidence-based classification of eating disorders : scientific findings for DSM-5 / edited by Ruth H. Striegel-Moore... [et al.]. — 1st ed.
   p. ; cm.
   Includes bibliographical references and index.
   ISBN 978-0-89042-666-1 (pbk. : alk. paper)
   1. Eating disorders—Classification. 2. Evidence-based medicine. I. Striegel-Moore, Ruth. [DNLM: 1. Diagnostic and statistical manual of mental disorders. 2. Eating Disorders—diagnosis. 3. Eating Disorders—classification. WM 175]
   RC552.E18D48 2011
   616.85'260012—dc22

                                                                    2010045316

British Library Cataloguing in Publication Data
A CIP record is available from the British Library.

CONTENTS

PART 1

Improving the Definition of Symptoms and Syndromes of Eating Disorders

PART 2
Empirical Approaches to Classification:
Methodological Considerations and
Research Findings

PART 3
Eating and Feeding Disorders in
Childhood and Adolescence

David B. Herzog, M.D.
Debra Katzman, M.D., FRCP(C)
Richard E. Kreipe, M.D.
Bryan Lask, M.D.
Daniel Le Grange, Ph.D.
James D. Lock, M.D., Ph.D.
Katharine L. Loeb, Ph.D.
Marsha D. Marcus, Ph.D.
Sloane Madden, M.B.B.S. (Hons.), FRANZP, CAPCert, FAED
Dasha Nicholls, M.B.B.S., MRCPsych, M.D.
Julie K. O'Toole, M.D., M.P.H.
Leora Pinhas, M.D.
Ellen Rome, M.D., M.P.H.
Mae Sokol-Burger, M.D.
Ulf Wallin, M.D., Ph.D.
Nancy Zucker, Ph.D.

Irene Chatoor, M.D.
Robert P. Hirsch, Ph.D.
Stephen A. Wonderlich, Ph.D.
Ross D. Crosby, Ph.D.

Julie K. O'Toole, M.D., M.P.H.
Janiece E. DeSocio, Ph.D., R.N., PMHNP-BC
Daniel J. Munoz, Ph.D.
Ross D. Crosby, Ph.D.

Marian Tanofsky-Kraff, Ph.D.
Susan Z. Yanovski, M.D.
Jack A. Yanovski, M.D., Ph.D.

PART 4

Cultural Considerations in the Classification
of Eating Disorders

CONTRIBUTORS

Stephanie Bauer, Ph.D.
Research Scientist, Center for Psychotherapy Research, University Hospital Heidelberg, Germany

Anne E. Becker, M.D., Ph.D., Sc.M.
Professor and Vice Chair, Department of Global Health and Social Medicine, Harvard Medical School; and Director, Eating Disorders Clinical and Research Program, Massachusetts General Hospital, Boston, Massachusetts

Terrill D. Bravender, M.D., M.P.H.
Chief, Adolescent Health, Nationwide Children's Hospital, Columbus, Ohio

Rachel Bryant-Waugh, M.Sc., D.Phil.
Joint Head, Feeding and Eating Disorders Service, Department of Child and Adolescent Health, Great Ormond Street Hospital, London, United Kingdom

Irene Chatoor, M.D.
Vice Chair, Department of Psychiatry, Children's National Medical Center; and Professor of Psychiatry and Pediatrics, The George Washington University, Washington, D.C.

Mark Chavez, Ph.D.
Chief of Eating Disorders Program, Chief of Side Effects of Psychiatric Therapeutics Program, and Associate Director of Research Training and Career Development, Division of Adult Translation Research and Treatment Development, National Institute of Mental Health, Rockville, Maryland

Heather L. Corliss, M.P.H., Ph.D.
Instructor in Pediatrics, Division of Adolescent/Young Adult Medicine, Department of Medicine, Children's Hospital Boston and Harvard Medical School, Boston, Massachusetts

Ross D. Crosby, Ph.D.
Director of Biomedical Statistics and Methodology, Department of Biostatistics, Neuropsychiatric Research Institute; and Clinical Professor, Department of Clinical Neuroscience, University of North Dakota School of Medicine and Health Sciences, Fargo, North Dakota

Scott J. Crow, M.D.
Professor, Department of Psychiatry, University of Minnesota, Minneapolis, Minnesota

Bruce Cuthbert, Ph.D.
Director, Division of Adult Translation Research, National Institute of Mental Health, Rockville, Maryland

Janiece E. DeSocio, Ph.D., R.N., PMHNP-BC
Associate Professor, Seattle University College of Nursing; Research Coordinator, Kartini Clinic for Pediatric Eating Disorders, Portland, Oregon

Faith-Anne Dohm, Ph.D.
Senior Associate Dean and Professor of Psychology, Graduate School of Education and Allied Professions, Fairfield University, Fairfield, Connecticut

Angela Celio Doyle, Ph.D.
Clinical Associate, Department of Psychiatry & Behavioral Neuroscience, Eating Disorders Program, The University of Chicago, Chicago, Illinois

Kamryn T. Eddy, Ph.D.
Assistant in Psychology, Department of Psychiatry, Massachusetts General Hospital, Boston, Boston, Massachusetts

Scott G. Engel, Ph.D.
Research Scientist, Department of Clinical Research, Neuropsychiatric Research Institute, School of Medicine and Health Sciences, University of North Dakota, Fargo, North Dakota

Manfred M. Fichter, M.D., Dipl.Psych.
Professor of Psychiatry, Department of Psychiatry, University of Munich; Professor of Psychiatry, Department of Behavioral Medicine, Schoen-Klinik Roseneck, Prien, Germany

Alison E. Field, Sc.D.
Associate Professor of Pediatrics, Division of Adolescent/Young Adult Medicine, Department of Medicine, Children's Hospital Boston and Harvard Medical School; Associate Epidemiologist, Channing Laboratory, Department of Medicine, Brigham and Women's Hospital and Harvard Medical School; and Associate Professor in the Department of Epidemiology, Harvard School of Public Health, Boston, Massachusetts

Erin L. Fink, M.S.
Doctoral Candidate, Department of Psychology, Florida State University, Tallahassee, Florida

Kathryn Gordon, Ph.D.
Assistant Professor, Department of Psychology, North Dakota State University, Fargo, North Dakota

Julie A. Gravener, M.A.
Graduate Student, Department of Psychology, University of Rochester, Rochester, New York

Alissa A. Haedt, M.A.
Doctoral Candidate, Department of Psychology, The University of Iowa, Iowa City, Iowa

David B. Herzog, M.D.
Director, Harris Center at Massachusetts General Hospital, Boston; and Endowed Professor of Psychiatry in the Field of Eating Disorders, Harvard Medical School, Boston, Massachusetts

Anja Hilbert, Ph.D.
Professor of Clinical Psychology, Department of Psychology, University of Fribourg, Fribourg, Switzerland

Robert P. Hirsch, Ph.D.
Professor of Epidemiology and Biostatistics, The George Washington University, Washington, D.C.

Jill Holm-Denoma, Ph.D.
Clinical Assistant Professor, Department of Psychology, University of Denver, Denver, Colorado

Nicholas J. Horton, Sc.D.
Associate Professor of Mathematics and Statistics, Department of Mathematics and Statistics, Smith College, Northampton, Massachusetts

Renee Rienecke Hoste, Ph.D.
Assistant Professor, Department of Psychiatry & Behavioral Neuroscience, Eating Disorders Program, The University of Chicago, Chicago, Illinois

Thomas E. Joiner, Ph.D.
Robert O. Lawton Distinguished Professor of Psychology, Department of Psychology, Florida State University, Tallahassee, Florida

Kirsten A. Kahler, B.A.
Department of Psychology, Concordia College; Department of Clinical Research, Neuropsychiatric Research Institute, School of Medicine and Health Sciences, University of North Dakota, Fargo, North Dakota

Debra Katzman, M.D., FRCP(C)
Head, Division of Adolescent Medicine, and Medical Director, Eating Disorders Program, The Hospital for Sick Children, University of Toronto; Associate Professor, Department of Pediatrics, University of Toronto; and Associate Scientist, Child Health Evaluative Services, Research Institute at The Hospital for Sick Children, University of Toronto, Toronto, Ontario, Canada

Pamela K. Keel, Ph.D.
Professor, Department of Psychology, Florida State University, Tallahassee, Florida

Haruka Konishi, B.A.
Research Assistant, Department of Psychology, College of Liberal Arts, Temple University in Japan, Tokyo

Richard E. Kreipe, M.D.
Professor, Department of Pediatrics, University of Rochester School of Medicine and Dentistry, Rochester, New York

Bryan Lask, M.D.
Emeritus Professor of Child and Adolescent Psychiatry, St. George's Hospital Medical School, University of London, London, United Kingdom; Research Director, Huntercombe Hospital Group and Oslo University Hospital, Oslo, Norway; and Honorary Consultant, Great Ormond Street Children's Hospital; Academic Director, Ellern Mede Center for Eating Disorders; and Consultant Child & Adolescent and Adult Psychiatrist, The Child and Family Practice, London, United Kingdom

Daniel Le Grange, Ph.D.
Professor, Department of Psychiatry and Behavioral Neuroscience; Director, Eating Disorders Clinic, The University of Chicago Medical Center, Chicago, Illinois

Olga Levin
Research Coordinator, Eating Disorders Clinical and Research Program, Massachusetts General Hospital, Boston, Massachusetts

James D. Lock, M.D., Ph.D.
Director, Stanford Child and Adolescent Eating Disorder Program, Department of Psychiatry and Behavioral Sciences, Stanford University School of Medicine, Stanford, California

Katharine L. Loeb, Ph.D.
Associate Professor, Department of Psychology, Farleigh Dickinson University, Madison, New Jersey; and Adjunct Associate Professor, Department of Psychiatry, Mount Sinai School of Medicine, New York, New York

Wesley C. Lynch, Ph.D.
Professor, Department of Psychology, Montana State University, Bozeman, Montana

Chad M. Lystad, M.S.
Research Associate, Department of Clinical Research, Neuropsychiatric Research Institute, School of Medicine and Health Sciences, University of North Dakota, Fargo, North Dakota

Sloane Madden, M.B.B.S. (Hons.), FRANZP, CAPCert, FAED
Head of Department, Psychological Medicine; Co-Director, Eating Disorder Service, The Children's Hospital at Westmead, Westmead, NSW, Australia

Marsha D. Marcus, Ph.D.
Professor of Psychiatry and Psychology and Chief, Behavioral Medicine Program, Western Psychiatric Institute and Clinic, University of Pittsburgh Medical Center, Pittsburgh, Pennsylvania

Traci McFarlane, Ph.D., C.Psych.
Psychologist and Team Leader, Eating Disorder Program, Department of Psychiatry, Toronto General Hospital, University Health Network; and Assistant Professor, Department of Psychiatry, University of Toronto, Toronto, Canada

James E. Mitchell, M.D.
Christoferson Professor and Chair, Department of Clinical Neuroscience; Chester Fritz Distinguished University Professor; and President and Scientific Director of Department of Clinical Research, Neuropsychiatric Research Institute, School of Medicine and Health Sciences, University of North Dakota, Fargo, North Dakota

Daniel J. Munoz, Ph.D.
Assistant Professor, School of Professional Psychology, Pacific University, Hillsboro, Oregon

Yoshikatsu Nakai, M.D., Ph.D.
Director, Kyoto Institute of Health Sciences, Kyoto, Japan

Dasha Nicholls, M.B.B.S., MRCPsych, M.D.
Joint Head of Feeding and Eating Disorders Service, Department of Child and Adolescent Mental Health, Great Ormond Street Hospital for Children, NHS Trust, London, United Kingdom

Marion P. Olmsted, Ph.D., C.Psych.
Director, Eating Disorder Program, Department of Psychiatry, Toronto General Hospital, University Health Network; and Professor, Department of Psychiatry, University of Toronto, Toronto, Canada

Julie K. O'Toole, M.D., M.P.H.
Medical Director, Kartini Clinic for Disordered Eating, Portland, Oregon

Carol B. Peterson, Ph.D.
Research Associate, Department of Psychiatry, University of Minnesota, Minneapolis, Minnesota

Kathleen M. Pike, Ph.D.
Professor of Psychology, College of Liberal Arts, Temple University in Japan, Tokyo, Japan

Leora Pinhas, M.D.
Psychiatric Director, Eating Disorders Program, Department of Psychiatry, The Hospital for Sick Children, University of Toronto, Toronto, Ontario, Canada

Norbert Quadflieg, Dipl.Psych.
Research Specialist, Department of Psychiatry, University of Munich, Munich, Germany

Ellen Rome, M.D., M.P.H.
Section Head, Adolescent Medicine, General Pediatrics, Cleveland Clinic, Cleveland, Ohio

Heather K. Simonich, M.A.
Research Coordinator, Department of Clinical Research, Neuropsychiatric Research Institute, School of Medicine and Health Sciences, University of North Dakota, Fargo, North Dakota

Hayley H. Skinner, M.P.H., M.Sc.
Doctoral Student, Department of Epidemiology, Harvard School of Public Health, Boston, Massachusetts

April R. Smith, M.S.
Doctoral Candidate, Department of Psychology, Florida State University, Tallahassee, Florida

Angela Smyth, M.D.
Clinical Associate, Department of Psychiatry & Behavioral Neuroscience, Eating Disorders Program, The University of Chicago, Chicago, Illinois

Mae Sokol-Burger, M.D.
Associate Professor, Departments of Psychiatry and Pediatrics, Creighton University School of Medicine, Omaha, Nebraska

Ruth H. Striegel-Moore, Ph.D.
Professor of Psychology and Walter A. Crowell University Professor of the Social Sciences, Wesleyan University, Middletown, Connecticut

Sonja A. Swanson, Sc.M.
Doctoral Candidate, Department of Epidemiology, Harvard School of Public Health, Boston, Massachusetts

Robyn Sysko, Ph.D.
Assistant Professor of Clinical Psychology in Psychiatry, Division of Clinical Therapeutics, New York State Psychiatric Institute; and Department of Psychiatry, College of Physicians and Surgeons of Columbia University, New York, New York

Marian Tanofsky-Kraff, Ph.D.
Assistant Professor, Department of Medical and Clinical Psychology, Uniformed Services University of the Health Sciences, Bethesda, Maryland

Jennifer J. Thomas, Ph.D.
Assistant Psychologist, Klarman Eating Disorders Center, McLean Hospital, Belmont; Assistant in Psychology, Eating Disorders Clinical and Research Program, Massachusetts General Hospital, Boston; and Instructor in Psychology, Department of Psychiatry, Harvard Medical School, Boston, Massachusetts

Lenny R. Vartanian, Ph.D.
Lecturer, School of Psychology, The University of New South Wales, Sydney, NSW, Australia

Ulf Wallin, M.D., Ph.D.
Head of Research and Development, Centre of Eating Disorders, Lund University Hospital, Lund, Sweden

B. Timothy Walsh, M.D.
Ruane Professor of Pediatric Psychopharmacology in Psychiatry, Department of Psychiatry, College of Physicians and Surgeons of Columbia University; and Director, Division of Clinical Therapeutics, New York State Psychiatric Institute, New York, New York

Denise E. Wilfley, Ph.D.
Professor of Psychiatry, Medicine, Pediatrics, and Psychology, Weight Management and Eating Disorders Research Lab, Washington University School of Medicine, St. Louis, Missouri

Stephen A. Wonderlich, Ph.D.
Chester Fritz Distinguished Professor and Associate Chairman, Department of Clinical Neuroscience, and Director of Clinical Research, Neuropsychiatric Research Institute, University of North Dakota School of Medicine and Health Sciences, Fargo, North Dakota

Yuko Yamamiya, Ph.D.
Adjunct Faculty, Department of Psychology, College of Liberal Arts, Temple University in Japan, Tokyo, Japan

Jack A. Yanovski, M.D., Ph.D.
Head, Unit on Growth and Obesity, Program in Developmental Endocrinology and Genetics, Eunice Kennedy Shriver National Institute of Child Health and Human Development, National Institutes of Health, Department of Health and Human Services, Bethesda, Maryland

Susan Z. Yanovski, M.D.
Co-Director, Office of Obesity Research, and Director, Obesity and Eating Disorders Program, National Institute of Diabetes and Digestive and Kidney Diseases, National Institutes of Health, Department of Health and Human Services, Bethesda, Maryland

Nancy Zucker, Ph.D.
Assistant Professor and Director, Duke Center for Eating Disorders, Department of Psychiatry and Behavioral Sciences, Duke University Medical Center, Durham, North Carolina

Disclosure of Competing Interests

The research conference series that produced this monograph was supported with funding from U.S. National Institutes of Health (NIH) Grant MH 81447 (Principal Investigator: Stephen A. Wonderlich, Ph.D.). Additional funding for the conference series was provided by the American Psychiatric Association. The conference series was not part of the official revision process for *Diagnostic and Statistical Manual of Mental Disorders,* Fifth Edition (DSM-5), but rather was a separate, rigorous research planning initiative meant to inform revisions of the psychiatric diagnostic classification of eating and feeding disorders. No private or industry sources provided funding for this research review. The monograph was produced with funding from and published by the American Psychiatric Association.

Coordination and oversight of the research conferences were provided by an Executive Steering Committee, which included Stephen A. Wonderlich, Ph.D. (chair), Ross D. Crosby, Ph.D., Thomas E. Joiner, Ph.D., James E. Mitchell, M.D., Darrel A. Regier, M.D., M.P.H., Ruth H. Striegel-Moore, Ph.D., and B. Timothy Walsh, M.D.

The Executive Committee gratefully acknowledges the important contributions of the following individuals: Mark Chavez, Ph.D., at the National Institute of Mental Health, for his guidance and support in conceiving of the initial conference series concept and its implementation; Chad M. Lystad, M.S., at the Neuropsychiatric Research Institute, Fargo, N.D., for his assistance with the logistical details of the conference; and Emily A. Kuhl, Ph.D., at the American Psychiatric Association, for her editorial assistance.

The following contributors to this book have indicated a financial interest in or other affiliation with a commercial supporter, a manufacturer of a commercial product, a provider of a commercial service, a nongovernmental organization, and/or a government agency, as listed below:

Scott J. Crow, M.D.—The author has received research support from Pfizer Pharmaceuticals and Novartis.

April R. Smith, M.S.—The author has received research support from the National Institute of Mental Health.

Robyn Sysko, Ph.D.—The author owns stock in Pfizer Pharmaceuticals.

The following contributors to this book do not have any conflicts of interest to disclose:

Stephanie Bauer, Ph.D.

Anne E. Becker, M.D., Ph.D., Sc.M.

Terrill D. Bravender, M.D., M.P.H.

Rachel Bryant-Waugh, M.Sc., D.Phil.

Irene Chatoor, M.D.

Heather L. Corliss, MPH, Ph.D.

Ross D. Crosby, Ph.D.

Janiece E. DeSocio, Ph.D., R.N.,
    PMHNP-BC

Faith-Anne Dohm, Ph.D.

Angela Celio Doyle, Ph.D.

Kamryn T. Eddy, Ph.D.

Scott G. Engel, Ph.D.

Manfred M. Fichter, M.D., Dipl.Psych.

Alison E. Field, Sc.D.

Erin L. Fink, M.S.

Kathryn Gordon, Ph.D.

Julie A. Gravener, M.A.

Alissa A. Haedt, M.A.

David B. Herzog, M.D.

Anja Hilbert, Ph.D.

Robert P. Hirsch, Ph.D.

Jill Holm-Denoma, Ph.D.

Nicholas J. Horton, Sc.D.

Renee Rienecke Hoste, Ph.D.

Thomas E. Joiner, Ph.D.

Kirsten A. Kahler, B.A.

Debra Katzman, M.D., FRCP(C)

Pamela K. Keel, Ph.D.

Haruka Konishi, B.A.

Richard E. Kreipe, M.D.

Bryan Lask, M.D.

Olga Levin

James D. Lock, M.D., Ph.D.

Katharine L. Loeb, Ph.D.

Wesley C. Lynch, Ph.D.

Chad M. Lystad, M.S.

Sloane Madden, M.B.B.S. (Hons.)

Marsha D. Marcus, Ph.D.

Traci McFarlane, Ph.D., C.Psych.

James E. Mitchell, M.D.

Daniel J. Munoz, Ph.D.

Yoshikatsu Nakai, M.D., Ph.D.

Dasha Nicholls, M.B.B.S.,
    MRCPsych, M.D.

Julie K. O'Toole, M.D., M.P.H.

Marion P. Olmsted, Ph.D., C.Psych.

Daniel Le Grange, Ph.D.

Carol B. Peterson, Ph.D.

Kathleen M. Pike, Ph.D.

Leora Pinhas, M.D.

Norbert Quadflieg, Dipl.Psych.

Ellen Rome, M.D., M.P.H.

Heather K. Simonich, M.A.

Hayley H. Skinner, M.P.H., M.Sc.

Angela Smyth, M.D.

Ruth H. Striegel-Moore, Ph.D.

Sonja A. Swanson, Sc.M.

Marian Tanofsky-Kraff, Ph.D.

Jennifer J. Thomas, Ph.D.

Lenny R. Vartanian, Ph.D.

Ulf Wallin, M.D., Ph.D.

B. Timothy Walsh, M.D.

Denise E. Wilfley, Ph.D.

Stephen A. Wonderlich, Ph.D.

Yuko Yamamiya, Ph.D.

Jack A. Yanovski, M.D., Ph.D.

Susan Z. Yanovski, M.D.

Nancy Zucker, Ph.D.

FOREWORD

Mark Chavez, Ph.D.
Bruce Cuthbert, Ph.D.

The chapters in this monograph reflect a commendable collaborative effort among eating disorders investigators from various countries to identify, share, analyze, and publish information from existing empirically derived data sets relevant to diagnostic and classification issues. Also noteworthy, the work was accomplished in a relatively short time frame with modest funding from the National Institute of Mental Health (NIMH). In addition to providing empirical information for the DSM-5 subcommittee tasked with addressing eating disorders nosology, the effort should be of value to the eating disorders research community at large.

Eating disorders are serious, often treatment-refractory conditions, with multiple medical complications and high mortality as well as high rates of psychiatric comorbidity. Research in a number of areas, including nosology, will be critical for advancing the clinical and scientific understanding of these disorders. Within the context of nosology, there are specific strengths in the current DSM classification systems for eating disorders, including the capacity to diagnose reliably via semi-structured or clinical interviews. Also, within the DSM classification system, anorexia nervosa (AN) and bulimia nervosa (BN) appear to demonstrate different longitudinal patterns within the context of recovery and mortality, and there is some evidence that AN and BN differ in regard to their cross-cultural and cross-historical representation. In contrast to these strengths, the current DSM classification has a number of well-described limitations. These include, in part, concerns about the validity of AN and BN subtype distinctions, the minimal justification for what constitutes the size and duration of clinically important binge episodes, and questions about the validity of the eating disorders not otherwise specified (EDNOS) category, into which approximately 60% of those with an eating disorder fall. Furthermore, other mental disorders, particularly mood and anxiety disorders, co-occur at rates much higher than would be expected by chance.

Many of these issues suggest that current diagnostic categories fail to capture fundamental dimensions of brain circuitry that implement particular kinds of behavior. In response to numerous such issues, Strategy 1.4 of the NIMH Strategic Plan

(National Institute of Mental Health 2008) calls for the development, for research purposes, of new ways of classifying psychopathology based on dimensions of observable behavior and neurobiological measures. The Research Domain Criteria project has been launched by NIMH to implement this strategy. In brief, the effort is to define basic dimensions of functioning and their implementing circuitry (such as reward circuitry and behavioral control systems) as studied across multiple levels of analysis, from genes to neural circuits to behaviors, cutting across disorder categories as traditionally defined. The project is designed to foster the study of psychopathology in terms of dysfunctions of normal processes, with the eating disorders serving as an excellent example. In this regard, conversations with the eating disorders research community will represent excellent opportunities for considering how a new viewpoint on brain-behavior relationships might provide important avenues for advances in our ability to treat and prevent these serious disorders.

Reference

National Institute of Mental Health: The National Institute of Mental Health Strategic Plan. Bethesda, MD, National Institute of Mental Health, 2008. Available at http://www.nimh.nih.gov/about/strategic-planning-reports/index.shtml. Accessed October 27, 2010.

INTRODUCTION

Stephen A. Wonderlich, Ph.D.
B. Timothy Walsh, M.D.
Ruth H. Striegel-Moore, Ph.D.
James E. Mitchell, M.D.

In June 2006, the National Institute of Mental Health (NIMH) sponsored a workshop on the classification and diagnosis of eating disorders in Arlington, Virginia. More than 30 scientists, clinicians, and students participated in 2 days of scientific presentations and discussions of key issues in the area of eating disorder diagnosis. The meeting was timely, because the DSM-5 Task Force was preparing to begin its work revising psychiatric disorder diagnoses, including the eating disorders.

Given the success of the workshop, a group of investigators (Drs. Striegel-Moore, Mitchell, Walsh, and Wonderlich) collaborated with a group of consultants (Drs. Crosby, Joiner, Regier, and Kupfer) to write an R13 grant application to NIMH to fund a series of meetings to present scientific analyses of data relevant to eating disorder classification. The first meeting was held in September 2008 and the second in March 2009. For each of these meetings, investigators and consultants from the grant interacted with scientists from around the world to review and discuss analyses of existing data sets that focused on examining classification and diagnostic issues. At each of these meetings, scientists presented the results of the studies to an audience composed of other researchers; officials from the National Institutes of Health, the American Psychiatric Association, and the American Psychological Association; students and early career researchers; and perhaps most importantly, members of the DSM-5 Eating Disorders Work Group. Scientific presentations focused on topics of significant interest to the Work Group, including the category of eating disorders not otherwise specified, the definition of binge eating, the latent structure of eating disorder diagnoses, eating and feeding disorders in children, the impact of culture on eating disorder classification, and the utility and validity of the binge eating disorder diagnosis. Interactions among the various participants provided a unique opportunity for discussions that had a significant impact on the ultimate formation of the DSM-5 eating disorder diagnoses. This monograph features summaries of research presentations and discussions of conceptual or methodological issues from these meetings.

We would like to express our appreciation to NIMH for the support and funding of this project. We are particularly indebted to Dr. Mark Chavez for his guidance and support throughout the process. Also, we extend our appreciation to our consultants, Drs. Ross Crosby, Thomas Joiner, Darrel Regier, and David Kupfer, for their astute observations and excellent work in the project. In particular, Dr. Crosby offered his extraordinary statistical talents and numerous hours of hard work in preparing various analyses of these data sets for the meetings. We gratefully acknowledge the logistical support provided by Chad Lystad at the Neuropsychiatric Institute in Fargo, North Dakota. Finally, we wish to extend our thanks to the American Psychiatric Association, and particularly the staff of the DSM-5 Task Force, for their assistance in all aspects of the meetings.

PART 1

IMPROVING THE DEFINITION OF SYMPTOMS AND SYNDROMES OF EATING DISORDERS

1

RETHINKING THE NOSOLOGY OF EATING DISORDERS

Robyn Sysko, Ph.D.
B. Timothy Walsh, M.D.

DSM-IV (American Psychiatric Association 1994) describes two specific categories for the diagnosis of eating disorders: anorexia nervosa (AN) and bulimia nervosa (BN). A residual category, designated eating disorder not otherwise specified (EDNOS), is provided for all other individuals with a clinically significant eating disorder. The appendix of DSM-IV also describes criteria for a provisional eating disorder diagnosis, binge eating disorder (BED), as a particular form of EDNOS and a category in need of further study. In recent years, problems with the EDNOS category have been described, including the high prevalence of this residual diagnosis in clinical settings (e.g., 50%–70%; Ricca et al. 2001; Turner and Bryant-Waugh 2004), heterogeneous symptom presentations, and limited data regarding the anticipated course, outcome, or treatment options for individuals with this diagnosis (Rockert et al. 2007).

Different solutions have been suggested to minimize the problem of classifying a large proportion of individuals with eating disorders in the residual EDNOS category. Proposals range from making limited changes to the existing diagnostic criteria (e.g., altering the wording of the criteria; Becker et al. 2009a) to adopting a

The project described was supported in part by award No. K23DK088532 to Dr. Sysko from the National Institute of Diabetes and Digestive and Kidney Diseases.

3

revised conceptual scheme for classifying eating disorders (e.g., the Broad Categories for the Diagnosis of Eating Disorders [BCD-ED] proposal; Walsh and Sysko 2009). This monograph presents a comprehensive overview of the latter proposal, including a description of the broad categories and subgroups, the integration of feeding and eating disorders in childhood into the scheme, and empirical data evaluating the proposal.

Overview of the Broad Categories for the Diagnosis of Eating Disorders Proposal

The BCD-ED scheme (Walsh and Sysko 2009) includes three groups of eating disorders based on the prototypes for AN, BN, and BED, arranged in hierarchical order and consisting of "anorexia nervosa and related conditions," "bulimia nervosa and related conditions," and "binge eating disorder and related conditions." All individuals classified using the BCD-ED system have symptoms that meet the fundamental conceptual definition of an eating disorder (Walsh and Sysko 2009)—that is, they experience a persistent disturbance of eating or eating-related behavior that results in the altered consumption or absorption of food and that significantly impairs physical health and/or psychosocial functioning. The disturbance is not secondary to any recognized general medical disorder or any other psychiatric disorder. Of note, this definition requires impairment related to the eating disturbance; distress is not sufficient, because the presence of distress appears to be particularly associated with help seeking rather than meeting criteria for a disorder (Angst et al., submitted). Subgroups are also provided within the BCD-ED scheme to more specifically describe clinical presentations observed among individuals in each of the three broad categories, including a "prototypical" or "classic" group.

Clinicians using the BCD-ED scheme to classify individuals into broad categories and subgroups would assess five domains: 1) body mass index, 2) frequency and size of episodes of eating characterized as being accompanied by a sense of loss of control, 3) frequency and nature of inappropriate compensatory behaviors (e.g., self-induced vomiting, laxative use), 4) level of concern about body shape and weight, and 5) degree of distress and impairment related to eating disorder symptoms. Comparisons would then be made between the reported symptoms and the descriptions that follow to determine the most appropriate diagnosis or condition. In descriptions of the BCD-ED scheme, the term *binge eating* refers to episodes that are characterized by the consumption of an objectively large amount of food in a discrete period of time while experiencing a sense of loss of control. Episodes called *out-of-control eating* include the experience of a sense of loss of control during the consumption of an amount of food that is not necessarily objectively large.

The version of BCD-ED described in this review adapts the categories and subgroups proposed by Walsh and Sysko (2009) in light of suggestions initiated by

Michael Phillips, M.D., of the DSM-5 Mood Disorders Work Group (see American Psychiatric Association 2010). The American Psychiatric Association (2010) proposal originated from concerns about the common use of the "not otherwise specified" category for mood disorders and also reflects changes in wording of some criteria recommended by the DSM-5 Work Group (www.dsm5.org). Thus, the term *condition* is used to refer to disorders about which there is limited information, and criteria are provided for a number of "conditions not elsewhere specified" about which evidence is insufficient to merit their being designated disorders.

Description of the Broad Categories and Subgroups Within the BCD-ED Proposal

ANOREXIA NERVOSA AND RELATED CONDITIONS (nnn.1)

The "anorexia nervosa and related conditions" section describes presentations that meet criteria for AN and conditions that closely resemble AN and satisfy the criteria for an eating disorder. In addition, within the broad category of AN, individuals are required to meet three criteria:

A. Restriction of food intake (e.g., severe self-imposed dieting) relative to caloric requirements resulting in the maintenance of a body weight less than minimally normal for age and height.
B. Resistance to maintaining a body weight at or above a minimally normal weight. Resistance may be expressed or otherwise apparent by observable behavior perpetuating or exacerbating low weight or inferred by lack of engagement in attempts to gain weight.
C. Maintenance of the inappropriately low weight is not better accounted for by another Axis I disorder or a general medical condition.

These criteria attempt to capture the core features of AN and variants of that syndrome. Criterion A requires the maintenance of an inappropriately low body weight but does not provide specific guidance about what constitutes "minimally normal," and Criterion B requires that the individual be making efforts to maintain the inappropriately low weight and resist weight gain (Becker et al. 2009b).

nnn.11 Anorexia Nervosa

The first subgroup within this broad category is "classic" AN, and the criteria for this group are similar to the DSM-IV criteria for AN:

A. Severe restriction of food intake relative to caloric requirements leading to the maintenance of a body weight below a minimally normal weight for an individual, taking into account age and height (e.g., 85% of that expected).
B. Resistance to maintaining a body weight at or above a minimally normal weight. Resistance may be expressed or otherwise apparent by observable behavior perpetuating or exacerbating low weight or inferred by lack of engagement in attempts to gain weight.
C. Disturbance in the way in which one's body weight or shape is experienced, undue influence of body shape or weight on self-evaluation, or denial of the seriousness of current low body weight.

Indicate current subtype: restricting type or binge-eating/purging

Within this subgroup, Criterion A has been altered to remove the word *refusal* from the DSM-IV criterion, because it was considered to be potentially pejorative and required an assessment of volition (Becker et al. 2009a). The proposed Criterion A requires a deficit in caloric intake relative to requirements; thus, an individual might qualify if caloric intake was within the normal range but energy requirements were above normal—for example, because of strenuous exercise. For weight, a guideline of 85% of expected is provided, as in DSM-IV and the proposed DSM-5 criteria (www.dsm5.org), but no definition of "expected" is given. Criterion B is similar to DSM-IV but eliminates the requirement that the individual express "fear of weight gain," in favor of requiring evidence of clear behavioral resistance to gaining weight. Therefore, this criterion can be satisfied if an individual who steadfastly denies fear of weight gain engages in behavior strongly suggesting he or she is afraid. Criterion C is unchanged from DSM-IV. Criterion D in DSM-IV, requiring amenorrhea, has been eliminated (see Attia and Roberto 2009). The subtyping scheme adopted in DSM-IV has been retained, but "current" has been added, consistent with the review by Peat et al. (2009).

Conditions Resembling Anorexia Nervosa Not Elsewhere Classified

The clinical presentations described in this section are considered conditions because they are known to exist and appear to be associated with a need for clinical attention; however, there is currently insufficient information to designate them as disorders (e.g., American Psychiatric Association 2010). As in the proposed changes to "depressive disorder not otherwise specified" (American Psychiatric Association 2010), the phrase *not otherwise specified* is replaced by *conditions not elsewhere classified,* and specific conditions are described and given diagnostic codes. In this way, clinicians and researchers are encouraged to provide information about specific conditions being assessed, treated, or studied. To avoid the inappropriate labeling of normal variants, such conditions include symptoms "associated with moderate to severe psychosocial dysfunction or distress" (American Psychiatric Association 2010). Consistent with this recommendation, to be classified in this section, individuals would be required to meet the criteria described earlier for an eating disorder and for the broad definition of AN and related conditions; these require impairment secondary to the eating problem. The category "conditions resembling anorexia nervosa not elsewhere classified" closely resembles the ICD-10 category of atypical AN (World Health Organization 2004). Hence, incorporation of this category would bring DSM and ICD into closer alignment.

nnn.12 Anorexia Nervosa Without Evidence of Distortions Related to Body Shape and Weight

---

A. Severe restriction of food intake relative to caloric requirements leading to the maintenance of a body weight below a minimally normal weight for an individual, taking into account age and height (e.g., 85% of that expected).
B. Resistance to maintaining a body weight at or above a minimally normal weight. Resistance may be expressed or otherwise apparent by observable behavior perpetuating or exacerbating low weight or inferred by lack of engagement in attempts to gain weight.
C. Does not meet criteria for nnn.11.

This condition describes individuals who meet all criteria for AN except that they do not endorse the psychological symptoms required by Criterion C. This condition has been described in a number of settings, but data on course, outcome, or other clinical validators are limited (see Becker et al. 2009a).

nnn.13 Anorexia Nervosa at or Above a Minimally Acceptable Weight

---

A. Severe restriction of food intake relative to caloric requirements in order to avoid weight gain.
B. Body weight at or above minimally normal for an individual, taking into account age and height.
C. Evidence of intense fear of gaining weight.
D. Disturbance in the way in which one's body weight or shape is experienced or undue influence of body shape or weight on self-evaluation.
E. Does not meet criteria for nnn.11 or nnn.12.

This condition describes individuals who meet all criteria for AN but whose weights, during this episode of illness, have not fallen below generally accepted levels for their age and height. This condition has been observed, for example, after bariatric surgery. Although there is little question that such individuals exist and occasionally present for treatment, very little information is available about their characteristics.

nnn.14 Conditions Similar to Anorexia Nervosa Not Elsewhere Classified

---

A. Severe restriction of food intake relative to caloric requirements leading to the maintenance of a body weight below a minimally normal weight for an individual, taking into account age and height (e.g., 85% of that expected).
B. Resistance to maintaining a body weight at or above a minimally normal weight. Resistance may be expressed or otherwise apparent by observable behavior perpetuating or exacerbating low weight or inferred by lack of engagement in attempts to gain weight.
C. Does not meet criteria for nnn.11, nnn.12, or nnn.13.

This condition describes individuals whose eating disturbance resembles AN but does not meet criteria for AN or any of the related conditions.

BULIMIA NERVOSA AND RELATED CONDITIONS (nnn.2)

The "bulimia nervosa and related conditions" category describes presentations that meet criteria for BN and conditions that closely resemble BN. As in the previous section, all presentations described in this section meet the criteria for an eating disorder. In addition, the following are required:

A. The individual engages in recurrent episodes of out-of-control eating and the recurrent use of inappropriate purging methods to control weight or shape and/or the absorption of food.
B. These behaviors are not better accounted for by another Axis I disorder (including AN) or a general medical condition.

Per this definition, individuals with a broadly defined BN diagnosis engage in recurrent out-of-control eating and recurrent purging and do not meet criteria for AN.

nnn.21 Bulimia Nervosa

A. Recurrent episodes of binge eating (the consumption of a large amount of food in a discrete period of time accompanied by a sense of loss of control).
B. Recurrent inappropriate compensatory purging behavior after binge eating to prevent weight gain (self-induced vomiting, abuse of laxatives, diuretics, or enemas).
C. The binge eating and inappropriate purging behavior both occur, on average, at least once a week for 3 months.
D. Self-evaluation is unduly influenced by body shape and weight.
E. Does not meet criteria for AN and related conditions.

These behaviors are not better accounted for by another Axis I disorder (including AN) or a general medical condition.

This definition of BN closely resembles that of DSM-IV and the proposed criteria for DSM-5. Although there are concerns about how best to identify binge eating (see review by Wolfe et al. [2009]), the definition of a binge eating episode is essentially unchanged from DSM-IV. In future versions of the criteria, it might be useful to add a criterion of distress about the binge eating episode to the definition, because this is implicit but not stated. Several features have been modified from DSM-IV on the basis of literature reviews. Specifically, the frequency criterion (C) was reduced from twice a week to once a week (Wilson and Sysko 2009), and the non-purging subtype was eliminated (van Hoeken et al. 2009).

Conditions Resembling Bulimia Nervosa Not Elsewhere Classified

As discussed earlier, per the American Psychiatric Association (2010) recommendations for depressive disorder not otherwise specified, this section comprises conditions resembling BN that are known to exist and appear to be associated, at least for some individuals, with a need for clinical attention. However, insufficient information is available to justify their being designated disorders. Similar to AN, the category "conditions resembling bulimia nervosa not elsewhere classified" closely resembles the ICD-10 category of atypical BN, and this category would bring DSM and ICD into closer alignment.

nnn.22 Bulimia Nervosa, Subthreshold Frequency

A. Recurrent episodes of binge eating (the consumption of a large amount of food in a discrete period of time accompanied by a sense of loss of control).

B. Recurrent inappropriate compensatory purging behavior after binge eating to prevent weight gain (self-induced vomiting, abuse of laxatives, diuretics, or enemas).
C. Self-evaluation is unduly influenced by body shape and weight.
D. Does not meet criteria for BN or for AN and related conditions.

The criteria for these conditions not elsewhere classified are identical to those for BN, except there is no specific frequency criterion. If the criteria for BN are not satisfied (Criterion D), individuals with this condition must be binge eating and/or purging less frequently than once weekly. Little is known about the characteristics of individuals meeting this definition, but these patients exist, and thus there should be a way to identify them.

nnn.23 Purging Disorder

A. Recurrent inappropriate compensatory purging behavior following episodes of out-of-control eating.
B. Self-evaluation is unduly influenced by body shape and weight.
C. Does not meet criteria for another eating disorder or condition.

There are several important issues related to purging disorder (for a review, see Keel and Striegel-Moore 2009). First, it is included as an atypical form of BN, even though some data suggest many individuals have psychological and behavioral characteristics resembling AN. The decision to group it with BN in the BCD-ED scheme is largely based on weight: if individuals meeting these criteria were underweight, they would meet criteria for AN. In this definition, the purging follows out-of-control eating. Some investigators do not believe this stipulation is appropriate. The requirement for out-of-control eating was added out of concern that without it, individuals who vomit simply secondary to anxiety would meet these criteria. In this definition, no frequency criterion is specified.

nnn.24 Conditions Similar to Bulimia Nervosa Not Elsewhere Classified

---

A. Recurrent out-of-control eating.
B. Recurrent use of inappropriate behaviors to control weight or shape and/or the absorption of food.
C. Does not meet criteria for nnn.21, nnn.22, or nnn.23.

This is a residual category/condition for conditions that resemble BN but are not described by previous categories. This condition might include individuals who experience loss of control over eating and recurrently induce vomiting after eating but deny overconcern with shape and weight.

BINGE EATING DISORDER AND RELATED CONDITIONS (nnn.3)

"Binge eating disorder and related conditions" includes presentations that meet criteria for BED and conditions that closely resemble BED. Presentations described in this section meet the criteria for an eating disorder. In addition, the following are required:

A. The individual engages in recurrent episodes of out-of-control eating.
B. These behaviors are not better accounted for by another Axis I disorder or condition (including AN and BN) or a general medical condition.

Per this definition, individuals with broadly defined BED engage in recurrent out-of-control eating and do not meet criteria for AN, BN, or related conditions.

nnn.31 Binge Eating Disorder

A. Recurrent episodes of binge eating (the consumption of a large amount of food in a discrete period of time accompanied by a sense of loss of control).
B. The binge eating occurs, on average, at least once a week for 3 months.
C. Does not meet criteria for AN, BN, or related conditions.

BED is proposed as a new disorder in DSM-5 (for a review, see Wonderlich et al. 2009a). The criteria for BED resemble those provided in the Appendix of DSM-IV, but several features have been modified on the basis of literature reviews. Specifically, the frequency criterion (B) was reduced from twice per week to once per week, and *binge eating episodes* rather than *binge-days,* an option described in DSM-IV, is used (Wilson and Sysko 2009). Thus, this criterion is parallel to the frequency criterion for BN.

The definition of an episode of binge eating is identical to that of BN, although there are concerns about how best to describe a "large amount of food" (see review by Wolfe et al. [2009]). As noted regarding the criteria for BN, it might be useful to add a criterion of distress about the binge eating episode to the definition, because this is implicit but not stated.

Two criteria for BED in DSM-IV have been eliminated. Criterion B described five behavioral indicators of loss of control over eating behavior; the determination that the eating episodes are associated with loss of control is an essential component of Criterion A, making Criterion B redundant. These behavioral indicators could be described in the text accompanying the BED criteria. Criterion C required marked distress about the binge eating. As suggested by Angst et al. (submitted), it seems likely that distress is particularly associated with help seeking rather than meeting criteria for a disorder. All individuals with an eating disorder, including BED, must meet the definition requiring impairment.

Conditions Resembling Binge Eating Disorder Not Elsewhere Classified

This section comprises conditions resembling BED that are known to exist and appear to be associated with a need for clinical attention. However, at this time, insufficient information is available to justify their being designated disorders. The inclusion of these conditions follows the recommendations for depressive disorder not otherwise specified (American Psychiatric Association 2010) as discussed earlier regarding the conditions resembling AN and BN.

nnn.32 Binge Eating Disorder, Subthreshold Frequency

A. Recurrent episodes of binge eating (the consumption of a large amount of food in a discrete period of time accompanied by a sense of loss of control).
B. Does not meet criteria for AN, BN, or related conditions or for BED.

The criteria for these conditions not elsewhere classified are identical to those for BED, except there is no specific frequency criterion. The fact that criteria for BED are not satisfied (Criterion B) indicates that individuals with this condition must be binge eating less frequently than once weekly. Little is known about the characteristics of individuals meeting this definition; however, these individuals do present for treatment, and thus this category allows for their classification in the BCD-ED scheme.

nnn.33 Recurrent Out-of-Control Eating

A. Recurrent episodes of out-of-control eating that do not involve the consumption of objectively large amounts of food.
B. Does not meet criteria for AN, BN, or related conditions or for BED or subthreshold BED.

Individuals meeting criteria for this condition describe recurrent episodes of out-of-control eating that do not involve the consumption of excessively large amounts of food. This pattern of behavior has been suggested to be associated with weight gain among youth at risk for obesity and adults after bariatric surgery (see review by Wolfe et al. [2009]). However, information about the frequency of this problem in the community and the characteristics of individuals who present with these criteria in clinical settings is very limited. These criteria do not include a minimum required frequency.

nnn.34 Night Eating Syndrome

A. The daily pattern of eating demonstrates a significantly increased intake in the evening and/or nighttime, as manifested by one or both of the following:

  1. At least 25% of food intake is consumed after the evening meal.
  2. At least two episodes of nocturnal eating per week.

B. Awareness and recall of evening and nocturnal eating episodes are present.

C. The clinical picture is characterized by at least three of the following features:

  1. Lack of desire to eat in the morning and/or breakfast is omitted on 4 or more mornings per week.
  2. Presence of a strong urge to eat between dinner and sleep onset and/or during the night.
  3. Sleep onset and/or sleep maintenance insomnia are present 4 or more nights per week.
  4. Presence of a belief that one must eat in order to initiate or return to sleep.
  5. Mood is frequently depressed and/or mood worsens in the evening.

D. The disordered pattern of eating has been maintained for at least 3 months.

E. The disorder is not better accounted for by another eating disorder, another psychiatric disorder, or a general medical disorder.

As reviewed by Striegel-Moore et al. (2009), a range of definitions have been employed to describe night eating syndrome. These criteria are slightly modified from those of Allison et al. (2009). In part because of the variability of definitions employed in the literature, insufficient information is available to recommend that night eating disorder be included as a disorder within the BCD-ED scheme. It may be problematic that out-of-control eating, which is required for the broad category in which this syndrome is included, is not explicitly required by the criteria.

nnn.35 Conditions Similar to Binge Eating Disorder Not Elsewhere Classified

---

A. Recurrent episodes of out-of-control eating.
B. Does not meet criteria for AN, BN, BED, or other related conditions.

This residual category would presumably be rarely used.

EATING DISORDER NOT ELSEWHERE CLASSIFIED

Clinically significant eating disorders that are consistent with the definition of an eating disorder but do not meet criteria for one of the three broad categories in the BCD-ED proposal would be described as eating disorders not elsewhere classified.

Feeding and Eating Disorders in Childhood

In DSM-IV, "Feeding and Eating Disorders of Infancy and Early Childhood" are included within the larger category of "Disorders Usually First Diagnosed in Infancy, Childhood, or Adolescence." In the proposed criteria for DSM-5, these disorders are grouped with the eating disorders under the category "Eating and Feeding Disorders" to reflect the fact that these disorders occur throughout the life span and do not always develop during infancy or childhood. This version of BCD-ED accommodates these proposed changes for DSM-5 by including three additional categories for feeding disorders: pica (nnn.4), rumination disorder (nnn.5), and avoidant/restrictive food intake disorder (nnn.6). The criteria for these disorders follow the suggestions of Bryant-Waugh et al. (2010).

Empirical Support for the BCD-ED Proposal

A literature review conducted by Walsh and Sysko (2009) examined three issues relevant to the BCD-ED proposal: 1) the proportion of individuals with an EDNOS according to DSM-IV would be reclassified using the BCD-ED scheme; 2) support for arranging categories of AN and related conditions, BN and related conditions, and BED and related conditions in hierarchical order, and 3) whether this scheme could result in overdiagnosis or an inappropriate number of individuals receiving an eating disorder diagnosis. Walsh and Sysko (2009) found significant empirical support for the BCD-ED proposal among existing studies and suggested that implementing BCD-ED would essentially eliminate the use of the DSM-IV EDNOS diagnosis.

Three empirical analyses of eating disorder symptoms have also provided support for the broad categories described in the BCD-ED proposal. Two of the papers used latent profile analysis among large samples of eating disorder patients (Crosby et al. 2009; Wonderlich et al. 2009b). Three clusters of symptoms were identified: a "binge-purge" class, a "binge" class, and a "restrictor" class. This type of classification was considered to be superior to DSM-IV with respect to demographic and clinical features and for avoiding the use of a residual diagnostic category (Wonderlich et al. 2009b); however, the empirical taxonomy performed less well than DSM-IV for mortality, recovery, and psychiatric status (Crosby et al. 2009). Peterson et al. (2009) utilized latent transition analysis to evaluate a longitudinal study of individuals with eating disorders and identified three classes similar to those in the Wonderlich et al. (2009b) and Crosby et al. (2009) analyses. Patients in the three empirical classes were less likely to demonstrate diagnostic crossover than patients classified using DSM-IV (Peterson et al. 2009). Thus, although the empirically derived groups in all three of these papers are not entirely consistent with BCD-ED, the findings suggest some utility of classifying patients into broader groups with characteristic symptoms similar to those described in BCD-ED.

More recently, we extended our previous review with a prospective study of individuals with a DSM-IV EDNOS diagnosis to determine the proportion that would be reclassified into a broad category using the BCD-ED scheme or the proposed DSM-5 criteria and the possibility for overdiagnosis of eating disorders among overweight individuals (Sysko and Walsh, in press). A total of 97 individuals with an EDNOS who had contacted a specialty clinic to inquire about treatment completed a brief phone interview assessing the six domains used for categorization within the BCD-ED scheme (height and weight, restriction of food intake, out-of-control eating, purging, concern about shape and weight, distress and functional impairment). With the proposed DSM-5 criteria, a total of 58 patients (59.8%) with DSM-IV EDNOS were assigned a diagnosis of AN, BN, or BED, and the other 39 individuals (40.2%) were still considered to have an EDNOS. After the BCD-ED scheme was applied to the individuals with DSM-IV EDNOS, 18 were classified as having a condition related to AN, 19 as having a condition related to BN, and 54 as having a condition related to BED; 6 still were assigned to the EDNOS category. The six individuals with an EDNOS diagnosis endorsed recurrent purging without a loss of control over eating. Thus, a total of 93.8% of patients with a DSM-IV EDNOS were reclassified into a broad category using the BCD-ED scheme. To evaluate the possibility of overdiagnosis, the BCD-ED scheme was also applied to 31 severely obese adolescents completing an in-person evaluation prior to bariatric surgery. Only four had an eating disorder diagnosis, all of whom had a DSM-IV EDNOS diagnosis (subthreshold BED). From these limited data, there was no evidence that the BCD-ED scheme increased the number of individuals classified with an eating disorder diagnosis among obese adolescents.

Conclusion

The BCD-ED scheme is appealing for a number of reasons, including its 1) offering the potential for significantly decreasing the number of individuals receiving an EDNOS diagnosis while preserving a system closely resembling that of DSM-IV, 2) facilitating the classification of individuals with eating disorders outside of specialist settings by providing broad categories that can be used even on the basis of relatively limited information, and 3) providing subgroups within the broad categories that could be used to inform clinical care and aid further research (Walsh and Sysko 2009). However, although this novel approach has potential advantages, there are also concerns related to its implementation. At this time, only limited data are available about the real-world implementation of this system (e.g., Sysko and Walsh, in press). In addition, the interpretation of existing data on course, outcome, or treatment response may be affected by adopting broader categories for AN, BN, and BED because these categories would be more heterogeneous than the current DSM-IV categories (Walsh and Sysko 2009). Finally, because data relevant to individuals classified as having EDNOS are limited, several of the proposed subgroups in the BCD-ED scheme were derived from clinical anecdote rather than established literature (Walsh and Sysko 2009).

References

Allison KC, Lundgren JD, O'Reardon JP, et al: Proposed diagnostic criteria for night eating syndrome. Int J Eat Disord 43:241–247, 2009

American Psychiatric Association: Diagnostic and Statistical Manual of Mental Disorders, 4th Edition. Washington, DC, American Psychiatric Association, 1994

American Psychiatric Association: Proposed revision to 311.00 depressive disorder not otherwise specified. Washington, DC, American Psychiatric Association, 2010. Available at http://www.dsm5.org/ProposedRevisions/Pages/proposedrevision.aspx?rid=47. Accessed March 10, 2010.

Angst J, Gamma A, Clarke DE, et al: The depression, bipolar, anxiety, panic, neurasthenia and insomnia severity spectra: distress, not diagnosis, predicts treatment seeking. Manuscript submitted for publication.

Attia E, Roberto CA: Should amenorrhea be a diagnostic criterion for anorexia nervosa? Int J Eat Disord 42:581–589, 2009

Becker AE, Eddy KT, Perloe A: Clarifying criteria for cognitive signs and symptoms for eating disorders in DSM-V. Int J Eat Disord 42:611–619, 2009a

Becker AE, Thomas JJ, Pike KM: Should non-fat-phobic anorexia nervosa be included in DSM-V? Int J Eat Disord 42:620–635, 2009b

Bryant-Waugh R, Markham L, Kreipe RE, et al: Feeding and eating disorders in childhood. Int J Eat Disord 43:98–111, 2010

Crosby RD, Fichter MM, Quadflieg N, et al: Validating eating disorder classification models with mortality and recovery data. Presented at the 15th annual meeting of the Eating Disorders Research Society, Brooklyn, NY, September 2009

Keel PK, Striegel-Moore RH: The validity and clinical utility of purging disorder. Int J Eat Disord 42:706–719, 2009

Peat C, Mitchell JE, Hoek H, et al: Validity and utility of sub-typing anorexia nervosa. Int J Eat Disord 42:590–594, 2009

Peterson CB, Crow SJ, Swanson SA, et al: Longitudinal stability of empirically derived vs. DSM-IV classification of eating disorder symptoms. Presentation at the 15th annual meeting of the Eating Disorders Research Society, Brooklyn, NY, September 2009

Ricca V, Mannucci E, Mezzani B, et al: Psychopathological and clinical features of outpatients with an eating disorder not otherwise specified. Eat Weight Disord 6:157–165, 2001

Rockert W, Kaplan AS, Olmsted MP: Eating disorder not otherwise specified: the view from a tertiary care treatment center. Int J Eat Disord 40:S99–S103, 2007

Striegel-Moore RH, Franko DL, Garcia J: The validity and clinical utility of night eating syndrome. Int J Eat Disord 42:720–738, 2009

Sysko R, Walsh BT: Does the Broad Categories for the Diagnosis of Eating Disorders (BCD-ED) scheme reduce the frequency of eating disorder not otherwise specified? Int J Eat Disord (in press)

Turner H, Bryant-Waugh R: Eating disorder not otherwise specified (EDNOS): profiles of clients presenting at a community eating disorder service. Eur Eat Disord Rev 12:18–26, 2004

van Hoeken D, Veling W, Sinke S, et al: The validity and utility of sub-typing bulimia nervosa. Int J Eat Disord 42:595–602, 2009

Walsh BT, Sysko R: Broad categories for the diagnosis of eating disorders (BCD-ED): an alternative system for classification. Int J Eat Disord 42:754–764, 2009

Wilson GT, Sysko R: Frequency of binge eating episodes in bulimia nervosa and binge eating disorder: diagnostic considerations. Int J Eat Disord 42:603–610, 2009

Wolfe BE, Baker CW, Smith AT, et al: Validity and utility of the current definition of binge eating. Int J Eat Disord 42:674–686, 2009

Wonderlich SA, Gordon KH, Mitchell JE, et al: The validity and clinical utility of binge eating disorder. Int J Eat Disord 42:687–705, 2009a

Wonderlich SA, Olmsted M, McFarlane T, et al: Empirical taxonomy of patients with eating disorders. Presented at the 15th annual meeting of the Eating Disorders Research Society, Brooklyn, NY, September 2009b

World Health Organization: International Statistical Classification of Diseases and Related Health Problems, 10th Revision, 2nd Edition. Geneva, World Health Organization, 2004

2

EATING DISORDER NOT OTHERWISE SPECIFIED

Theoretical and Empirical Advances Since the Publication of a Meta-Analysis Covering 1987–2007

Jennifer J. Thomas, Ph.D.
Lenny R. Vartanian, Ph.D.

When the DSM-5 Eating Disorders Work Group first convened in mid-2007, one of the most vexing criticisms of DSM-IV (American Psychiatric Association 1994) eating disorder diagnostic criteria was the preponderance of patients presenting for treatment who did not meet full criteria for anorexia nervosa (AN) or bulimia nervosa (BN). Such patients—estimated to constitute 40% (Rockert et al. 2007) to 60% (Fairburn et al. 2007) of treatment seekers at eating disorder specialty clinics and up to 90% of eating disorder patients in general psychiatric settings (Zimmerman et al. 2008)—could only be diagnosed with eating disorder not otherwise specified (EDNOS). In anticipation of the pending 2013 publica-

Portions of this manuscript were presented at the National Institute of Mental Health–sponsored R-13 conference for the DSM-5 Eating Disorders Work Group at the American Psychiatric Association Headquarters in Arlington, Virginia. The original meta-analytic results were published in Thomas et al. 2009, which is cited in the reference list.

We would like to thank the Klarman Family Foundation for funding this project through a postdoctoral research fellowship to Jennifer J. Thomas.

tion of DSM-5, the eating disorder research community produced several innovative but distinct proposals for redistributing EDNOS into more clinically useful diagnostic categories. These solutions ranged from expanding the diagnostic criteria for AN and BN (Andersen et al. 2001) to identifying new disorders such as purging disorder (Keel et al. 2005) and night eating syndrome (Allison et al. 2005) to moving toward a transdiagnostic (Fairburn and Bohn 2005) or even a dimensional (Williamson et al. 2005) system.

The starting point for choosing among or creatively combining these proposed solutions is a strong empirical base. Fortunately, a wealth of data on EDNOS subtypes had been published since the 1987 debut of the EDNOS category in the official psychiatric nomenclature (i.e., DSM-III-R; American Psychiatric Association 1987). However, conflicting findings, low statistical power, and different definitions of EDNOS across studies had hindered the ability of this literature to foster consensus on suggested revisions. Meta-analytic techniques are designed to overcome many of these methodological and interpretive difficulties by pooling effect sizes across studies and enhancing statistical power to determine the magnitude and statistical significance of overall effects. Meta-analysis also capitalizes on heterogeneity in study design by identifying study level characteristics (moderator variables) that are systematically associated with larger versus smaller effects. Therefore, we conducted a systematic review and meta-analysis of studies published from 1987 to 2007, each of which compared EDNOS with the officially recognized eating disorder categories with regard to eating pathology, general psychopathology, and physical health (Thomas et al. 2009). Since the closing of our meta-analytic literature search in early 2007, the number of high-quality studies focusing on EDNOS has greatly increased, and the DSM-5 Work Group has published its draft criteria online with an invitation for public comment. Thus the aims of the present chapter are threefold: 1) to summarize the results of our original meta-analysis (covering studies published in 1987–2007), 2) to discuss how the findings of more recent studies (published in 2007–2010) compare with our original results, and 3) to comment on the recently published DSM-5 draft criteria from the perspective of both our meta-analytic findings as well as recent advances in the eating disorder field.

Summary of Original Meta-Analytic Findings (1987–2007)

Our original meta-analysis featured studies that compared individuals with officially recognized DSM-IV eating disorders (i.e., AN and BN) with individuals with EDNOS. We also included binge eating disorder (BED) as an "officially recognized" eating disorder for comparison purposes because this disorder had been heavily researched in the years leading up to our meta-analysis and is still actively being considered for inclusion in DSM-5. The outcomes that we examined included eating pathology (e.g., Eating Disorder Inventory scores, body checking, dieting), general psychopathology (e.g., Beck Depression Inventory scores, comorbid Axis I diagnoses), and physical health (e.g., gastrointestinal disorders, bone mineral density). These outcome measures were selected because of their relevance to clinical practice.

The primary aim of our meta-analysis was to provide a comprehensive, quantitative summary of the differences in eating pathology, general psychopathology, and physical health between EDNOS and each of the officially recognized eating disorders. In addition to examining overall group differences, we were also interested in identifying potential moderators of these group differences, such as the specific diagnostic features of EDNOS subgroups. Much of the discourse regarding eating disorder diagnosis had focused on the utility and validity of specific diagnostic criteria (e.g., amenorrhea in AN, binge frequency in BN). Therefore, whenever the available data permitted, we compared EDNOS groups that were missing specific diagnostic criteria with their full-criteria counterparts.

METHOD

In order to obtain an exhaustive list of EDNOS studies, we conducted a comprehensive search of the available literature comparing EDNOS with the officially recognized eating disorders using a four-step process. First, we searched electronic databases for articles related to "eating disorder not otherwise specified," "EDNOS," and numerous other terms used by researchers to refer to individuals who do not meet full diagnostic criteria for AN, BN, or BED (e.g., atypical, partial, subclinical; for a full listing of search terms, see Thomas et al. 2009). Second, we reviewed the reference sections of each identified article to search for additional relevant articles. Third, we hand-searched the table of contents of four journals identified by the SCOPUS database as publishing the highest number of eating disorder–related articles (*International Journal of Eating Disorders, European Eating Disorders Review, Eating and Weight Disorders,* and *American Journal of Psychiatry*). Finally, we sought to identify unpublished work by searching for relevant dissertations and theses and by contacting the corresponding authors of eligible studies to obtain unpublished or in-press work.

To ensure a minimum standard of methodological quality and comparability among studies included in the meta-analysis, we required that studies meet certain specific inclusion criteria. For example, eating disorder diagnoses must have been established by clinical interview or by means of well-validated questionnaires that specifically operationalized diagnostic criteria (e.g., Eating Disorder Examination Questionnaire), and diagnoses were required to reflect current (rather than past or lifetime) symptoms (see Thomas et al. 2009 for complete details). We identified a total of 125 studies that met our inclusion criteria.

RESULTS

Table 2–1 summarizes the overall effects for the analyses comparing AN, BN, and BED with EDNOS on each of the outcome measures. All effects are reported as Cohen's *d,* with positive effects indicating that individuals with officially recognized eating disorders exhibited greater pathology than individuals with EDNOS on the outcome of interest.

Overall, individuals with EDNOS did not differ from individuals with AN or BED in terms of either eating pathology or general psychopathology. Individuals with BN did, however, score higher than individuals with EDNOS on measures of eating pathology and general psychopathology. Far fewer studies had examined indices of physical health, but results indicated that individuals with EDNOS did not differ from individuals with AN on physical health outcomes, whereas individuals with EDNOS actually exhibited significantly worse physical health than did individuals with BN.

We next conducted a series of moderator analyses comparing specific subgroups of individuals with EDNOS with their full-criteria counterparts on measures of eating pathology. For AN, these subgroups included individuals with AN who did not meet the DSM-IV weight guideline of less than 85% of expected body weight (high-weight AN), individuals with AN who did not have amenorrhea (AN with menses), and individuals with AN who did not endorse intense fear of gaining weight or becoming fat (non-fat-phobic AN [NFP-AN]). For BN, the subgroups included individuals who did not meet the binge-frequency criterion of twice per week for at least 3 months (low-binge-frequency BN) and individuals for whom the binges were not objectively large (purging disorder). For BED, the only available subgroup included individuals who did not meet the binge frequency criterion of twice per week for at least 6 months (low-binge-frequency BED).

Table 2–2 summarizes the results of the moderator analyses. With respect to AN, individuals with menses and individuals who were above the weight threshold did not differ from individuals with full-criteria AN. However, individuals with full-criteria AN showed significantly greater eating pathology than did individuals with NFP-AN. For BN, individuals who did not meet the binge frequency criterion did not differ from individuals with full-criteria BN, but individuals with purging disorder showed significantly lower levels of eating pathology. Finally, with respect to BED, individuals who did not meet the binge frequency criterion did not differ significantly from their full-criteria counterparts.

SUMMARY AND CONCLUSIONS

Overall, our meta-analytic findings indicated that individuals with EDNOS exhibited a level of pathology similar to that observed among individuals with officially recognized eating disorders. Specifically, EDNOS did not differ from AN

TABLE 2–1. Summary of effect sizes comparing eating disorder not otherwise specified with anorexia nervosa, bulimia nervosa, and binge eating disorder

	Number of effects	Cohen's d	SE	P
Anorexia nervosa				
Eating pathology	73	0.09	0.06	0.09
General psychopathology	53	0.02	0.05	0.68
Physical health	11	0.14	0.16	0.40
Bulimia nervosa				
Eating pathology	82	0.39	0.05	<0.001
General psychopathology	62	0.19	0.03	<0.001
Physical health	14	−0.18	0.08	0.03
Binge eating disorder				
Eating pathology	29	0.17	0.09	0.06
General psychopathology	24	0.03	0.07	0.66

Note. In the literature search for the original meta-analysis, we did not identify any studies comparing eating disorder not otherwise specified with binge eating disorder on indices of physical health.

TABLE 2–2. Comparison of the eating pathology of specific eating disorder not otherwise specified subgroups to full-criteria anorexia nervosa, bulimia nervosa, and binge eating disorder

	Number of effects	Cohen's d	SE	P
EDNOS-AN subgroup				
High-weight anorexia nervosa	2	−0.02	0.19	0.93
AN with menses	4	0.20	0.20	0.32
NFP-AN	5	0.74	0.23	0.001
EDNOS–bulimia nervosa subgroup				
Low-binge-frequency bulimia nervosa	5	0.10	0.14	0.49
Purging disorder	5	0.39	0.11	<0.001
EDNOS–binge eating disorder subgroup				
Low-binge-frequency binge eating disorder	3	0.28	0.32	0.37

Note. EDNOS = eating disorder not otherwise specified; NFP-AN = non-fat-phobic anorexia nervosa.

and BED in terms of eating pathology or general psychopathology. Individuals with BN did, however, show more severe levels of eating pathology and general psychopathology than did individuals with EDNOS. Of particular importance to the issues of diagnosis and classification is the identification of the specific diagnostic criteria (if any) that best differentiate EDNOS from full-criteria eating disorders. Our moderator analyses found that certain criteria fail to differentiate individuals with EDNOS from their full-criteria counterparts (amenorrhea and body weight in AN, frequency of binge eating in BN and BED), suggesting that these criteria could be omitted or revised in DSM-5. In contrast, other criteria did differentiate individuals with EDNOS from their full-criteria counterparts (fat phobia in AN, binge size in BN), suggesting that these criteria should be retained as important diagnostic features of those disorders in DSM-5.

Based on the results of our meta-analysis, we offered the following suggestions for revisions to future editions of DSM:

1. Several of the diagnostic criteria for AN, BN, and BED could be revised or omitted without sacrificing the homogeneity of diagnostic categories, which would serve to reduce clutter in an overpopulated EDNOS category.
2. In addition to the currently recognized eating disorders, there are other identifiable, uniquely defined disorders that exhibit clinically significant levels of pathology but that also differ from full-criteria presentations in important ways (e.g., severity of eating pathology). Identifying and clearly describing such disorders would further serve to refine the EDNOS category, reserving that diagnosis for truly atypical cases.
3. A somewhat more radical recommendation might be the creation of a two-tiered approach to eating disorder classification, similar to what is observed in the classification of mood disorders. The first-tier disorders would include AN (with relaxed criteria for menses and weight), BN (with relaxed criteria for binge frequency), and BED (with relaxed criteria for binge frequency). The second tier would be reserved for clinically significant eating disorders that are clearly and uniquely defined but exhibit a level of psychopathology that is less severe than the first-tier disorders. These second-tier disorders could include, for example, purging disorder and NFP-AN.

Our meta-analysis also allowed us to identify theoretical and methodological limitations in the literature, and we offered a number of suggestions for future EDNOS research. These recommendations included 1) clearer identification of diagnostic features of the EDNOS groups, 2) adherence to a consistent (even if provisional) nomenclature, 3) the adoption of innovative study methodologies and statistical techniques, and 4) greater statistical power. Recent research on EDNOS has shown major improvements in each of these domains. For example, several studies have transcended univariate group comparisons in favor of latent class (Pinheiro et al. 2008), latent profile (Eddy et al. 2009), and latent transition (Cain et al. 2010) analyses and incorporated interesting new validators for EDNOS subgroups such as neuroendocrine abnormalities (Jimerson et al. 2009; Keel et al. 2007), treatment response (Dalle Grave et al. 2008a; Santonastaso et al. 2009), and diagnostic crossover (Stice et al. 2009; Zanarini et al. 2010). Unfortunately, low statistical power continues to plague empirical approaches to eating disorder classification given the low base rate of specific EDNOS presentations in clinical settings (e.g., NFP-AN; Carter and Bewell-Weiss 2010; Dalle Grave et al. 2008b). In the next section, we review the literature that has been published since 2007 in order to determine how the results of recent studies compare with our original findings.

Findings of Recent Empirical Studies (2007–2010)

In our original systematic review, the sample sizes for moderator analyses examining the validity of individual DSM-IV diagnostic criteria for AN, BN, and BED were quite small. Eligible studies featuring EDNOS subgroups in which all participants were missing only a single diagnostic criterion for an officially recognized eating disorder ranged from just two to five studies per comparison. Because these modestly powered single-criterion analyses arguably represent those most critical to the DSM-5 decision-making process, we have taken this opportunity to conduct a qualitative update to our original quantitative review in order to highlight studies published in the past 3 years that would have met our meta-analytic inclusion criteria. Findings suggest that the majority of recent cross-sectional investigations examining eating pathology, general psychopathology, and physical health have provided additional empirical support for our original diagnostic recommendations. A new generation of studies tracking treatment response and longitudinal outcome—which had not yet been published by the time we concluded our meta-analytic literature search—have, however, diverged somewhat from our original results.

ANOREXIA NERVOSA

Recent cross-sectional studies comparing individuals with DSM-IV AN to those with subthreshold AN variants meeting all but one diagnostic criterion have largely supported our conclusion that the weight and amenorrhea criteria could be revised or omitted without sacrificing diagnostic homogeneity, whereas the fat phobia criterion should be retained in light of its robust association with eating pathology.

High-Weight Anorexia Nervosa

Two studies comparing patients with DSM-IV AN with those meeting all criteria for AN except for weighing more than 85% expected body weight have confirmed our meta-analytic finding that these two groups exhibit similar levels of eating pathology (Santonastaso et al. 2009), general psychopathology (Santonastaso et al. 2009), and physical health (Peebles et al. 2010). Thus both are consistent with our original recommendation that the example weight criterion for AN be omitted or made more lenient in DSM-5. In contrast, a treatment outcome study reported superior response to outpatient cognitive-behavioral therapy in high-weight AN versus DSM-IV AN (Santonastaso et al. 2009), raising the possibility that the weight criterion may have predictive—if not concurrent—validity, at least with regard to a treatment modality that depends in part on patients' ability to participate cognitively in the intervention.

Anorexia Nervosa With Menses

One study replicated our meta-analytic finding of commensurate levels of eating pathology in individuals who met all criteria for AN except amenorrhea compared with DSM-IV AN (Santonastaso et al. 2009), whereas another reported lower levels of eating pathology in AN with menses (Dalle Grave et al. 2008a). However, both of these studies identified comparable levels of general psychopathology between DSM-IV AN and menstruating AN (Dalle Grave et al. 2008a; Santonastaso et al. 2009) and extended our cross-sectional findings by reporting similar response to inpatient (Dalle Grave et al. 2008a) and outpatient (Santonastaso et al. 2009) cognitive-behavioral therapy. Taken together, these results are consistent with our meta-analytic recommendation that amenorrhea be dropped from the diagnostic criteria for AN.

Non-Fat-Phobic Anorexia Nervosa

All recent studies comparing NFP-AN with DSM-IV AN have confirmed our original report of milder eating pathology in NFP-AN (Carter and Bewell-Weiss 2010; Dalle Grave et al. 2008b; Lee et al. 2010; Santonastaso et al. 2009). Furthermore, a second meta-analysis extended our findings to reveal that differences in eating pathology remained large and significant even when analyses were restricted to only those measures with no potential for conceptual overlap with fat phobia (Becker et al. 2009). Also consistent with our meta-analysis, another study reported similar rates of medical complications between NFP-AN and DSM-IV AN (Peebles et al. 2010). Although we originally found no difference in general psychopathology between DSM-IV AN and NFP-AN, two recent studies reported lower levels of general psychopathology in NFP-AN (Carter and Bewell-Weiss 2010; Santonastaso et al. 2009), which provides additional support for our recommendation to retain the fat phobia criterion for AN in DSM-5. In summary, recent cross-sectional findings have provided additional empirical support for the concurrent validity of fat phobia as a central diagnostic feature of AN.

In contrast to cross-sectional comparisons, three treatment outcome studies have reported similar treatment response in NFP-AN and DSM-IV AN (Carter and

Bewell-Weiss 2010; Dalle Grave et al. 2008b; Santonastaso et al. 2009). The similarity between AN and NFP-AN at the longitudinal level appears to contradict the dissimilarity between AN and NFP-AN at the cross-sectional level and is therefore illustrative of Wonderlich et al.'s (2007) argument that different empirical validators may promote conflicting conclusions about the validity of diagnostic categories.

BULIMIA NERVOSA

Recent cross-sectional and longitudinal studies comparing individuals with DSM-IV BN with those with subthreshold BN meeting all except one diagnostic criterion have provided mixed support for our conclusion that the twice-weekly binge frequency criterion does not distinguish well between these groups. New investigations on purging disorder, however, have largely confirmed the clinical distinctiveness of this presentation as well as our meta-analytic recommendation that it be recognized as a disorder for further study in DSM-5.

Low-Binge-Frequency Bulimia Nervosa

Although our original meta-analysis found no difference in eating pathology between individuals with DSM-IV BN and those who met all criteria except the twice-weekly binge frequency criterion, more recent findings have been mixed. Consistent with our meta-analysis, two studies reported no differences in psychosocial impairment (Spoor et al. 2007) or physical health (Peebles et al. 2010) among individuals who met the twice-weekly binge-purge threshold versus those who did not. In contrast, two other studies identified milder eating pathology among individuals who binged and purged just once weekly (Roberto et al. 2009; Rockert et al. 2007). Notably, in both studies, individuals with low-binge-frequency BN still scored in the clinical range on measures of eating pathology (Roberto et al. 2009; Rockert et al. 2007), suggesting that lowering the binge-purge frequency criterion to once per week would probably not introduce undue heterogeneity into DSM-5 BN.

Purging Disorder

Recent findings have largely confirmed the clinical distinctiveness of purging disorder in comparison with DSM-IV BN, in keeping with our meta-analytic recommendation to retain the objectively large binge requirement for BN in DSM-5. Specifically, two studies identified lower levels of disordered eating attitudes in purging disorder compared with DSM-IV BN (Roberto et al. 2009; Rockert et al. 2007), and an 8-year longitudinal study identified minimal diagnostic crossover between the two syndromes (Stice et al. 2009), thus providing further support for both concurrent and predictive validity of objectively large binges. However, a study reporting similar rates of a wide variety of eating disorder–related medical complications in purging disorder compared with DSM-IV BN (Peebles et al. 2010) highlighted the clinical significance of purging disorder in its own right. Given our meta-analytic recommendation that purging disorder be recognized as a second-tier eating disorder in DSM-5, we were pleased to see that since the closing of our meta-analytic literature search, several studies have investigated the optimal frequency of compensatory behaviors to define the purging disorder diagnosis. This was beyond the scope of our original meta-analysis, because comparing purging disorder with subthreshold purging disorder represents an EDNOS-with-EDNOS comparison in DSM-IV terms. Echoing our meta-analytic findings for BN and BED, recent studies have found no difference in eating pathology (Roberto et al. 2009), general psychopathology (Haedt and Keel 2010; Roberto et al. 2009), or psychosocial impairment (Haedt and Keel 2010; Spoor et al. 2007) between individuals who purge at least twice weekly versus those who purge less frequently. Thus once-weekly purging may prove to be the optimal minimum threshold for purging disorder in DSM-5 (Haedt and Keel 2010; Roberto et al. 2009).

BINGE EATING DISORDER

Very few recent studies have investigated the validity of individual diagnostic criteria for BED. However, one study has provided additional empirical support for our meta-analytic finding that the twice-weekly binge frequency criterion does not distinguish well between DSM-IV and subthreshold BED, and other investigations have extended our original findings by highlighting the uniqueness of BED in comparison to other forms of EDNOS.

Low-Binge-Frequency Binge Eating Disorder

One study found similar levels of eating pathology and general psychopathology among individuals with DSM-IV BED versus those who met all criteria except for binge eating less than twice per week (Roberto et al. 2009). This finding is consistent with our meta-analytic recommendation to lower the binge frequency threshold for BED (e.g., to once per week) in DSM-5.

Binge Eating Disorder Versus Purging Disorder

Since the conclusion of our meta-analytic literature search, two studies have examined whether BED can be differentiated from another distinct form of EDNOS that shares only minor overlap in behavioral features: purging disorder. Both studies identified higher levels of dietary restraint in purging disorder versus BED (Keel et al. 2010; Roberto et al. 2009), thus providing further support for the heterogeneity of EDNOS and the possibility of highlighting BED and purging disorder as distinct syndromes in DSM-5.

SUMMARY AND CONCLUSIONS

The past 3 years of cross-sectional data have largely corroborated our original meta-analytic findings. Recent studies have provided additional empirical support for our original recommendations to relax the weight guideline, drop the amenorrhea criterion, and retain the fat phobia criterion for AN; retain the objectively large binge size criterion for BN; and reduce the binge frequency criterion for BED. Support for reducing the binge frequency criterion for BN has been mixed; however, confirmation that individuals with low-binge-frequency BN still exhibit clinical-range psychopathology suggests that a conservative reduction (i.e., from twice to once weekly) would probably not reduce the construct validity of this diagnostic group.

DSM-5 Draft Criteria

The DSM-5 Eating Disorders Work Group published their original DSM-5 draft criteria online in February 2010 with an invitation for public comment and posted revised versions of these criteria in April 2010, and again in October 2010, after considering the feedback they received. Consistent with the Work Group's stated commitment to base DSM-5 criteria on a strong empirical foundation, nearly all of the proposed revisions are consistent with our original meta-analytic findings and with subsequent scientific advances in the eating disorder field.

ANOREXIA NERVOSA

The proposed revisions for DSM-5 AN serve to make the individual diagnostic criteria more lenient and the overall diagnosis more inclusive. Such revisions are consistent with the small, nonsignificant differences between AN and EDNOS that we identified in our original meta-analysis and are also reflective of our single-criterion meta-analytic moderator analyses.

Criterion A (Body Weight)

Consistent with our finding that the 85% expected body weight guideline does not distinguish well between full and subthreshold AN, the DSM-5 Work Group has dropped the 85% example from the diagnostic criteria in favor of the more general requirement of "significantly low body weight." Rather than providing an example guideline in the official criteria, the Work Group recommends that low weight be "defined as a weight that is less than minimally normal, or, for children and adolescents, less than that minimally expected" (American Psychiatric Association 2010), with the possibility for further specific guidance in the supporting text.

Criteria B (Fear of Weight Gain) and C (Body Image Disturbance)

The cognitive criteria for AN have been retained, but the Work Group added the clarification that "persistent behavior that interferes with weight gain, even though at significantly low weight" could be substituted for "intense fear of gaining weight" (American Psychiatric Association 2010). The retention of the fat phobia criterion is consistent with the large and highly replicable differences in eating pathology that we observed between AN and NFP-AN both in our original meta-analysis and in more recent empirical findings. Moreover, the Work Group's decision to retain the requirement for a "disturbance in the way in which one's body weight or shape is experienced, undue influence of body weight or shape on self-evaluation, or persistent lack of recognition of the seriousness of the current low body weight" (American Psychiatric Association 2010) appears prudent because we could identify no studies that evaluated the validity of this particular criterion, and it shares substantial conceptual overlap with fat phobia.

Criterion D (Amenorrhea)

The Work Group's recommendation to drop the amenorrhea criterion (American Psychiatric Association 2010) dovetails with our meta-analytic finding that individuals who meet all criteria for AN except amenorrhea exhibit similar levels of psychopathology in comparison with those with DSM-IV AN, as well as more recent empirical work that has replicated this meta-analytic result.

BULIMIA NERVOSA

In contrast to the substantial revisions suggested for DSM-5 AN, the Work Group has recommended that the criteria for BN remain quite similar between DSM-IV and DSM-5. This conservative approach is consistent with the significant, small- to medium-sized differences that we observed between BN and EDNOS in our meta-analysis and subsequent literature review, which provides strong support for the construct validity of DSM-IV BN.

Criterion A (Objectively Large Binge Episodes)

The DSM-5 criteria for BN will continue to require "recurrent episodes of binge eating," which are "characterized by...eating...an amount of food that is definitely larger than most people would eat during a similar period of time and under similar circumstances" (American Psychiatric Association 2010). The retention of the requirement for objectively large binge episodes will prevent individuals with purging disorder from being diagnosed with BN and is consistent with the results of our meta-analysis as well as more recent empirical work highlighting important differences between the two presentations.

Criterion B (Compensatory Behaviors)

Compensatory behaviors will continue to be viewed as a core symptom of DSM-5 BN (American Psychiatric Association 2010), which will ensure that individuals with BED—who binge but do not purge—will not receive a diagnosis of BN. This decision is consistent with our meta-analytic recommendation to promote BED to an officially recognized first-tier eating disorder.

Criterion C (Binge Frequency)

The Work Group has recommended that the frequency threshold for binge eating and compensatory behaviors be reduced from twice weekly to "at least once a week for 3 months" (American Psychiatric Association 2010). Although more recent findings have been mixed, this revision is consistent with our original meta-analytic finding of no difference between individuals with DSM-IV BN and those who meet all criteria except the binge-purge frequency criterion and dovetails with more recent findings suggesting that individuals with low-frequency BN nonetheless score in the clinical range on measures of eating pathology.

Criterion D (Overvaluation of Weight and Shape)

The Work Group has recommended that overvaluation of weight and shape remain in the diagnostic criteria for DSM-5 BN (American Psychiatric Association 2010). This recommendation seems prudent because we were unable to locate any studies—in our original meta-analysis or subsequent qualitative update—comparing individuals with DSM-IV BN with those meeting all criteria except overvaluation and therefore have no data on which to base any suggested modifications.

BINGE EATING DISORDER

The Work Group has recommended that BED be promoted to an officially recognized eating disorder, which is consistent with our treatment of BED as a separate disorder in our original meta-analysis. The individual diagnostic criteria will remain very much the same, which appears appropriately conservative given the small number of studies comparing DSM-IV BED with subthreshold BED in both our original quantitative review and later qualitative update.

Criterion D (Binge Frequency)

Consistent with our moderator analyses and with subsequent empirical findings, the Work Group has elected to reduce the binge frequency criterion from twice per week to "at least once a week for 3 months" (American Psychiatric Association 2010). This will confer the added benefit of making the DSM-5 binge frequency criterion for BED comparable with the newly recommended once-weekly binge-purge frequency criterion for DSM-5 BN.

EATING DISORDER NOT OTHERWISE SPECIFIED

Lastly, the Work Group has recommended that the heretofore heterogeneous ED-NOS category be replaced with brief descriptions of specific syndromes of potential clinical significance. These new syndromes—including purging disorder and night eating syndrome, among others—will fall under the new umbrella term "Feeding and Eating Conditions Not Elsewhere Classified (FECNEC; American Psychiatric Association 2010). Of note, the inclusion of these subtypes under the FECNEC moniker is in keeping with the two-tiered approach we suggested in our original meta-analysis, in which the first tier would consist of more inclusive definitions of AN, BN, and BED, and the second tier would comprise truly unqiue eating disorder presentations. We anticipate that the identification and description of these atypical syndromes in DSM-5 will catalyze clinical detection and research efforts.

Conclusion

The DSM-5 revision process highlighted eating disorder not otherwise specified as an important area for concentrated study and, as a consequence, high-quality research in this area has proliferated in the past several years. True to their commitment to base revisions on empirical evidence, the DSM-5 Eating Disorders Work Group has made conservative recommendations that appear quite sound from the perspective of our meta-analytic results and more recent empirical advances. Recent studies have strengthened a number of the arguments and suggestions we made in our original meta-analysis. Newer work has highlighted additional variables—such as biological factors, treatment outcome, and diagnostic crossover—that may prove to be important diagnostic validators in DSM-6 and beyond. Continued efforts to validate and refine eating disorder phenotypes are certain to enhance not only clinical communication and treatment planning but also epidemiological inquiry, primary prevention, and basic research.

References

Allison KC, Grilo CM, Masheb RM, et al: Binge eating disorder and night eating syndrome: a comparative study of disordered eating. J Consult Clin Psychol 73:1107–1115, 2005

American Psychiatric Association: Diagnostic and Statistical Manual of Mental Disorders, 3rd Edition, Revised. Washington, DC, American Psychiatric Association, 1987

American Psychiatric Association: Diagnostic and Statistical Manual of Mental Disorders, 4th Edition. Washington, DC, American Psychiatric Association, 1994

American Psychiatric Association: DSM-5 proposed diagnostic criteria for eating disorders. Washington, DC, American Psychiatric Association, 2010. Available at: http://www.dsm5.org/ProposedRevisions/Pages/EatingDisorders.aspx. Accessed November 15, 2010.

Andersen AE, Bowers WA, Watson T: A slimming program for eating disorders not otherwise specified: reconceptualizing a confusing, residual diagnostic category. Psychiatr Clin North Am 24:271–280, 2001

Becker AE, Thomas JJ, Pike KM: Should non-fat-phobic anorexia nervosa be included in DSM-V? Int J Eat Disord 42:620–635, 2009

Carter JC, Bewell-Weiss CV: Nonfat phobic anorexia nervosa: clinical characteristics and response to inpatient treatment. Int J Eat Disord June 28, 2010 [Epub ahead of print]

Cain AS, Epler AJ, Steinley D, et al: Stability and change in patterns of concerns related to eating, weight, and shape in young adult women: a latent transition analysis. J Abnorm Psychol 119:255–267, 2010

Dalle Grave R, Calugi S, Marchesini G: Is amenorrhea a clinically useful criterion for the diagnosis of anorexia nervosa? Behav Res Ther 46:1290–1294, 2008a

Dalle Grave R, Calugi S, Marchesini G: Underweight eating disorder without over-evaluation of shape and weight: atypical anorexia nervosa? Int J Eat Disord 41:705–712, 2008b

Eddy KT, Crosby RD, Keel PK, et al: Empirical identification and validation of eating disorder phenotypes in a multisite clinical sample. J Nerv Ment Dis 197:41–49, 2009

Fairburn CG, Bohn K: Eating disorder NOS (EDNOS): an example of the troublesome "not otherwise specified" (NOS) category in DSM-IV. Behav Res Ther 43:691–701, 2005

Fairburn CG, Cooper Z, Bohn K, et al: The severity and status of eating disorder NOS: implications for DSM-V. Behav Res Ther 45:1705–1715, 2007

Haedt AA, Keel PK: Comparing definitions of purging disorder on point prevalence and associations with external validators. Int J Eat Disord 43:433–439, 2010

Jimerson DC, Wolfe BE, Carroll DP, et al: Psychobiology of purging disorder: reduction in circulating leptin levels in purging disorder in comparison with controls. Int J Eat Disord August 31, 2009 [Epub ahead of print]

Keel PK, Haedt A, Edler C: Purging disorder: an ominous variant of bulimia nervosa? Int J Eat Disord 38:191–199, 2005

Keel PK, Wolfe BE, Liddle RA, et al: Clinical features and physiological response to a test meal in purging disorder and bulimia nervosa. Arch Gen Psychiatry 64:1058–1066, 2007

Keel PK, Holm-Denoma JM, Crosby RD: Clinical significance and distinctiveness of purging disorder and binge eating disorder. Int J Eat Disord March 2010 [Epub ahead of print]

Lee S, Ng KL, Kwok K, et al: The changing profile of eating disorders at a tertiary psychiatric clinic in Hong Kong (1987–2007). Int J Eat Disord 43:307–314, 2010

Peebles R, Hardy KK, Wilson JL, et al: Are diagnostic criteria for eating disorders markers of medical severity? Pediatrics 125:e1193–e1201, 2010

Pinheiro AP, Bulik CM, Sullivan PF, et al: An empirical study of the typology of bulimic symptoms in young Portuguese women. Int J Eat Disord 41:251–258, 2008

Roberto CA, Grilo CM, Masheb RM, et al: Binge eating, purging, or both: eating disorder psychopathology findings from an Internet community survey. Int J Eat Disord October 27, 2009 [Epub ahead of print]

Rockert W, Kaplan AS, Olmsted MP: Eating disorder not otherwise specified: the view from a tertiary care treatment center. Int J Eat Disord 40:S99–S103, 2007

Santonastaso P, Bosello R, Schiavone P, et al: Typical and atypical restrictive anorexia nervosa: weight history, body image, psychiatric symptoms, and response to outpatient treatment. Int J Eat Disord 42:464–470, 2009

Spoor ST, Stice E, Burton E, et al: Relations of bulimic symptom frequency and intensity to psychosocial impairment and health care utilization: results from a community-recruited sample. Int J Eat Disord 40:505–514, 2007

Stice E, Marti CN, Shaw H, et al: An 8-year longitudinal study of the natural history of threshold, subthreshold, and partial eating disorders from a community sample of adolescents. J Abnorm Psychol 118:587–597, 2009

Thomas JJ, Vartanian LR, Brownell KD: The relationship between eating disorder not otherwise specified (EDNOS) and officially recognized eating disorders: meta-analysis and implications for DSM. Psychol Bull 135:407–433, 2009

Williamson DA, Gleaves DH, Stewart TM: Categorical versus dimensional models of eating disorders: an examination of the evidence. Int J Eat Disord 37:1–10, 2005

Wonderlich SA, Crosby RD, Mitchell JE, et al: Testing the validity of eating disorder diagnoses. Int J Eat Disord 40:S40–S45, 2007

Zanarini MC, Reichman CA, Frankenburg FR, et al: The course of eating disorders in patients with borderline personality disorder: a 10-year follow-up study. Int J Eat Disord 43:226–232, 2010

Zimmerman M, Francione-Witt C, Chelminski I, et al: Problems applying the DSM-IV eating disorders diagnostic criteria in a general psychiatric outpatient practice. J Clin Psychiatry 69:381–384, 2008

3

CURRENT AND FUTURE DIRECTIONS FOR THE ASSESSMENT OF THE COGNITIVE CRITERIA FOR ANOREXIA NERVOSA

April R. Smith, M.S.
Erin L. Fink, M.S.
Thomas E. Joiner, Ph.D.

Anorexia nervosa (AN) is presently conceptualized in DSM-IV (American Psychiatric Association 1994) using four criteria: 1) refusal to maintain a body weight that is at or above approximately 85% of what would be expected given one's age and height; 2) fear surrounding potential weight gain even while underweight; 3) disturbance in the way one evaluates one's body, placing over-importance on weight or shape during self-evaluation, or denial of the serious nature of low weight; and 4) amenorrhea in those who otherwise would be expected to menstru-

This study was funded, in part, by National Institute of Mental Health grant F31MH083382 to A.R. Smith (under the sponsorship of T.E. Joiner). The content of this paper is solely the responsibility of the authors and does not necessarily represent the official views of the National Institute of Mental Health or the National Institutes of Health.

ate. Diagnostic schemes such as those used in DSM-IV present inherent problems for the diagnosis of mental disorders generally and AN specifically.

Becker et al. (2009) suggested that a main difficulty in correctly diagnosing AN is due to the cognitive nature of many of the criteria. By conducting a thorough literature review regarding the difficulties of clinical evaluation of cognitive symptoms of eating disorders, the authors highlighted several main issues. Relating to Criterion A—refusal to maintain body weight—the authors first pointed out the problematic nature of the word "refusal," in that it connotes defiance. There is no clear evidence that those with AN are defiantly "refusing" to maintain a healthy weight; rather, they may have an inability, or lack the skills, to regulate their weight properly. Further, Becker and colleagues advised that using such a term can set up a client-clinician relationship in which a clinician is attempting to force a client into a behavior while the client is openly rejecting the clinician's advice. Clearly, such an oppositional situation is not beneficial for client-clinician rapport. Furthermore, Mitchell et al. (2005) pointed out that the 85% weight cutoff present in Criterion A was not originally intended to be a steadfast percentage but rather was included as a rough guideline indicative of significant weight loss. Even though this criterion was not established using empirical methods, it is frequently misused as a strict cutoff when diagnosing AN.

In regard to Criterion B—intense fear surrounding weight gain—Becker et al. (2009) referred to several studies that described a partial-syndrome group of individuals who meet all criteria for AN except Criterion B. At present, it is not known how this group of individuals differs from those with full-threshold AN, if at all. However, the possibility remains that such a group could represent a diagnostic variant of AN. Additionally, Mitchell et al. (2005) related that an intense fear of weight gain may be applicable to the presentation of AN in Western cultures, but that this criterion—which has a largely sociocultural basis—may hold little diagnostic utility in other cultures.

Similarly, Criterion C is not endorsed by all individuals who may experience other symptoms of AN, and such an endorsement may depend largely on extant social norms. Becker and colleagues (2009) pointed out that self-evaluation varies largely cross-culturally (i.e., from country to country) as well as within cultures (i.e., between genders). Clearly, some societies place a premium on the physical appearance and body shape of an individual. It stands to reason that individuals in this type of society would place a large emphasis on body shape and size when self-evaluating. On the other hand, other regions may place more importance on successful social relationships. In this type of culture, individuals would likely be more inclined to self-evaluate using social rather than physical criteria. Furthermore, differences on self-evaluation can occur within cultures, as men and women often value disparate characteristics in self-schemas. For these reasons, Criterion C may be bound largely by cultural norms rather than descriptive of a behavior that is pathognomonic of anorexia.

Several diagnostic issues relating to Criterion D—amenorrhea—have been noted in recent years (Abraham et al. 2005; Grave et al. 2008; Roberto et al. 2008). For example, Garfinkel et al. (1996) compared a group of women diagnosed with AN (full syndrome), a group of women who met all criteria of AN except for amenorrhea (partial syndrome), and a healthy comparison group on a variety of indices. Their results indicated that the full- and partial-syndrome AN groups were quite similar on measures of comorbidity, bulimic behaviors, family histories, and past abuse and that both groups differed significantly from the comparison group on a host of measures. Thus, the authors concluded that the amenorrhea criterion may lack diagnostic utility.

In addition to the specific problems with the criteria, a broader issue with the diagnosis of AN is the cognitive nature of the symptoms described in DSM. Even if Criteria A–C describe a syndrome best characterized as AN, Becker et al. (2009) pointed out that these criteria are not easily observable, nor quantified, and largely depend upon the accurate self-report of clients. Clinicians are met with a dilemma in that they heavily depend upon a client to disclose these symptoms. Clients may be motivated to knowingly avoid disclosure for several reasons. First, in order to appear more socially desirable and/or avoid stigmatization, individuals may choose to withhold symptoms even if they are experiencing them. This may be especially true for men, who may resist reporting symptoms for fear of being labeled "womanly" (Smith et al. 2010). Additionally, clients may recognize these symptoms but think that they serve a useful purpose in their lives, and therefore prefer to deny a particular symptom. Whereas some patients willingly deny symptoms, other patients—particularly younger clients—may simply lack insight into the symptoms they are experiencing. This would result in nondisclosure of symptoms—not necessarily because a client actively chooses to avoid telling a clinician about his or her symptoms, but rather because he or she lacks the ability to recognize them. Clearly, these issues with disclosure of symptoms can put clinicians in a bind. If clinicians suspect AN but clients do not endorse some of the criteria, clinicians then have two choices, neither of which are particularly desirable: 1) they can diagnose AN based on their intuition and risk diagnosing a disorder the client is not actually experiencing, or 2) they can accept the client's report at face value and fail to diagnose a condition that may actually exist. In order to remediate some of these issues, eating disorder researchers have proposed some changes to the criteria necessary for an AN diagnosis in the upcoming DSM-5.

Proposed Changes to the DSM-5 Anorexia Nervosa Criteria

The first proposed change to DSM-IV by the Eating Disorders Work Group is a clarification of the word "refusal" in criterion A. It is suggested that the term "refusal" be removed in order to avoid the negative intention on the part of a client that this word may connote. Instead, the Work Group has initially recommended a more behavioral phrasing, specifically "restriction of food intake relative to caloric requirements leading to the maintenance of a body weight less than a minimally normal weight for age and height." A behavior such as restriction may be easier to identify for clinicians because it can more readily be said to be either present or absent. On the other hand, the term "refusal" requires a clinician not only to ascertain that restriction was present but also to deem *why* this behavior was present (i.e., the client was not simply restricting calories but rather was "refusing," by choice, to consume a sufficient amount of calories).

In terms of Criterion B—intense fear of weight gain—the Work Group again recommends adding a more behavioral component to supplement the existing cognitive component of intense fear. The recommended behavioral component is "persistent behavior to avoid weight gain, even though underweight." This criterion demarcates a symptom that is more readily observable than "fear," which can be denied, minimized, or unrecognized by a client. A further suggested revision involves Criterion C and changes the word "denial" to "persistent lack of recognition of the seriousness of the current low body weight." Similar to changing the word "refusal," changing the wording of Criterion C clarifies the connotation of this symptom, in that an individual may not be purposefully denying the seriousness of the problem but rather is unable to recognize it.

Finally, the DSM Work Group has proposed a removal of Criterion D—amenorrhea—from DSM-5. Although they point out that bone health may be worse in AN individuals who experience amenorrhea, they also note that some individuals experience all other symptoms of AN except for amenorrhea and, according to the current diagnostic system, would not be diagnosed with AN. As Mitchell et al. (2005) noted, those experiencing AN without amenorrhea appear to experience accompanying problems and a course that is quite similar to those with amenorrhea. The Work Group also suggests that Criterion D be removed because it is not possible to assess this criterion in several groups of people, including females who are prepubertal, those taking hormonal contraceptives, and males.

Innovative Cognitive Assessment and Diagnosis

Despite these changes, it will likely still be difficult for clinicians to make diagnostic decisions regarding AN, owing to the fact that the remaining cognitive symptoms can be particularly hard to assess for the reasons discussed earlier, such as denial, minimization, or failure to report symptoms because of associated stigma or lack of insight. Thus it may be fruitful to explore other ways to test for the presence of the disordered cognitions that are believed to be important to the symptom presentation of individuals with AN. One promising alternative to assessing for self-reported attitudes is to assess for more implicit cognitions or attitudes.

IMPLICIT ATTITUDES

Broadly speaking, attitudes are judgments about something else. For example, how you like a steak cooked and whether you like rock music are attitudes. *Explicit attitudes,* such as "I like my steak cooked medium-well," are controlled and conscious evaluative responses (Baumeister and Bushman 2008). *Implicit attitudes,* however, are automatic thoughts not under conscious control. It is possible that one's explicit and implicit attitudes agree—for example, in the case of explicitly saying one likes rock music and unconsciously preferring it—but it is also possible for a person's implicit attitude to conflict with his or her explicit attitude: this is referred to as having "dual attitudes" (Baumeister and Bushman 2008). Often, implicit attitudes diverge from explicit attitudes in domains of morality. For example, a person may claim to hold egalitarian views, yet show racism at an implicit level (e.g., Devine 1989; Dovidio et al. 1997). Furthermore, implicit attitudes are believed to be more affected by early experiences, affective experiences, and cultural biases than are explicit attitudes (Rudman 2004). For example, Rudman and colleagues (2007) found that smokers' implicit attitudes about smoking, which were mostly negative, were associated with their earliest memories about smoking, whereas their explicit attitudes about smoking, which were mostly positive, corresponded to their most recent smoking experience. Moreover, Greenwald et al. (1998) found that Japanese and Korean American students showed implicit biases toward the other group (historically, there is antagonism between Japanese and Koreans) and that the strength of the bias was associated with how immersed in either Japanese or Korean culture the participant was. An important strength of using implicit attitudes is that because they are outside of conscious control, they are not susceptible to the problems inherent in the measurement of explicit attitudes, such as self-report bias and demand expectancies.

IMPLICIT ATTITUDES AND ANOREXIA NERVOSA

Leading cognitive theories of AN (e.g., Fairburn et al. 1998) hold that extreme overvaluation of shape and weight is central to the disorder. Disordered cognitions and cognitive biases are believed to play a major role in the development and maintenance of AN (e.g., Cooper 1997, 2005; Shafran et al. 2007). Specifically, cognitive theories of AN posit that people with this disorder hold dysfunctional beliefs about their eating habits, shape, and weight. These core beliefs perpetuate negative automatic thoughts and attentional biases in the processing of information (e.g., attending only to information regarding one's body size). These negative automatic thoughts and attentional biases tend to be outside of conscious control and thus are more difficult to assess with explicit measures; however, they should be evident in cognitive tasks assessing for implicit cognitions and attitudes.

In order to assess for the presence of these implicit attitudes and cognitions, one needs implicit tests. We envision that implicit tests could be used in conjunction with more traditional explicit measures, such as structured clinical interviews, as a way to aid in the often difficult process of diagnosis among people believed to have AN. We would like to note, however, that because (to our knowledge) no such implicit diagnostic assessments have been developed, the discussion of such assessment tools at the current time must remain speculative.

Before discussing the potential use for implicit assessments in AN, we first review some existing research on the usefulness of these types of tasks. Generally speaking, tasks measuring implicit attitudes use response latencies as the outcome measure. For example, after being primed with a particular construct, a participant might be told to try to distinguish letter strings as real words or nonwords as quickly and accurately as possible. The researcher then measures the participant's reaction times to words of interest. Because the participant is generally unaware of the prime (if used) and the response latencies of interest, these tasks allow researchers to measure evaluations that are less likely to be consciously controlled.

Crucially, research has demonstrated that controlled versus automatic processes can differentially predict behavior. For example, in a classic study (Dovidio et al. 1997), participants' explicit attitudes—but not implicit attitudes—about race predicted their decisions in a simulated trial, such that participants who outwardly endorsed more egalitarian views were more likely to find a black defendant not guilty. However, participants' implicit attitudes about race predicted nonverbal behaviors, such as blinking and eye contact, as well as their performance on a spontaneous word-completion task. In another study, participants' implicit attitudes predicted spontaneous behavior, whereas their explicit attitudes regarding food predicted deliberate behavior (Perugini 2005). Specifically, positive implicit attitudes toward snacks versus fruits predicted whether a participant spontaneously chose to eat a snack or a fruit, respectively. Moreover, explicit attitudes about fruits versus snacks were significantly associated with self-reports regarding the quantities of fruits and snacks participants ate in a week.

Research has also demonstrated that implicit cognitions can predict psychopathology. For instance, using an implicit association task (described in more detail in the following section), Teachman et al. (2001) found that individuals with spider fears responded more quickly when spider stimuli were paired with negative descriptors than when snake stimuli were paired with negative descriptors. This same pattern of results (i.e., faster responding when snake stimuli were paired with negative descriptors) held for individuals with snake fears. Importantly, by using the outcomes of several cognitive tasks measuring implicit associations, these researchers were able to correctly identify 92% of participants as either spider- or snake-fearful. This is a level of discrimination above and beyond many self-report scales. Among participants with body dysmorphic disorder, Buhlmann et al. (2009) found that implicit beliefs regarding self-esteem and attractiveness predicted overall symptom severity, distress during a mirror exposure, and avoidance during a mirror exposure. Furthermore, Nock and Banaji (2007) found that among self-injurers, an implicit association between "cutting" and "me" better predicted self-injury than typical self-report measures.

A few of these types of tasks have also been used to differentiate participants at risk of developing an eating disorder from those who are not at risk. For example, Ferraro et al. (2003) found that individuals who were at risk for developing an eating disorder were faster at responding to fat-related words (e.g., "heavy," "plump," "cellulite") than words unrelated to fat, whereas control subjects were faster at recognizing "nonfat" words than "fat" words. Additionally, Ahern et al. (2008) found that participants who had positive implicit attitudes toward images of underweight women had higher drive-for-thinness scores on the Eating Disorder Inventory–2 and chose lower ideal body sizes than did participants who had more positive implicit attitudes toward normal-weight models.

Major Assessment Strategies for Implicit Attitudes

The Implicit Association Task (IAT; Greenwald et al. 1998), which is a computerized task that measures the strength of the association between constructs of interest, is one such task that could potentially be adapted to assess for disordered cognitions among people with AN. The IAT is currently the most widely used assessment of implicit attitudes. The strength of an automatic association is believed to be represented by the speed with which participants classify related and unrelated concepts; thus, the main variable of interest in an IAT is the difference in the average response time between these two types of categorizations (Teachman et al. 2001). For example, participants might decide whether pictures of typing, sunbathing, sitting in meetings, and traveling on a boat belong to the category "work" or "vacation." Additionally, in an IAT the categories of "work" and "vacation" are simultaneously paired on the computer screen with qualitative categories, such as "pleasant" and "unpleasant." For example, in one critical trial block, "vacation" and "pleasant" will both be displayed on the left side of the screen, and "work" and "unpleasant" will be displayed on the right side of the screen. Next, words or images that could belong to any of the four classes are randomly displayed on the screen, and participants are asked to categorize them (e.g., press the left key for stimuli that belong to either the vacation or pleasant category and the right key for stimuli that belong to either the work or unpleasant category). The task would then be switched such that "vacation" and "unpleasant" are paired on the same side of the screen and "work" and "pleasant" are paired on the other side of the screen. People tend to categorize the stimuli faster when they are in line with the way they evaluate or associate the categories in memory, and they are slower when the categories are incongruent. Thus, participants who consider vacation to be more pleasurable than work would be expected to classify "sunbathing" more quickly into the vacation category when it is paired with "pleasant."

Another task that is commonly used to measure implicit associations between constructs is the Lexical Decision Task (LDT). The basic task for a participant completing an LDT is to classify letter strings as real words or nonwords. The basic premise of the LDT is that people are quicker at classifying a concept (e.g., doctor) after seeing a related concept (e.g., hospital) than they are at classifying a concept (e.g., ham) after seeing an unrelated concept (e.g., board). For example, a participant may be primed with "dessert" by watching a clip of someone making cakes. The participant would next be asked to classify letter strings as real words or nonwords. The types of real words the participant would be asked to classify would belong to certain categories, for example, "good" words (e.g., happy, friendly) and "bad" words (e.g., mean, terrible). If dessert is associated with "good" in the participant's memory structures, then he or she should be faster at recognizing "good" words than "bad" words. Because LDTs are a parsimonious and direct way to test for the presence of associations, they have also been used extensively in cognitive and social psychology.

Applying Implicit Attitude Assessments to Eating Disorder Diagnostics

We present an example of a cognitive assessment that might aid in the assessment of the part of Criterion C related to disturbance in the experience of body weight. The example presented is modeled off Nock and Banaji's (2007) self-injury identity IAT and would aim to test the strength of the association an individual holds between thinness and him- or herself. In this task, participants would be presented with a series of images that are related to either thinness (i.e., pictures of thin people) or average weight (i.e., pictures of average-weight individuals), and participants would then be asked to classify these images as quickly as possible as representing the concept "thin" or "average weight." (Additionally, images related to "overweight" could also be used, but we are not including this comparison group in the current example.) Participants would also be presented with words that are either self-relevant (e.g., "I," "mine") or other-relevant (e.g., "they," "them") and would be asked to classify these as quickly as possible as representing the attributes "me" or "not me."

In this example, critical test blocks would consist of trials in which the participants are instructed to press the same computer key in response to both "thin" and "me" stimuli (thus pairing stimuli related to thinness and oneself) and another computer key for "average weight" and "not me" stimuli. For the second critical test block, the opposite sorting would be performed (i.e., pairing stimuli related to "thin" and "not me" as well as pairing stimuli related to "average weight" and "me"). The relative strength of the association between thinness and oneself could be indexed by calculating a standardized D score for each participant by subtracting the mean response latency for the thin/me test block from the mean response latency of the thin/not me test block and dividing by the standard deviation of the response latency for all trials. Thus, positive D scores reflect slower responding (i.e., weaker associations) when thinness and oneself are paired, whereas negative D scores reflect faster responding (i.e., stronger associations) when thinness and oneself are paired.

If AN participants do in fact experience cognitive distortions in the way they perceive their bodies, one would expect that they would more closely identify with the average-weight bodies than with the thin bodies, despite being dangerously underweight. Specifically, the following predictions could be made: 1) participants will be faster at pairing average-weight bodies with self-relevant concepts, 2) participants will be slower at pairing thin bodies with self-relevant concepts, 3) participants will be faster at pairing thin bodies and other-relevant concepts, and 4) participants will be slower at pairing average-weight bodies and other-relevant concepts. Support for one or more of these hypotheses would provide some evidence for a distortion in the way a participant's body is experienced.

Another example of an implicit task that could be piloted is one that would aim to assess implicit attitudes about fear over gaining weight (Criterion B). We describe the use of an LDT in testing for this type of implicit attitude. As mentioned, LDTs operate under the assumption that after being primed with a particular construct, people will be faster at responding to related constructs. Thus, in order to assess for an association between fear and weight gain, one could prime AN participants with the concept of weight gain. This could be done in a number of ways, but one way would be to have the participants write about gaining 15 pounds (more specific instructions might be to write about how this weight gain would make the person feel, what parts of his or her body would be affected, and how his or her life would be changed). After priming the participants with weight gain, one would next want to test for the association with fear, which could be done by using an LDT that incorporated various word types, such as fear words, neutral words, calm words, and negatively valenced words (we suggest the addition of negatively valenced words to rule out the possibility that weight gain makes participants feel "bad" rather than fearful). Faster responses to fear-related words as opposed to neutral, calm, or negatively valenced words would provide evidence that the participant did in fact have fear about gaining weight.

These are but a few examples of the types of tasks that could be designed to aid in the assessment of cognitive symptoms of AN. Some implicit tasks have already been used in populations with eating disorders; however, it remains to be determined whether these types of tests can improve diagnostic accuracy, predict group membership, and/or demonstrate convergent validity when a patient's explicit and implicit attitudes align. Making accurate diagnostic decisions is critical to treatment and research; unfortunately, diagnostic accuracy can be compromised by many factors. In the case of AN, diagnostic difficulties may arise when a person's self-report seems to conflict with his or her actual thoughts, feelings, and behavior.

Specifically, individuals with AN may deny the presence of cognitive symptoms for a variety of reasons; however, their denial does not mean that the symptoms do not exist. When making diagnostic decisions, clinicians and researchers are encouraged to pull from multiple sources. We have suggested that a potentially useful source of information is implicit attitudes and cognitions. We believe that assessing for the presence of certain types of cognitions and attitudes has the potential to aid in making diagnostic decisions. These assessments could further be used for making treatment recommendations as well as to monitor progress.

References

Abraham S, Pettigrew B, Boyd C, et al: Usefulness of amenorrhea in the diagnoses of eating disorder patients. J Psychosom Obstet Gynaecol 26:211–215, 2005

Ahern A, Bennett K, Hetherington M: Internalization of the ultra-thin ideal: positive implicit associations with underweight fashion models are associated with drive for thinness in young women. Eat Disord 16:294–307, 2008

American Psychiatric Association: Diagnostic and Statistical Manual of Mental Disorders, 4th Edition. Washington, DC, American Psychiatric Association, 1994

Baumeister R, Bushman B: Social Psychology and Human Nature. Belmont, CA, Thomson Wadsworth, 2008

Becker A, Eddy K, Perloe A: Clarifying criteria for cognitive signs and symptoms for eating disorders in DSM-V. Int J Eat Disord 42:611–619, 2009

Buhlmann U, Teachman B, Naumann E, et al: The meaning of beauty: implicit and explicit self-esteem and attractiveness beliefs in body dysmorphic disorder. J Anxiety Disord 23:694–702, 2009

Cooper M: Cognitive theory of anorexia nervosa and bulimia nervosa: a review. Behav Cogn Psychother 25:113–145, 1997

Cooper M: Cognitive theory in anorexia nervosa and bulimia nervosa: progress, development and future directions. Clin Psychol Rev 25:511–531, 2005

Devine P: Automatic and controlled processes in prejudice: the role of stereotypes and personal beliefs, in Attitude Structure and Function. Edited by Pratkanis AR, Breckler SJ, Greenwald AG. Hillsdale, NJ, Erlbaum, 1989, pp 181–212

Dovidio J, Kawakami K, Johnson C, et al: On the nature of prejudice: automatic and controlled processes. J Exp Soc Psychol 33:510–540, 1997

Fairburn C, Shafran R, Cooper Z: A cognitive behavioral theory of anorexia nervosa. Behav Res Ther 37:1–13, 1998

Ferraro F, Andres M, Stromberg L, et al: Processing fat-related information in individuals at risk for developing an eating disorder. J Psychol 137:467–475, 2003

Garfinkel P, Lin E, Goering P, et al: Should amenorrhea be necessary for the diagnosis of anorexia nervosa? Evidence from a Canadian community sample. Br J Psychiatry 168:500–506, 1996

Grave R, Calugi S, Marchesini G: Is amenorrhea a clinically useful criterion for the diagnosis of anorexia nervosa? Behav Res Ther 46:1290–1294, 2008

Greenwald A, McGhee D, Schwartz J: Measuring individual differences in implicit cognition: the implicit association test. J Pers Soc Psychol 85:197–216, 1998

Mitchell J, Cook-Myers T, Wonderlich S: Diagnostic criteria for anorexia nervosa: looking ahead to DSM-V. Int J Eat Disord 37:S95–S97, 2005

Nock M, Banaji M: Assessment of self-injurious thoughts using a behavioral test. Am J Psychiatry 164:820–823, 2007

Perugini M: Predictive models of implicit and explicit attitudes. Br J Soc Psychol 44:29–45, 2005

Roberto C, Steinglass J, Mayer L, et al: The clinical significance of amenorrhea as a diagnostic criterion for anorexia nervosa. Int J Eat Disord 41:559–563, 2008

Rudman L: Sources of implicit attitudes. Curr Dir Psychol Sci 13:79–82, 2004

Rudman L, Phelan J, Heppen J: Developmental sources of implicit attitudes. Pers Soc Psychol Bull 33:1700–1713, 2007

Shafran R, Lee M, Cooper Z, et al: Attentional bias in eating disorders. Int J Eat Disord 40:369–380, 2007

Smith A, Hawkeswood S, Joiner T: The measure of a man: associations between digit ratio and disordered eating in males. Int J Eat Disord 43:543–548, 2010

Teachman B, Gregg A, Woody S: Implicit associations for fear-relevant stimuli among individuals with snake and spider fears. J Abnorm Psychol 110:226–235, 2001

4

CHARACTERIZATION, SIGNIFICANCE, AND PREDICTIVE VALIDITY OF BINGE SIZE IN BINGE EATING DISORDER

Anja Hilbert, Ph.D.
Denise E. Wilfley, Ph.D.
Faith-Anne Dohm, Ph.D.
Ruth H. Striegel-Moore, Ph.D.

Patients with binge eating disorder (BED) present with heterogeneity in core symptoms, binge eating, and associated psychopathology (Wolfe et al. 2009). Variability has been found in the size of binge eating episodes (Raymond et al. 2007; Sysko et al. 2007; Walsh and Boudreau 2003; Yanovski et al. 1992), which may frequently not be unambiguously large (Greeno et al. 2000; Hilbert and Tuschen-Caffier 2007). The clinical relevance of different binge sizes in BED, however, remains largely unclear.

We would like to thank our collaborators Drs. Kathleen M. Pike, Christopher G. Fairburn, G. Terence Wilson, W. Stewart Agras, and Brunna Tuschen-Caffier for their support of the current paper. Funding sources for datasets presented in this paper include National Institutes of Health grants K24MH070446, R29MH51384 (Dr. Wilfley), R01MH064153 (Drs. Wilfley, Wilson, Agras), R01MH52348 (Dr. Striegel-Moore), and grants TU78/3–1 and 3–3 (Dr. Tuschen-Caffier) from the German Research Foundation.

In DSM-IV (American Psychiatric Association 1994) *binge eating* is defined as 1) consumption of a large amount of food, 2) a sense of loss of control (LOC) over eating, and 3) occurrence within a discrete period of time. Beyond objective bulimic episodes (OBEs), outlined in DSM, subjective bulimic episodes (SBEs) have been described as another type of binge eating (Fairburn and Cooper 1993). SBEs involve the consumption of an amount of food that is not unambiguously large but is subjectively perceived as large and is accompanied by a sense of LOC over eating. Binge eating episodes at any size or episodes of LOC eating include both OBEs and SBEs.

In the community, both OBEs and SBEs have been found to be clinically relevant and associated with increased eating disorder psychopathology, whereas associations with general psychopathology have been inconsistent (Colles et al. 2008; Elder et al. 2008; Mond et al. 2006). The co-occurrence of both types of episodes accounted for higher psychopathology than SBEs or OBEs alone (Mond et al. 2006), whereas the presence of OBEs accounted for greater body mass index (BMI; Colles et al. 2008; Mond et al. 2006). In a clinical sample of BED patients, there were no differences in the associations between the number of OBEs versus SBEs and eating disorder and general psychopathology (Niego et al. 1997), as was found in patients with bulimic or mixed symptomatology (Latner et al. 2007; Pratt et al. 1998). In a latent class analysis on a clinical sample with BED, the highest-severity eating disorder and general psychopathology was detected in patients with the most frequent SBEs and OBEs (Sysko et al. 2010). These patients benefited most from interpersonal psychotherapy (IPT) compared with guided self-help and behavioral weight loss, likely owing to IPT's greater efficacy for depressive symptoms. In addition, SBEs were found to be more persistent after self-help treatment (Loeb et al. 2000) and slower to decrease during psychotherapy (Niego et al. 1997). Because evidence on the convergent validity of binge size assessment by clinical interviews or self-report questionnaires is limited (Bartholome et al. 2006), validation using concurrent assessment methodologies such as self-monitoring and laboratory test meals is warranted. Thus, our overall goal in this chapter was to elucidate the construct of binge size in BED regarding clinical significance, predictive validity, and convergent validity by reanalyzing data from several community-based and clinical studies.

Clinical Significance

Binge size and concurrent clinical outcomes were examined using the data set of the New England Women's Health Project (NEWHP; Pike et al., unpublished data; Striegel-Moore et al. 2005). The NEWHP includes well-characterized, nonclinical samples of individuals with BED ($n=154$) and bulimia nervosa (BN; $n=61$), and a clinical sample of individuals with anorexia nervosa (AN; $n=70$). Eating disorder diagnosis was based on an abbreviated diagnostic version of the Eating Disorder Examination (EDE; Fairburn and Cooper 1993), and items assessing the frequency of

SBEs and OBEs over the previous 3 months were used in the analyses. Further measures included the Eating Disorder Examination Questionnaire (EDE-Q; Fairburn and Beglin 1994), for assessment of eating disorder psychopathology (subscales of restraint, eating concern, shape concern, and weight concern and the global severity score); the Brief Symptom Inventory, for assessment of general psychopathology (global severity index; Derogatis 1991); the Structured Clinical Interview for DSM-IV Axis I Disorders, for comorbid psychiatric diagnosis (First et al. 1997); and participants' self-reported health care utilization (i.e., number of health care visits in the past year). Data analysis was based on univariate General Linear Model (GLM) analyses for repeated measures for comparison of OBE versus SBE frequencies, on univariate GLM or χ^2 tests for comparison of concurrent clinical outcomes by binge status (OBEs only vs. OBEs and SBEs), and on correlation analyses ($\alpha < 0.05$).

BINGE SIZE ACROSS THE EATING DISORDERS

OBEs occurred more frequently than SBEs in individuals with BED (18.11 ± 13.02 OBEs/month over the past 3 months vs. 6.34 ± 12.00 SBEs/month; $F_{1,153} = 64.62$, $P < 0.001$). The same pattern emerged for BN (25.98 ± 21.95 vs. 7.52 ± 19.09; $F_{1,60} = 22.99$, $P < 0.001$); however, there was no such difference in frequency of OBEs and SBEs in AN (14.31 ± 27.08 vs. 15.79 ± 28.64; $F_{1,69} = 0.10$, $P = 0.750$). Categorically, more BED patients reported only OBEs as compared with both OBEs and SBEs (99/154, 64.3% vs. 55/154, 35.7%; binomial test, $P < 0.05$; see Table 4–1). The same pattern of binge status emerged in BN (41/61, 67.2% OBEs only vs. 20/61, 32.8% OBEs and SBEs; $P < 0.05$). In AN, binge eating symptomatology was more varied, with 8 participants reporting OBEs only (out of 70, 11.4%), 22 OBEs and SBEs (31.4%), and 17 SBEs only (24.3%), whereas one-third ($n = 23$) did not have any episodes of LOC eating (32.9%), but rates of occurrence did not differ ($P > 0.05$). in an analysis of the number of LOC episodes by binge status, those with SBEs and OBEs had a greater number of LOC episodes than those with OBEs only in the BED group (see Table 4–1) and in the BN group (OBEs only: 25.73 ± 23.12 LOC episodes/month; OBEs and SBEs: 49.43 ± 31.07; $F_{1,59} = 11.22$, $P = 0.001$). In AN, the number of LOC episodes over the past 3 months did not differ between those with OBEs only and those with OBEs and SBEs, but the number of LOC episodes was greater in those with OBEs and SBEs than in those with SBEs only (OBEs only: 48.75 ± 41.64; OBEs and SBEs: 58.45 ± 42.79; SBEs only: 25.33 ± 34.84; no LOC: 0.00 ± 0.00; $F_{3,66} = 13.10$, $P < 0.001$, post hoc Tukey honestly significant difference tests, $P < 0.05$). To summarize, these results show that SBEs are present in one-third of BED cases. Those with SBEs in addition to OBEs experienced about twice as many LOC episodes as those with OBEs only. Although a similar pattern of results emerged for BN, binge eating symptomatology in AN was more varied.

TABLE 4–1. Concurrent psychopathology by binge status in a nonclinical sample of binge eating disorder patients ($N=154$)

	OBEs only ($n=99$)		OBEs and SBEs ($n=55$)		$F_{1,149-152}$	P	n OBEs, r	n SBEs, r	n LOC, r
	M	SD	M	SD					
OBEs	18.79	14.22	16.90	10.53	0.75	0.389	—		
SBEs	0.00	0.00	17.76	14.19			−0.05	—	
LOC episodes	18.79	14.22	34.66	17.59	37.05	<0.001**	0.72**	0.66**	—
EDE-Q Restraint	1.89	1.42	2.59	1.44	8.94	0.003**	−0.17*	0.24**	0.03
EDE-Q Eating Concern	2.54	1.24	3.15	1.22	8.14	0.005**	0.15	0.31**	0.32**
EDE-Q Shape Concern	4.04	1.40	4.65	1.07	7.33	0.008**	0.02	0.26**	0.20**
EDE-Q Weight Concern	3.68	1.37	4.34	1.08	8.97	0.003**	0.00	0.26**	0.18*
EDE-Q Global Score	3.04	1.12	3.68	0.93	12.95	<0.001**	−0.01	0.33**	0.22**
BSI Global Severity Index	68.78	21.76	71.34	19.24	0.31	0.576	−0.02	0.11	0.06
Health care use	1.67	0.82	1.96	1.01	3.38	0.068	−0.03	0.08	0.03
	n	%	n	%	χ^2_1	P			
SCID any Axis I disorder	83	53.9	48	31.2	0.33	0.567	−0.02	0.08	0.02

Note. Objective bulimic episodes (OBEs), subjective bulimic episodes (SBEs), and episodes of loss of control (LOC) over eating were assessed using the Eating Disorder Examination (EDE); average episode frequencies per month (over the past 3 months) are displayed. Data analysis included general linear model or χ^2 tests, or Spearman Brown correlation coefficients.

BSI=Brief Symptom Inventory T scores (higher scores indicating less favorable conditions); EDE-Q=Eating Disorder Examination—Questionnaire (range 0–6); health care use=number of health care visits in past year; SCID=Structured Clinical Interview for DSM-IV.

*$P<0.05$; **$P<0.01$.

BINGE SIZE AND CONCURRENT CLINICAL OUTCOMES

When we focus on the associated psychopathology by binge status in BED, individuals with BED who reported both OBEs and SBEs revealed greater eating disorder psychopathology than those with OBEs only ($P<0.05$), whereas there were no differences in general psychopathology, psychiatric comorbidity, and health care use ($P>0.05$; see Table 4–1). Addressing the association of binge eating frequency with psychopathology, we found that the number of SBEs, but not OBEs, was significantly associated with greater eating disorder psychopathology across all indicators of the EDE-Q ($P<0.05$; see Table 4–1). While the number of SBEs was positively associated with restraint, the number of OBEs was negatively associated with it ($P<0.05$). In contrast, the number of OBEs and SBEs was unrelated to general psychopathology, psychiatric comorbidity, and health care use ($P>0.05$). In these analyses, it was unnecessary to control for association between OBEs and SBEs because their frequencies were not significantly related ($P>0.05$). In addition, age or measured BMI (kg/m^2) did not differ by binge status ($P>0.05$). However, although a higher proportion of black individuals reported only OBEs compared with OBEs and SBEs (44/154, 77.2% vs. 13/154, 22.8%), similar proportions of white individuals reported only OBEs or OBEs and SBEs (55/154, 56.7% vs. 42/154, 43.3%; $\chi^2_{1,154}=6.57$, $P=0.010$). Including race as a covariate did not modify the results on greater eating disorder psychopathology in those with OBEs and SBEs compared with those with OBEs only (all $P<0.05$). However, when race was controlled for, the associations between the number of OBEs or SBEs and restraint became insignificant (partial correlations, $P>0.05$). To summarize, these results show that the presence and frequency of SBEs accounted for increased eating disorder psychopathology in BED, and vice versa. In contrast, a greater number of OBEs was associated with less restraint over eating. Black individuals were less affected by SBEs than were white individuals.

Predictive Validity

Data from two psychological treatment trials were reanalyzed to determine the prognostic validity of binge size.

COGNITIVE-BEHAVIORAL THERAPY VERSUS INTERPERSONAL PSYCHOTHERAPY

In a randomized controlled trial comparing the effectiveness of group cognitive-behavioral therapy (CBT) and group IPT (Wilfley et al. 2002), outcome by pretreatment binge status, prognostic validity of binge status, and binge status outcome at 1-year follow-up were analyzed. Assessment of OBEs, SBEs, and LOC episodes (for the past 28 days) was based on the EDE, as well as assessment of restraint, composite shape/weight concern, and the global score of eating disorder psychopathology. General psychopathology was measured using the global severity index of the Symptom Checklist–90—Revised (Derogatis 1977). From a total of 162 patients, 161 patients for whom baseline SBE data were available were included in the analyses. Data analysis was based on assessment completers; assessment noncompletion rates were low (Wilfley et al. 2002). First, the time course of numbers of OBEs, SBEs, and LOC episodes was analyzed in a repeated measures GLM of Binge Status (OBEs only, OBEs and SBEs) × Time (pretreatment, posttreatment, 1-year follow-up). In additional steps, treatment condition (CBT, IPT) was included as a factor, and measured BMI was used as a covariate. Second, logistic regression analyses were used to predict abstinence from OBEs, the primary outcome criterion in treatment studies of BED, and abstinence from LOC eating at posttreatment and 1 year following treatment cessation from pretreatment binge status. Additionally, logistic regression analyses were rerun, controlling for BMI and treatment condition. Third, in order to cross-sectionally examine the psychopathology by binge status 1 year following treatment cessation, univariate GLM analyses by binge status (no LOC, SBEs only, OBEs only, OBEs and SBEs) were calculated ($\alpha < 0.05$).

The time course of binge eating episodes by pretreatment binge status is depicted in Figure 4–1. The number of OBEs, SBEs, and LOC episodes decreased significantly from pretreatment to posttreatment and remained decreased from pretreatment to 1-year follow-up in patients who had OBEs only or both OBEs and SBEs prior to treatment (repeated measures GLM of Binge Status × Time, post hoc least significant difference tests, $P < 0.05$). Patients with OBEs and SBEs revealed a stronger decrease in LOC episodes than patients with OBEs only from pretreatment to posttreatment (post hoc Tukey honestly significant difference test, $P < 0.05$). For both patients with OBEs only and patients with OBEs and SBEs prior to treatment, there was a significant increase in OBEs and LOC episodes (post hoc least significant difference tests, $P < 0.05$), but not in SBEs ($P > 0.05$), from posttreatment to 1-year follow-up. Including treatment condition as a factor or BMI as a covariate did not modify the results.

Concerning the prediction of OBE and LOC abstinence from pretreatment binge status, logistic regression analyses, summarized in Table 4–2, revealed that the initial presence of SBEs predicted better treatment response in terms of abstinence from OBEs and from LOC episodes at posttreatment ($P < 0.05$) but not at 1-year follow-up ($P > 0.05$). In these analyses, adjustment by treatment condition or BMI did not modify the results.

Concerning psychopathology by binge status 1 year following treatment cessation, as illustrated in Figure 4–2, the presence of SBEs at 1-year follow-up was an indicator of greater eating disorder psychopathology when compared with no LOC (cross-sectional GLM by binge status at follow-up [no LOC, SBEs only, OBEs only, OBEs and SBEs], post hoc Tukey honestly significant difference tests,

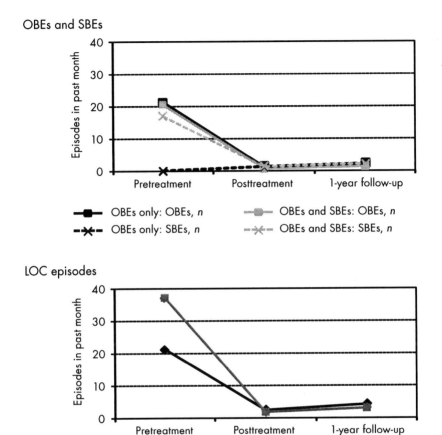

FIGURE 4–1. Number of binge eating episodes by binge status before psychological treatment of binge eating disorder, after treatment end, and 1 year following treatment cessation (N=161).

Objective bulimic episodes (OBEs), subjective bulimic episodes (SBEs), and episodes of loss of control (LOC) over eating determined using the Eating Disorder Examination. Repeated measures general linear model of binge status (OBEs only, OBEs and SBEs) × time (pretreatment, posttreatment, 1-year follow-up): Number of OBEs—binge status: $F_{1,140}=1.02$, $P=0.315$; time: $F_{1,166}=330.39$, $P<0.001$; interaction: $F_{1,166}=3.43$, $P=0.884$. Number of SBEs—binge status: $F_{1,136}=45.95$, $P<0.001$; time: $F_{2,211}=37.35$, $P<0.001$; interaction: $F_{2,211}=56.16$, $P<0.001$. LOC episodes—binge status: $F_{1,140}=16.15$, $P<0.001$; time: $F_{1,202}=303.48$, $P<0.001$; interaction: $F_{1,202}=31.28$, $P<0.001$.

TABLE 4–2. Abstinence from objective bulimic episodes (OBEs) and from loss-of-control (LOC) episodes following cognitive-behavioral therapy and interpersonal psychotherapy of binge eating disorder and 1 year after treatment cessation, by pretreatment binge status ($N=161$)

	OBEs only (n=75)	OBEs and SBEs (n=86)	B	SE	Wald χ^2_1	P	R^2
Abstinence from OBEs							
Posttreatment, n (%)	50 (68.5)	72 (85.7)	1.02	0.40	6.41	0.011*	0.06
1-year follow-up, n (%)	44 (63.8)	55 (75.3)	0.55	0.37	2.23	0.135	0.02
Abstinence from LOC episodes							
Posttreatment, n (%)	35 (47.9)	56 (66.7)	0.78	0.33	5.54	0.019*	0.05
1-year follow-up, n (%)	35 (50.7)	43 (58.9)	0.33	0.34	0.96	0.328	0.01

Note. OBEs, subjective bulimic episodes (SBEs), and episodes of LOC over eating were assessed with the Eating Disorder Examination. Results of logistic regression analysis are presented.
*$P<0.05$; **$P<0.01$.

$P<0.05$), although the pattern of association was not completely consistent and did not apply to restraint ($P>0.05$). The presence of OBEs at 1-year follow-up emerged as an indicator of general psychopathology when compared with no LOC ($P<0.05$). Binge status did not show any significant association with percent weight change from pretreatment to 1-year follow-up nor with BMI at 1-year follow-up ($P>0.05$). Inclusion of treatment condition or control by BMI and further pretreatment scores did not modify the results. As opposed to the results from the nonclinical NEWHP population described earlier, there were no differences between patients with OBEs and those with OBEs and SBEs ($P>0.05$) in this clinical population of BED individuals 1 year after treatment cessation; however, trends were in the same direction with small to medium effect sizes (EDE Global Score: $\eta^2=0.04$, EDE Shape/Weight Concern: $\eta^2=0.04$, Restraint: $\eta^2=0.01$).

To summarize, both SBEs and OBEs showed significant and long-lasting decreases through psychological treatment. Whereas OBEs increased slightly but significantly during the 1-year follow-up period, this was not the case for SBEs. SBEs at pretreatment emerged as a positive prognostic indicator of short-term, but not long-term, treatment success. While LOC after treatment indicated increased eating disorder and general psychopathology, no LOC was associated with less psychopathology.

INTERPERSONAL PSYCHOTHERAPY, GUIDED SELF-HELP, AND BEHAVIORAL WEIGHT LOSS

Using data from a randomized trial comparing the effectiveness of individual IPT, guided self-help, and behavioral weight loss (Wilson et al. 2010), prognostic validity of binge status and binge status outcome at 2-year follow-up were analyzed ($N=205$). Assessment of OBEs, SBEs, LOC episodes, and associated eating disorder psychopathology was based on the EDE (for the past 28 days), and depressive symptoms were measured using the Beck Depression Inventory (Beck et al. 1961). Data analysis followed the same rationale as described earlier.

Concerning the prediction of OBE and LOC abstinence, logistic regression analyses, displayed in Table 4–3, revealed a tendency of pretreatment SBEs to predict better treatment in terms of abstinence from OBEs at posttreatment only ($P=0.058$). Adjustment for treatment condition, intervention site, and BMI did not modify the results. As shown in Figure 4–3, the presence of OBEs 2 years following treatment cessation was an indicator of greater shape/weight concern and global eating disorder psychopathology when compared with the presence of SBEs only or no LOC ($P<0.05$) and also of greater restraint and depression than no LOC ($P<0.05$). Binge status did not show any significant association with BMI change from pretreatment or BMI at 2-year follow-up ($P>0.05$). Inclusion of treatment condition, intervention site, or control by BMI and further pretreatment scores did not modify the results. Thus, the presence of SBEs at pretreatment emerged as a

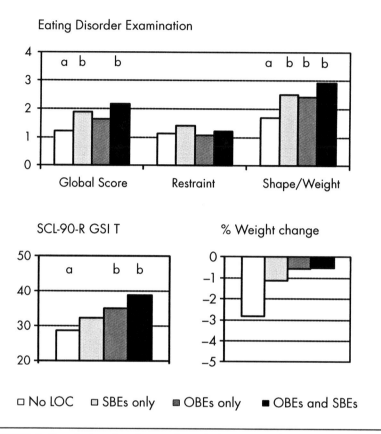

FIGURE 4–2. Eating disorder psychopathology, general psychopathology, and weight change by binge status 1 year following cognitive-behavioral therapy or interpersonal psychotherapy of binge eating disorder (*N*=161).

Objective bulimic episodes (OBEs), subjective bulimic episodes (SBEs), and episodes of loss of control (LOC) over eating determined using the Eating Disorder Examination. Univariate general linear model analyses of binge status (no LOC, SBEs only, OBEs only, OBEs and SBEs): Eating Disorder Examination Global Score, $F_{3,135}=6.62$, $P<0.001$; Restraint, $F_{3,135}=0.38$, $P=0.770$; Shape/Weight Concern, $F_{3,135}=6.61$, $P<0.001$. SCL-90-R GSI, $F_{3,118}=6.31$, $P<0.001$; percent weight change from pretreatment, $F_{3,136}=0.81$, $P=0.492$. Letters *a* and *b* indicate significant post hoc Tukey honestly significant difference tests, $P<0.05$.

SCL-90-R GSI=Global Severity Index of the Symptom Checklist–90–Revised.

TABLE 4–3. Abstinence from objective bulimic episodes (OBEs) and from loss-of-control (LOC) episodes after interpersonal psychotherapy, guided self-help, and behavioral weight loss treatment of binge eating disorder and 2 years following treatment cessation, by pretreatment binge status (N=177)

	OBEs only (n=92)	OBEs and SBEs (n=85)	B	SE	Wald χ^2_1	P	R^2
Abstinence from OBEs							
Posttreatment, n (%)	57 (62.0)	64 (75.3)	0.63	0.33	3.59	0.058	0.03
2-year follow-up, n (%)	58 (69.0)	57 (77.0)	0.41	0.36	1.26	0.262	0.01
Abstinence from LOC episodes							
Posttreatment, n (%)	46 (50.0)	42 (49.4)	–0.02	0.30	0.01	0.938	0.00
2-year follow-up, n (%)	40 (47.6)	35 (47.3)	–0.01	0.32	0.00	0.968	0.00

Note. OBEs, subjective bulimic episodes (SBEs), and episodes of LOC over eating were assessed with the Eating Disorder Examination. Results of logistic regression analysis are presented.
*$P<0.05$; **$P<0.01$.

trendwise positive prognostic indicator of posttreatment abstinence from OBEs, which is consistent with results gathered in the trial of CBT and IPT in BED.

Convergent Validity

Concerning the validity of the EDE-derived binge size distinction of SBEs and OBEs, data from three separate studies using food diaries, Ecological Momentary Assessment, and test meal assessments were analyzed.

FOOD DIARY STUDY

In a food diary study (Hilbert and Tuschen-Caffier, unpublished data), 20 individuals with BED were recruited from the community and diagnosed using the EDE and an established psychiatric interview for DSM-IV (Margraf 1994). Participants were asked to concurrently monitor the type and quantity of all foods and drinks they consumed over 4 consecutive days and to indicate whether they considered each eating episode a binge. Food intake was converted into kilocalorie intake and kilocalorie intake from macronutrients using nutritional software. For the comparison of food intake and meal patterns by binge status and nonparametric correlation analyses, it was decided to report effects of at least medium size (point biserial or Spearman $r \geq 0.30$), because of the limited sample size. Raw data were reported; changes through adjustment by BMI were reported in addition.

As presented in Figure 4–4, individuals with OBEs only reported a greater average kilocalorie intake during self-identified binges than those with OBEs and SBEs ($r=0.30$), which coincided with a greater intake of macronutrient fat ($r=0.30$). Overall caloric intake per day was more than 1,000 kcal greater in those with OBEs only than in those with OBEs and SBEs ($r=0.32$). This greater intake was attributable to increased intake during binge eating episodes, because there were no differences by binge status in caloric and macronutrient intake during regular episodes of eating ($r<0.30$). Furthermore, associations were determined between the number of EDE-reported OBEs, SBEs, and LOC episodes and self-monitored intake. The number of OBEs and LOC episodes showed associations of at least medium size with the monitored kilocalorie intake per binge ($r=0.50$ and 0.40, respectively), while the number of SBEs was unrelated to kilocalorie intake per binge ($r<0.30$). Concerning meal patterns, the presence of OBEs and SBEs led to a smaller number of regular meals per day when compared with the presence of OBEs only ($r=0.36$; see Table 4–4).

ECOLOGICAL MOMENTARY ASSESSMENT STUDY

Data from an Ecological Momentary Assessment study (Hilbert and Tuschen-Caffier 2007) were reanalyzed for confirmation of findings from the food diary study, fol-

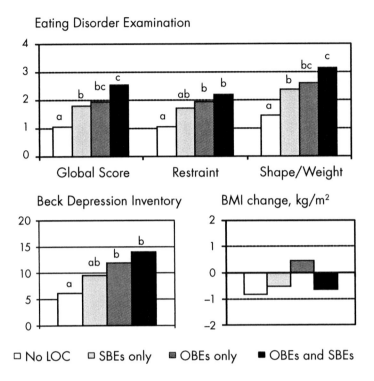

FIGURE 4–3. Eating disorder psychopathology, general psychopathology, and change in body mass index by binge status 2 years following interpersonal psychotherapy, guided self-help, and behavioral weight loss treatment of binge eating disorder (*N*=205).

Objective bulimic episodes (OBEs), subjective bulimic episodes (SBEs), and episodes of loss of control (LOC) over eating determined using the Eating Disorder Examination. Univariate general linear model analyses of binge status (no LOC, SBEs only, OBEs only, OBEs and SBEs): Eating Disorder Examination Global Score, $F_{3,154}=21.66$, $P<0.001$; Restraint, $F_{3,154}=6.27$, $P<0.001$; Shape/Weight Concern, $F_{3,154}=16.24$, $P<0.001$. Beck Depression Inventory, $F_{3,150}=8.18$, $P<0.001$. BMI change from pretreatment, $F_{3,154}=0.84$, $P=0.475$. Letters *a, b,* and *c* indicate significant post hoc Tukey honestly significant difference tests, $P<0.05$.

BMI = body mass index.

Food diary study

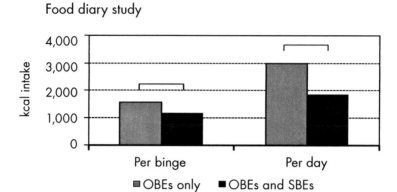

Ecological momentary assessment

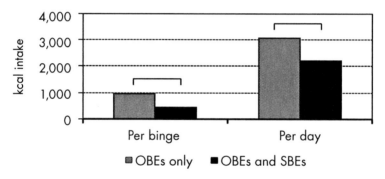

FIGURE 4–4.   Food intake per binge and day in a food diary study and in an Ecological Momentary Assessment study of binge eating disorder (*N*=20 each).

Objective bulimic episodes (OBEs) and subjective bulimic episodes (SBEs) determined using the Eating Disorder Examination. *Brackets* indicate differences of at least medium effect size ($r \geq 0.30$).

lowing the same data analytic procedure. In this study, 20 individuals with BED were recruited from the community. Diagnosis and assessment of OBEs, SBEs, and LOC episodes (for the previous 4 weeks) were based on the EDE. For an assessment period of 2 consecutive days, probands were supplied with minicomputers for random sampling of mood and cognitions in the naturalistic environment. In addition, they were instructed to monitor all types and quantities of foods consumed and to indicate whether they considered an eating episode a binge.

TABLE 4–4.   Meal patterns in a food diary study and in an Ecological Momentary Assessment study of binge eating disorder ($N=20$ each)

	OBEs only		OBEs and SBEs		
	Mean	SD	Mean	SD	r
Food diary					
n Regular meals/day[a]	4.08	1.20	3.11	1.44	0.36
n Binge eating episodes/day	1.21	1.05	0.96	0.83	–0.12
Ecological momentary assessment					
n Regular meals/day[a]	3.38	0.75	3.72	1.17	–0.13
n Binge eating episodes/day	1.13	0.48	1.66	0.93	0.25

Note.   Objective bulimic episodes (OBEs) and subjective bulimic episodes (SBEs) determined through the Eating Disorder Examination.
[a]Four or five meals/day are normative in Germany (Deutsche Gesellschaft für Ernährung, www.dge.de).

The results confirmed a larger energy intake in those with OBEs only than in those with OBEs and SBEs per self-identified binge ($r=0.72$) and per day ($r=0.41$), which was due to greater consumption of all macronutrients ($0.43 \le r \le 0.68$). In this study, those with OBEs only also had a greater intake during regular meals than those with OBEs and SBEs ($r=0.56$). The number of SBEs and of LOC episodes showed negative associations with the monitored kilocalorie intake per binge ($r=-0.30$ and -0.42, respectively), whereas the number of OBEs was unrelated to kilocalorie intake per binge ($r<|0.30|$). The associations of regular meal patterns with binge status had lower than medium effect sizes ($r<0.30$; see Table 4–4). Of note is that individuals with BED who endorsed OBEs and SBEs on the EDE showed a trend of more self-identified binge eating episodes than those with OBEs only ($r=-0.25$).

TEST MEAL STUDY

In a randomized component analysis, 24 patients with BED underwent a laboratory test meal before and 4 months after cessation of CBT with exposure-based versus cognitive interventions on body image (Hilbert and Tuschen-Caffier 2004). Patients were offered a three-course standard dinner to be selected from a menu (850 kcal total) and were asked to eat as much as they liked. Pre- and postconsumption weight and food were determined, and food intake in grams was converted into kilocalorie intake and kilocalorie intake from macronutrients using nutritional software. For the comparison by binge status, point biserial r was computed, and partial correlations were calculated for adjustment by pretreatment binge status and BMI ($\alpha<0.05$).

As shown in Figure 4–5, patients who had OBEs with or without SBEs 4 months following CBT, as determined by the EDE, showed a significantly greater kilocalorie intake at the test meal than those who did not have any LOC episodes or who had SBEs only ($r=0.66$, $P<0.05$), which was attributable to greater intake of all macronutrients (all $r \ge 0.56$). These group differences were independent from pretreatment binge status and BMI ($P>0.05$).

Conclusion

The results underscore that SBEs are a common and clinically significant experience affecting about one-third of individuals with BED. This pattern of occurrence and the frequencies of OBEs and SBEs in BED were similar to those in BN, whereas binge eating symptomatology in AN was more varied, likely related to the absence of an OBE threshold for diagnosis. The number of LOC episodes was twice as high in BED individuals with SBEs in addition to OBEs than in those with OBEs only, amounting to more than one LOC episode per day. This more generalized sense of

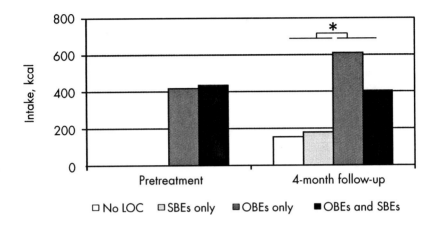

FIGURE 4–5. Food intake in a laboratory test meal study of binge eating disorder prior to and 4 months following cessation of cognitive-behavioral therapy (*N*=24).

Objective bulimic episodes (OBEs) and subjective bulimic episodes (SBEs) determined using the Eating Disorder Examination.

*Point biserial correlations, *P*<0.05.

LOC=loss of control.

LOC coincided with a more pervasive dysregulation of meal patterns and with greater eating disorder psychopathology, but not with greater general psychopathology or health care use, consistent with previous research (Mond et al. 2006). As opposed to Mond et al.'s (2006) results in a community sample with lower BMI, BMI did not differ by binge status in our nonclinical and clinical datasets of BED, although those with OBEs only revealed a greater energy intake by day than those with OBEs and SBEs or SBEs/no LOC. Because SBEs have been associated with low stability in BED (Grilo et al. 2004), fluctuations in binge status could—among other factors—account for this absence of difference in BMI.

The binge size distinction had convergent validity and corresponded to binge size assessed in food diaries, ecological momentary assessment, and test meal assessment, confirming initial evidence (Bartholome et al. 2006); however, the threshold for distinction between unambiguously and subjectively large amounts of food remains unclear (see Raymond et al. 2003). Nevertheless, there was evidence to suggest that SBEs and OBEs may be maintained differentially (Agras and Telch 1998; Latner and Clyne 2008). The more individuals with BED gave up on restricting food intake, the more they experienced OBEs and vice versa, while SBEs may be maintained differentially through failure of attempts at strict dieting, similar to that found in patients with BN (Kerzhnerman and Lowe 2002). These associations with restraint were interestingly explained by race; a greater proportion of white individuals than black individuals with BED reported SBEs.

Both OBEs and SBEs showed significant and long-lasting improvements after specialist treatment of BED. That SBEs did not emerge as more resistant to treatment is opposed to the results of a self-help treatment study (Loeb et al. 2000). It should, however, be noted that the specialist treatment IPT was found to be more potent than nonspecialist guided self-help in cases of greater eating disorder psychopathology (Wilson et al. 2010), which has been linked to more frequent SBEs. Unlike OBEs, SBEs did not show a significant relapse through follow-up. Moreover, pretreatment SBEs seemed to make patients with BED more responsive to treatment in the short term; consistently, the presence of more pretreatment SBEs but fewer OBEs was found to be significantly associated with placebo response (Jacobs-Pilipsky et al. 2007). Notwithstanding, further evidence is needed to clarify the course (Hildebrandt and Latner 2006; Niego et al. 1997) and mechanisms of change of SBEs versus OBEs during treatment. In addition, SBEs are warranted to be considered in the definition of treatment outcome: As eating disorder psychopathology was significantly greater with LOC non-abstinence than with LOC abstinence, LOC abstinence represented a more stringent outcome criterion than the commonly used abstinence from OBEs as an indicator of eating disorder psychopathology. However, OBE abstinence indicated less general psychopathology and test meal overeating, making it the more comprehensively relevant outcome criterion.

Overall, the results underscore the importance of assessing SBEs in addition to OBEs in BED. Both types of episodes are clinically relevant, but OBEs even more so because of their association with poorer treatment response, more general residual symptomatology, and greater tendency to relapse. Based on the current findings, it is recommended that DSM-5 include a scheme for determining the presence and frequency of both SBEs and OBEs over the diagnostic time period, in order to begin tracking and evaluating this information systematically in BED as well as other syndromal and subsyndromal eating disorders. Careful characterization of binge size in psychopathology, course, and treatment studies will allow for further clarification of the nature and clinical significance of binge size across the eating disorder spectrum.

References

Agras WS, Telch CF: The effects of caloric deprivation and negative affect on binge-eating in obese binge-eating disordered women. Behav Ther 29:491–503, 1998

American Psychiatric Association: Diagnostic and Statistical Manual of Mental Disorders, 4th Edition. Washington, DC, American Psychiatric Association, 1994

American Psychiatric Association: Diagnostic and Statistical Manual of Mental Disorders, 4th Edition, Text Revision. Washington, DC, American Psychiatric Association, 2000

Bartholome LT, Raymond NC, Lee SS, et al: Detailed analysis of binges in obese women with binge eating disorder: comparisons using multiple methods of data collection. Int J Eat Disord 39:685–693, 2006

Beck AT, Ward CH, Mendelson M, et al: An inventory for measuring depression. Arch Gen Psychiatry 4:561–571, 1961

Colles SL, Dixon JB, O'Brien PE: Loss of control is central to psychological disturbance associated with binge eating disorder. Obesity 16:608–614, 2008

Derogatis LR: SCL-90-R: Administration, Scoring and Procedures Manual-I for the Revised Version. Baltimore, MD, Johns Hopkins School of Medicine, 1977

Derogatis LR: Brief Symptom Inventory. Baltimore, MD, Clinical Psychometric Research, 1991

Elder KA, Paris M Jr, Anez LM, et al: Loss of control over eating is associated with eating disorder psychopathology in a community sample of Latinas. Eat Behav 9:501–503, 2008

Fairburn CG, Beglin SJ: Assessment of eating disorders: interview or self-report questionnaire? Int J Eat Disord 16:363–370, 1994

Fairburn CG, Cooper Z: The Eating Disorder Examination (12th edition), in Binge Eating: Nature, Assessment and Treatment. Edited by Fairburn CG, Wilson GT. New York, Guilford, 1993, pp 317–360

First MB, Spitzer RL, Gibbon M, et al: Structured Clinical Interview for DSM-IV Axis I Disorders, Research Version, Patient Edition With Psychotic Screen. New York, Biometrics Research, New York State Psychiatric Institute, 1997

Greeno CG, Wing RR, Shiffman S: Binge antecedents in obese women with and without binge eating disorder. J Consult Clin Psychol 68:95–102, 2000

Grilo CM, Masheb RM, Lozano-Blanco C, et al: Reliability of the Eating Disorder Examination in patients with binge eating disorder. Int J Eat Disord 35:80–85, 2004

Hilbert A, Tuschen-Caffier B: Body image interventions in cognitive-behavioural therapy of binge-eating disorder: a component analysis. Behav Res Ther 42:1325–1339, 2004

Hilbert A, Tuschen-Caffier B: Maintenance of binge eating through negative mood: a naturalistic comparison of binge eating disorder and bulimia nervosa. Int J Eat Disord 40:521–530, 2007

Hildebrandt T, Latner JD: Effect of self-monitoring on binge eating: treatment response or "binge drift"? Eur Eat Disord Rev 14:17–22, 2006

Jacobs-Pilipski MJ, Wilfley DE, Crow SJ, et al: Placebo response in binge eating disorder. Int J Eat Disord 40:204–211, 2007

Kerzhnerman I, Lowe MR: Correlates of subjective and objective binge eating in binge-purge syndromes. Int J Eat Disord 31:220–228, 2002

Latner JD, Clyne C: The diagnostic validity of the criteria for binge eating disorder. Int J Eat Disord 41:1–14, 2008

Latner JD, Hildebrandt T, Rosewall JK, et al: Loss of control over eating reflects eating disturbances and general psychopathology. Behav Res Ther 45:2203–2211, 2007

Loeb KL, Wilson GT, Gilbert JS, et al: Guided and unguided self-help for binge eating. Behav Res Ther 38:259–272, 2000

Margraf J: Mini-DIPS: Diagnostisches Kurzinterview psychischer Störungen. Berlin, Germany, Springer, 1994

Mond J, Hay P, Rodgers B, et al: Use of extreme weight control behaviors with and without binge eating in a community sample: implications for the classification of bulimic-type eating disorders. Int J Eat Disord 39:294–302, 2006

Niego SH, Pratt EM, Agras WS: Subjective or objective binge: is the distinction valid? Int J Eat Disord 22:291–298, 1997

Pratt EM, Niego SH, Agras WS: Does the size of a binge matter? Int J Eat Disord 24:307–312, 1998

Raymond NC, Neumeyer B, Warren CS, et al: Energy intake patterns in obese women with binge eating disorder. Obes Res 11:869–879, 2003

Raymond NC, Bartholome LT, Lee SS, et al: A comparison of energy intake and food selection during laboratory binge eating episodes in obese women with and without a binge eating disorder diagnosis. Int J Eat Disord 40:67–71, 2007

Striegel-Moore RH, Fairburn CG, Wilfley DE, et al: Toward an understanding of risk factors for binge-eating disorder in black and white women: a community-based case-control study. Psychol Med 35:907–917, 2005

Sysko R, Devlin MJ, Walsh BT, et al: Satiety and test meal intake among women with binge eating disorder. Int J Eat Disord 40:554–561, 2007

Sysko R, Hildebrandt T, Wilson GT, et al: Heterogeneity moderates treatment response among patients with binge eating disorder. J Consult Clin Psychol 78:681–690, 2010

Walsh BT, Boudreau G: Laboratory studies of binge eating disorder. Int J Eat Disord 34(suppl):S30–S38, 2003

Wilfley DE, Welch RR, Stein RI, et al: A randomized comparison of group cognitive-behavioral therapy and group interpersonal psychotherapy for the treatment of overweight individuals with binge-eating disorder. Arch Gen Psychiatry 59:713–721, 2002

Wilson GT, Wilfley DE, Agras WS, et al: Psychological treatments of binge eating disorder. Arch Gen Psychiatry 67:94–101, 2010

Wolfe BE, Baker CW, Smith AT, et al: Validity and utility of the current definition of binge eating. Int J Eat Disord 42:674–686, 2009

Yanovski SZ, Leet M, Yanovski JA, et al: Food selection and intake of obese women with binge-eating disorder. Am J Clin Nutr 56:975–980, 1992

5

EATING BEHAVIOR IN OBESE BINGE EATING DISORDER, OBESE NON–BINGE EATING DISORDER, AND NON-OBESE CONTROL PARTICIPANTS

A Naturalistic Study

Scott G. Engel, Ph.D.
Kirsten A. Kahler, B.A.
Chad M. Lystad, M.S.
Ross D. Crosby, Ph.D.
Heather K. Simonich, M.A.
Stephen A. Wonderlich, Ph.D.
Carol B. Peterson, Ph.D.
James E. Mitchell, M.D.

Reprinted from *Behaviour Research and Therapy*, Vol. 47, Engel SG, Kahler KA, Lystad CM, et al.: "Eating Behavior in Obese BED, Obese non-BED, and Non-obese Control Participants: A Naturalistic Study," pp. 897–900, 2009, with permission from Elsevier.

We thank the National Eating Disorders Association for providing funding for the current project.

Binge eating disorder (BED) is characterized in DSM-IV (American Psychiatric Association 1994) by the consumption of an objectively large amount of food coupled with a sense of loss of control (LOC) and not accompanied by compensatory behaviors. BED patients are commonly obese and also experience more impaired emotional functioning, lower quality of life, and poorer physical health compared with non-BED obese individuals (de Zwaan et al. 2002). This population also may have higher rates of impairment and distress due to the increased presence of comorbid psychopathology (Wilfley et al. 2000). Furthermore, the behavior of binge eating has been shown to be associated with weight gain and subsequent obesity (de Zwaan 2001; Fairburn et al. 2001).

Objective evidence that the eating behavior of BED patients differs from that of obese individuals without BED would add support to the validity of the diagnosis (Walsh and Boudreau 2003). However, data from two different assessment methodologies are contradictory. Several laboratory studies have shown that obese BED individuals eat significantly more than comparable obese non-BED participants in simulation of a binge eating episode. When asked to "binge eat" or "let themselves go when eating," BED participants eat markedly more than non-BED participants. This finding appears in the laboratory consistently, regardless of whether participants are given an array of food (e.g., Yanovski et al. 1992) or a single-item test meal (e.g., Sysko et al. 2007).

Field studies have attempted to examine binge eating patients in their natural settings (e.g., Wegner et al. 2002) by employing a methodology called *ecological momentary assessment* (EMA). Two EMA-based field studies are particularly relevant to the current investigation. Contrary to the laboratory findings, Greeno et al. (2000) found that both BED and non-BED groups reported binge eating frequencies that well exceeded the minimum of two binge eating episodes per week required for diagnosis and that the caloric content of the participant-identified binge eating episodes did not differ between the BED and non-BED groups (800 vs. 792 calories, respectively). A second EMA study (le Grange et al. 2001) found that binge eating frequency did not significantly differ between the BED and non-BED groups.

These two EMA studies used a combination of self-identified behaviors (i.e., after a participant engaged in an eating episode, he or she labeled the eating episode as a "binge" or as something else) and food logs. Both of these techniques have proven useful in clinical settings as well as in several recent empirical studies; however, they have several limitations, not the least of which are the subjectivity of the participant-labeled behaviors and the questionable validity of the food logs due to poor compliance and retrospective recall biases (Engel et al. 2005). Furthermore, the use of traditional food logs likely limits the validity of comparisons of caloric intake across groups. Regardless of the specific reasons for the contradictory findings in the literature, reconciling this discrepancy will provide extremely useful information about the BED diagnosis.

In the current study, we attempt to circumvent those limitations by employing a novel adaptation of EMA. As described in more detail later, we couple EMA techniques with a standardized computer dietary recall system that minimizes reliance on retrospective recall, avoids relying on participant definitions of behaviors, and enables us to place EMA and eating information in correct temporal space. With this more comprehensive assessment method, we hypothesized that both groups of obese samples (with and without BED) would have greater rates of binge eating and overeating compared with non-obese control subjects while in their natural environment. Also, we hypothesized that the BED group would have greater rates of binge eating compared with the non-BED obese group.

Methods

PARTICIPANTS

Participants included 40 individuals recruited through community and university flyers and by referral from an eating disorders treatment facility. Flyers posted in the community and local universities sought individuals who were "normal weight or overweight and over the age of 18." Because we were primarily looking to recruit BED patients from the eating disorders treatment facility, clinicians were told that we were seeking individuals who were obese, binge ate, and did not engage in compensatory behaviors. Two participants were excluded from the analyses because they provided EMA data that appeared to be invalid. Of the remaining 38 participants, 16 were non-obese control subjects (body mass index [BMI] 20–25 and no eating disorder as determined by the Structured Clinical Interview for DSM-IV Axis I Disorders [SCID-I; First et al. 1995]), 13 were obese non-BED subjects (BMI>30 and no eating disorder diagnosis as determined by the SCID-I), and 9 were obese BED subjects (BMI>30 and a diagnosis of BED as determined by the SCID-I). Participants with a BMI of 25–30 were excluded from the study. Participants could be male or female, and all participants were over the age of 18. Exclusion criteria included being pregnant or currently breastfeeding; having a current diagnosis of a psychotic disorder; having previous gastrointestinal surgery; having any medical illness requiring dietary modification; using any medication associated with weight or eating change; having suicidal ideation; purging; and being unable to read English. Participants were compensated $100 for participation in the study, with the potential to earn another $50 for compliance by attending all scheduled appointments. This protocol was approved by the University of North Dakota Institutional Review Board.

Demographic information for the sample is summarized in Table 5–1.

MEASURES

Phone Screening

The eating disorder module of SCID-I was administered by phone to determine eligibility and diagnosis and was used to determine group membership. The phone screening was also supplemented with probes from the Eating Disorder Examination (EDE; Fairburn and Cooper 1993). This phone screening was the primary instrument used to diagnose the presence of BED in each participant and was conducted by a SCID-I/EDE-trained master's-level assessor.

Ecological Momentary Assessment

For the EMA protocol, each participant carried a handheld computer for 7 days and was asked to rate mood, stress, hunger, and level of control over eating just before he or she began any eating episode. Ratings for LOC were made on a one- to five-point Likert-type scale. A rating of one on the scale signified "no control" and a five signified "complete control."

Eating Behavior

The Nutritional Data System for Research (NDS-R) was used to gather nutritional intake data on each of the eating episodes recorded by participants (Schakel et al. 1988). The NDS-R is a Windows-based, interviewer-administered assessment that allows for the nutrient intake calculation of foods eaten over a 24-hour time interval. It is considered by many to be the gold standard method of assessment of food intake (Feskanich et al. 1999) and has been used successfully with research on overweight and obese samples (e.g., Ebbeling et al. 2004). NDS-R reports of caloric intake also correlate significantly with doubly labeled water data, suggesting the instrument is a valid assessment of eating behavior (Raymond et al. 2003). Caloric data were collected for each eating episode recorded on the handheld computer. Each eating episode was classified by caloric amount into the categories of less than 1,000 calories, overeating, and binge eating.

Past research findings show that 1,000 calories or more exceeds what most people would consume in a typical eating episode (Keel et al. 2002; Mitchell et al. 1998). Therefore, *overeating* was defined as consuming 1,000 calories or more in one eating episode. Consistent with the DSM-IV definition, *binge eating* was defined as consuming 1,000 calories or more and a sense of LOC. *Loss of control* was defined as a rating of one to three on the one- to five-point Likert-type scale for LOC.

PROCEDURES

After the phone screening, qualified participants attended an informational meeting at the research facility. At this meeting, participants first gave their informed con-

TABLE 5–1. Demographics and eating behavior of study sample, by group

	BED, mean (SE)	Non-BED, mean (SE)	NOC, mean (SE)	P	Effect size	Post hoc
Body mass index	42.3 (3.4)	36.5 (1.9)	23.1 (0.3)	0.001	0.637[a]	BED, non-BED > NOC
Age	37.3 (4.9)	34.6 (2.8)	22.7 (1.0)	0.001	0.337[a]	BED, non-BED > NOC
Caucasian, %	100	84.6	92.9	0.51	0.382[b]	
Never married, %	44.4	38.5	68.8	0.02	0.748[b]	BED, non-BED < NOC
Eating episodes per day	3.5 (0.2)	3.0 (0.2)	4.0 (0.2)	<0.001	0.059[a]	Non-BED < NOC
Kilocalories per day	2,536.0 (136.1)	2,005.0 (107.3)	1,606.0 (103.3)	<0.001	0.083[a]	BED > non-BED > NOC
Kilocalories per eating episode	837.6 (53.3)	739.4 (42.0)	414.6 (40.4)	<0.001	0.135[a]	BED, non-BED > NOC
Loss of control	3.51 (0.07)	3.55 (0.06)	4.18 (0.06)	<0.001	0.040[a]	BED, non-BED < NOC
Overeating, %	0.24 (0.03)	0.16 (0.02)	0.04 (0.01)	<0.001	0.077[a]	BED > non-BED > NOC
Binge eating, %	0.16 (0.02)	0.09 (0.02)	0.01 (0.01)	<0.001	0.170[a]	BED > non-BED > NOC

Note. All reported means are age-corrected.

BED = binge eating disorder; NOC = non-obese control subjects.

[a]Proportion of variance explained.

[b]Phi coefficient.

sent. Participants next provided descriptive and demographic information. Each participant was given thorough instruction on how to use the handheld computer and completed a 1-day practice period to ensure understanding of EMA procedures. Practice data were not included in the analyses.

Participants came to the research facility every day during the data collection period. At that time, information from the handheld computer was uploaded and monitored for compliance, and feedback was provided by the research coordinator to the participant about the quality of data. The eating recordings were then used to interview the participants about their dietary intake. The time points of each eating episode were entered into the NDS-R system, and participants were asked to recall the details of each episode as well as whether they had forgotten to report any eating episode. Following each NDS-R interview, the nutritional data of interest were merged with the EMA data to create a temporal picture of the eating and LOC ratings for the previous day. At the final visit, participants returned their handheld computer, completed a payment form, and were debriefed.

STATISTICAL ANALYSIS

Because groups were found to differ by age ($P=0.001$), with non-obese control participants being younger than BED and non-BED participants, all inferential statistics were performed using age as a covariate, and means reported are corrected for age. Binge eating, overeating, and LOC variables were examined using one-way analysis of covariance, with age as a covariate. The three groups were compared on overeating (1,000 calories in one eating episode) and binge eating episodes (1,000 calories and LOC in an eating episode) by means of a two-level hierarchical generalized linear model based on a binomial sampling distribution (Raudenbush and Bryk 2002). Level 1 observations were represented by momentary reports of overeating and binge eating behaviors. Level 2 observations were represented by the group variable: non-obese control, non-BED, and BED. Analyses were performed using SPSS Version 16.0.1 (SPSS for Windows 2008) and HLM Version 5.04 (Raudenbush et al. 2001). Pairwise age-adjusted, Bonferroni-corrected contrasts were used for post hoc comparisons.

Results

LOSS OF CONTROL

When LOC immediately before any eating episode was examined, a significant effect for group was identified ($F_{2,928}=28.03$, $P<0.001$) (see Table 5–1 for details).

EATING BEHAVIOR

Table 5–1 shows the number of eating episodes per day, the number of kilocalories per day, and the number of kilocalories per eating episode (all age-corrected) for each of the three groups. Analyses showed a significant group difference in the number of eating episodes per day ($F_{2,280} = 9.25$, $P = 0.001$) as well as the total number of kilocalories reported eaten each day ($F_{2,280} = 12.68$, $P = 0.001$) and the number of kilocalories eaten at each eating episode ($F_{2,280} = 19.99$, $P = 0.001$).

Participants reported a total of 131 overeating episodes (> 1,000 kcal in an eating episode). After controlling for age, there was a significant effect for group on frequency of overeating (Wald $\chi^2 = 51.69$, $P = 0.001$). A total of 57 binge eating episodes (> 1,000 kcal in an eating episode and LOC) were reported by all participants in the study. After controlling for age, there was a significant effect for group on frequency of binge eating (Wald $\chi^2 = 52.47$, $P = 0.001$).

Discussion

In the current study, we found a number of important differences between the obese participants (BED and non-BED) and the non-obese control group. Furthermore, we found several differences between BED and non-BED participants and, importantly, showed that the BED group reported more overeating and binge eating than the non-BED group.

We believe that the findings of the current study help clarify the contradictory conclusions of laboratory studies (e.g., Yanovski et al. 1992) and field studies (Greeno et al. 2000; le Grange et al. 2001). Despite the modest sample size, we were able to find significant group differences between BED and non-BED groups in overeating and binge eating. We believe this suggests the assessment strategy used in the current study is more sensitive than the assessment strategies previously used in field studies (e.g., food logs and binge eating episodes identified by participants). Although those assessments have proven useful clinically, we believe the method used in the current study may be more objective.

An obvious limitation of the current study is the modest sample size. However, in spite of the small number of participants per group, we had adequate power to detect the hypothesized group differences. Related to this concern, one must consider the representativeness of the small sample sizes in the current study. Another limitation is that although we consider the dietary recall data collected to be more objective and less reliant on recall biases and interpretation than data from past field studies, these data are still based on self-report.

According to Walsh and Boudreau (2003), demonstrating that individuals with and without BED differ on more objective measures of binge eating would provide important support for the validity of the diagnostic category. We would add that demonstrating that these differences exist in the participants' natural environment further adds to the validity of the construct of BED. Taken together with the recent evidence that the BED diagnosis tends to have a familial heritability (Hudson et al. 2006) and may be relatively stable over time (Pope et al. 2006), the present data provide further support for the validity of the BED construct. Empirical support of the construct of BED may have important clinical implications for the revision of eating disorder diagnoses in DSM-5.

References

American Psychiatric Association: Diagnostic and Statistical Manual of Mental Disorders, 4th Edition. Washington, DC, American Psychiatric Association, 1994

de Zwaan M: Binge eating disorder and obesity. Int J Obes Relat Metab Disord 25:S51–S55, 2001

de Zwaan M, Mitchell JE, Howell LM, et al: Two measures of health-related quality of life in morbid obesity. Obes Res 10:1143–1151, 2002

Ebbeling CB, Sinclair KB, Pereira MA, et al: Compensation for energy intake from fast food among overweight and lean adolescents. JAMA 291:2828–2833, 2004

Engel SG, Wonderlich SA, Crosby RD: Ecological momentary assessment, in The Assessment of Patients With Eating Disorders. Edited by Mitchell JE, Peterson C. New York, Guilford, 2005, pp 203–220

Fairburn CG, Cooper Z: The Eating Disorder Examination (12th Edition), in Binge Eating: Nature, Assessment and Treatment. Edited by Fairburn CG, Wilson GT. New York, Guilford, 1993, pp 317–360

Fairburn C, Cooper Z, Doll H, et al: The natural course of bulimia nervosa and binge eating disorder in young women. Arch Gen Psychiatry 57:659–665, 2001

Feskanich D, Sielaff BH, Chong K, et al: Computerized collection and analysis of dietary intake information. Comput Methods Programs Biomed 30:47–57, 1999

First MB, Spitzer RL, Gibbon M, et al: Structured Clinical Interview for DSM-IV Axis I Disorders (SCID-IP). Washington, DC, American Psychiatric Press, 1995

Greeno CG, Wing RR, Shiffman S: Binge antecedents in obese women with and without binge eating disorder. J Consult Clin Psychol 68:95–102, 2000

Hudson JI, Lalonde JK, Berry JM: Binge eating disorder as a distinct familial phenotype in obese individuals. Arch Gen Psychiatry 63:313–319, 2006

Keel PK, Cogley CB, Ghosh S, et al: What constitutes an unusually large amount of food for defining binge episodes? Paper presented at the Academy for Eating Disorders 10th International Conference on Eating Disorders, Boston, MA, April 2002

le Grange D, Gorin A, Catley D, et al: Does momentary assessment detect binge eating in overweight women that is denied at interview? Eur Eat Disord Rev 9:309–324, 2001

Mitchell JE, Crow S, Peterson CB, et al: Feeding laboratory studies in patients with eating disorders: a review. Int J Eat Disord 24:115–124, 1998

Pope HG Jr, Lalonde JK, Pindyck LJ, et al: Binge eating disorder: a stable syndrome. Am J Psychiatry 163:2181–2183, 2006

Raudenbush SW, Bryk AS: Hierarchical Linear Models: Applications and Data Analysis Methods, 2nd Edition. Thousand Oaks, CA, Sage, 2002

Raudenbush S, Bryk AS, Cheong YF, et al: HLM 5: Hierarchical Linear and Nonlinear Modeling. Lincolnwood, IL, Scientific Software International, 2001

Raymond NC, Neumeyer B, Warren CS, et al: Energy intake patterns in obese women with binge eating disorder. Paper presented at the annual Eating Disorder Research Society meeting, Port Douglas, Australia, September 2003

Schakel SF, Sievert YA, Buzzard IM: Sources of data for developing and maintaining a nutrient database. J Am Diet Assoc 88:1268–1271, 1988

SPSS for Windows, Release 16.0.1. Chicago, IL, SPSS Inc, 2008

Sysko R, Devlin MJ, Walsh BT, et al: Satiety and test meal intake among women with binge eating disorder. Int J Eat Disord 40:554–561, 2007

Walsh BT, Boudreau G: Laboratory studies of binge eating disorder. Int J Eat Disord 24:S30–S38, 2003

Wegner KE, Smyth JM, Crosby RD, et al: An evaluation of the relationship between mood and binge eating in the natural environment using ecological momentary assessment. Int J Eat Disord 32:352–361, 2002

Wilfley DE, Friedman MA, Dounchis JZ, et al: Comorbid psychopathology in binge eating disorder: relation to eating disorder severity at baseline and following treatment. J Consult Clin Psychol 68:641–649, 2000

Yanovski SZ, Leet M, Flood M, et al: Food intake and selection of obese women with and without binge eating disorder. Am J Clin Nutr 56:975–980, 1992

6

LOSS-OF-CONTROL EATING AS A PREDICTOR OF WEIGHT GAIN AND THE DEVELOPMENT OF OVERWEIGHT, DEPRESSIVE SYMPTOMS, BINGE DRINKING, AND SUBSTANCE USE

Alison E. Field, Sc.D.
Heather L. Corliss, M.P.H., Ph.D.
Hayley H. Skinner, M.P.H., M.Sc.
Nicholas J. Horton, Sc.D.

Although commonly used, the DSM-IV (American Psychiatric Association 1994) criteria for eating disorders have been widely questioned (Herzog et al. 1996; le Grange et al. 2006; Sullivan et al. 1998; Wilfley et al. 2007; Wonderlich et al. 2007). One problem with the current classification scheme is that in both clinical and gen-

The analysis was supported by a research grant (MH087786-01) from the National Institutes of Health.

eral population samples, the majority of individuals with eating disorders meet some but not all of the criteria for anorexia nervosa (AN) or bulimia nervosa (BN) and thus fall into the category of eating disorder not otherwise specified (EDNOS) (Eddy et al. 2008; Field et al. 2008; le Grange et al. 2006; Patton et al. 2008). In order to create a more accurate classification system that will result in fewer people in the EDNOS category, it is essential that there be empirical evidence for the utility of each of the criteria.

In DSM-IV, binge eating disorder (BED), a subtype of EDNOS, and BN both require that an individual engage in frequent episodes of binge eating. A *binge* is defined as eating a large amount of food in a relatively short amount of time and feeling out of control during the episode. Both the frequency threshold and the importance of the control criteria have been hotly debated. The decision to require someone to binge eat, on average, twice per week was not based on research that found differences in comorbidity, treatment, or outcome among those who engaged in bulimic behaviors less or more frequently. In fact, several studies have found that females who binge and purge less than once a week exhibit high levels of eating concerns (le Grange et al. 2006), comorbid disorders, and personality traits (Steiger and Bruce 2007) as well as functional impairment (Mond et al. 2006). Therefore, it is essential to determine empirically whether a lower frequency is justified in the diagnostic criteria, particularly because DSM-5 is likely to lower the frequency threshold to at least once a week.

At present there is debate regarding whether the focus should be on size (objective vs. subjective binges) or the perception of being out of control during the episode. The DSM-IV and draft DSM-5 criteria require both objectively large binges and feeling out of control during the binge, but this decision was not evidence based. Because it is not entirely clear what the threshold should be for classifying an eating episode as large, particularly in the United States, where portion sizes are often extremely large, it is of great importance to determine whether it is the consumption of a large amount of food or feeling out of control during the episode that is the more important criterion.

The aim of the present investigation was to assess whether loss of control during an overeating episode is predictive of adverse outcomes, including becoming overweight or obese, starting to use drugs, starting to binge drink frequently, and developing high levels of depressive symptoms. Our secondary aim was to assess how the risk of adverse outcomes varied by frequency of binge eating or overeating without a loss of control. To assess these aims, we used seven follow-up assessments over 9 years of more than 7,200 females in the Growing Up Today Study (GUTS) who were 9–15 years of age at baseline.

Methods

GUTS was established in 1996 by recruiting children of women participating in the Nurses' Health Study II (NHS II). The NHS II was established in 1989 and consists of 116,608 female nurses, ages 25–43 years at entry. Follow-up questionnaires have been sent to participants biennially since 1989. Additional details about the cohort have been reported elsewhere (Solomon et al. 1997). Using the NHS II data, we identified mothers who had children ages 9–14. We wrote a detailed letter to the mothers, explaining the purpose of GUTS and seeking parental consent to enroll their children. Children whose mothers gave us consent to invite them to participate were mailed an invitation letter and a questionnaire. Additional details have been reported previously (Field et al. 2001). Approximately 68% of the females (*n* = 9,039) and 58% of the males (*n* = 7,843) returned completed questionnaires, thereby assenting to participate in the cohort. The participants have been sent questionnaires every 12–18 months. The study was approved by the Human Subjects Committee at Brigham and Women's Hospital, and the analyses presented in this chapter were approved by the Institutional Review Boards at Brigham and Women's Hospital and Children's Hospital Boston.

SAMPLE

Participants were excluded from the analysis if they did not return at least two contiguous assessments (e.g, 1996 and 1997, 1998 and 1999). Because binge eating was less common among the males, we did not have sufficient power to detect associations between binge eating and adverse outcomes and therefore excluded males from the analysis. Sample sizes varied by outcome. In all analyses, females who had reported overeating episodes at baseline (i.e., prevalent cases) were excluded, and once a female reported the outcome of interest, she was censored from analyses using subsequent time periods. After these exclusions, 7,260 females remained for the analyses predicting becoming overweight or obese, 7,289 females remained for the analyses predicting starting to binge drink, 4,882 females remained for the analyses predicting starting to use drugs, and 3,672 females remained for the analyses predicting developing high levels of depressive symptoms.

MEASURES

Questionnaires Completed by GUTS Participants

In the fall of 1996 through 2003, GUTS participants received a questionnaire every 12–18 months assessing a variety of factors. Self-reported weight and height were assessed on all questionnaires. The validity of weight change based on serial self-reported measures of weight has been assessed by Field et al. (2007) using data from 1,671 females and 1,613 males in the National Longitudinal Study of Adolescent

Health, a prospective study that has both measured and obtained self-reported weights and heights at two time points approximately 5 years apart. Field and colleagues observed that both males and females slightly underreported their weights but were consistent in their underreporting. As a result, weight change based on self-reported weights at waves II and III underestimated weight change based on measured weights by only an average of 2.1 lb, and the correlation between weight change based on self-report versus measured weights was $r=0.8$. The discrepancy between weight change based on self-reported versus measured weights was not significantly associated with known predictors of weight change: being African American or Hispanic, weight change efforts, activity level, and time spent watching television.

Weight Status

Body mass index (BMI: weight [kg]/height [m²]) was calculated using self-reported weight and height. Children were classified as overweight or obese based on the International Obesity Task Force cutoffs (Cole et al. 2000), which are age- and gender-specific and provide comparability in assessing overweight and obesity from adolescence to adulthood.

Weight Control Behaviors and Binge Eating

Weight control behaviors and binge eating have been assessed on all questionnaires (i.e, 1996, 1997, 1998, 1999, 2000, 2001, 2003, and 2005). Weight control behaviors were assessed with questions adapted from the Youth Risk Behavior Surveillance System questionnaire (Kann et al. 1996). Purging was assessed with two questions: "During the past year, how often did you make yourself throw up to keep from gaining weight?" and "During the past year, how often did you take laxatives to keep from gaining weight?" Binge eating was assessed with a two-part question. Participants were first asked about the frequency during the past year of eating a very large amount of food. Children who reported at least occasional episodes of overeating were directed to a follow-up question that asked whether they felt out of control during these episodes, as though they could not stop eating even if they wanted to stop. *Binge eating* was defined as eating a very large amount of food in a short amount of time at least monthly and feeling out of control during the eating episode. Both the binge eating and the purging questions have been validated in the GUTS cohort. Among the girls, the specificity and negative predictive values of self-reported purging and binge eating were high, thereby demonstrating that the questionnaire did an excellent job at classifying females who did not purge (Field et al. 2004).

Participants who reported that they engaged in binges at least twice a week and did not engage in purging were classified as having BED, whereas those who reported engaging in binges at least once a week and not engaging in purging were classified as having subthreshold BED. In addition, participants were classified as binge eaters or overeaters regardless of purging status. Females who reported weekly episodes of overeating and having a loss of control during the eating episode were classified as weekly bingers, whereas females who reported weekly episodes of overeating but did not report a loss of control were classified as weekly overeaters. Similar definitions were used to classify females as monthly bingers and monthly overeaters.

Binge Drinking

A question on binge drinking was added in 1998 and appeared on the 1998, 1999, 2000, 2001, and 2003 questionnaires. Children who reported that they had ever consumed alcohol were asked a series of questions about their drinking behavior. One of those questions asked about the frequency in the past year of drinking four or more drinks over a few hours, which was our definition of binge drinking among females. Participants who reported at least 12 episodes of binge drinking in the past year were classified as frequent binge drinkers.

Drug Use

Questions on drug use were added in 1999 and also were included on the 2001 and 2003 questionnaires. Participants were asked a series of questions about drug use. The questions regarding illicit drug use asked whether they had used marijuana or hashish, cocaine, crack (1999 and 2001), heroin, ecstasy, phencyclidine (PCP; 1999 and 2001), γ-hydroxybutyrate (GHB; 1999 and 2001), lysergic acid diethylamide (LSD), mushrooms, ketamine (1999 and 2001), or amphetamines. Because of an expected strong cross-sectional association between overeating episodes and marijuana and hashish use, we did not include marijuana or hashish in our drug use outcome. Participants who reported using cocaine, crack, heroin, ecstasy, PCP, GHB, LSD, mushrooms, ketamine, or amphetamines and had never reported using any of those drugs at an earlier time period were classified as incident drug use cases.

Depressive Symptoms

Depressive symptoms were assessed with the six-item validated scale of the McKnight Risk Factor Survey IV (Shisslak et al. 1999). All responses were scored on a five-point Likert scale ranging from never to always. Participants in the top quintile of depressive symptoms were considered cases; thus incident cases of high levels of depressive symptoms were females who were in one of the bottom four quintiles of depressive symptoms on one assessment but in the top quintile on the next assessment.

STATISTICAL ANALYSIS

We modeled the log odds of the hazard rate for four different outcomes—becoming overweight or obese, starting to binge drink frequently, starting to use drugs other than marijuana, and developing high levels of depressive symptoms. Predictors were lagged so that outcomes at a given time point were modeled as a function of predictors from the previous time point. The models were fitted by means of generalized estimating equations (Zeger and Liang 1986) with an exchangeable working covariance matrix and empirical variance estimator in order to address the dependence between children who shared the same mother. The analyses were performed using PROC GENMOD (SAS Version 8.2). All analyses were adjusted for age.

Results

At baseline, the mean age of the participants was approximately 12 years (Table 6–1). During 9 years of follow-up, approximately 20% became overweight or obese, 27% started to binge drink frequently, 10% started to use drugs, and 22% developed high levels of depressive symptoms.

As can be seen in Figure 6–1, binge eating increased over time as the girls aged, but the prevalence of overeating remained constant. Although binge eating was more common than overeating without a loss of control, both were predictive of becoming overweight or obese over the subsequent 1–2 years. The association was strongest with females who engaged in binge eating at least once a week but did not purge (i.e., BED). Females classified as having subthreshold BED according to DSM-IV (or BED in DSM-IV) had 2.3 times the odds (95% CI = 1.5–3.7) of becoming overweight or obese in the next 1–2 years compared with their peers who did not binge eat. The association was slightly lower (Table 6–2), but still significant, with weekly binges (irrespective of purging status) and weekly overeating episodes without a loss of control. When the frequency cutoff was changed from at least weekly to at least monthly episodes of binge eating or overeating without a loss of control, a different pattern emerged. For binge eating, the association with becoming overweight or obese was extremely similar for weekly and monthly binge eating, whereas for overeating without a loss of control, the association with weekly episodes was stronger than that with monthly episodes.

Binge drinking became increasingly prevalent with age. Both weekly and monthly binge eating were predictive of starting to binge drink. Females who engaged in weekly binge eating episodes had two times higher odds of starting binge drinking frequently over the following 1–2 years (OR = 2.1; 95% CI = 1.5–2.8) compared with their peers who did not binge eat. However, having weekly episodes of overeating without a loss of control was not predictive of starting to binge drink frequently (Table 6–3), which may reflect a lack of statistical power due to the relatively small number of females who engaged in weekly episodes of overeating.

Only 9.8% of females started to use drugs other than marijuana; thus our power to detect associations was somewhat limited, particularly for predictors with low prevalence rates such as BED. Although there was a suggestion of an association between subthreshold BED and starting to use drugs other than marijuana in the

TABLE 6–1. Prevalence of overweight, binge drinking, and doing drugs at baseline among 7,260 adolescent girls in the Growing Up Today Study

Age, years[a]	12.1 (1.6)
Body mass index (kg/m²)[a]	19.0 (3.3)
Overweight or obese at baseline, %	20.1
Binge eating ≥ weekly at baseline, %	0.9
Overeating without loss of control ≥ weekly at baseline, %	0.4
Binge drinking frequently,[b] %	2.1
Using drugs other than marijuana,[c] %	9.1
High level of depressive symptoms,[c,d] %	18.8

[a]Mean (SD).
[b]First assessed in 1998. At least 12 episodes in the past year.
[c]First assessed in 1999.
[d]Top quintile of depressive symptoms on the McKnight Risk Factor Survey IV six-item scale.

next 2 years (Table 6–4), the association was not significant. However, females who engaged in binge eating weekly (OR=1.9; 95% CI=1.1–3.3) or monthly (OR=2.0; 95% CI=1.4–2.9) were significantly more likely to start using drugs. At both frequency cutoffs (weekly and monthly), the associations were stronger with binge eating than with overeating without a loss of control.

Weekly binge eating was strongly predictive of developing high levels of depressive symptoms over the following 2 years. Subthreshold BED cases (OR=2.7; 95% CI=1.3–5.7) and females classified as engaging in weekly binge eating, regardless of purging status (OR=3.0; 95% CI=1.7–5.3) were significantly more likely to develop high levels of depressive symptoms. The associations between overeating without a loss of control and depressive symptoms were weaker than those with binge eating (Table 6–5).

Discussion

Among more than 7,200 female adolescents and young adults in GUTS, followed for up to 9 years, we observed that binge eating increased with age but that overeating did not. Moreover, binge eating was a stronger predictor than overeating without a loss of control of starting to binge drink frequently, starting to use drugs, or developing high levels of depressive symptoms. However, both binge eating and overeating without a loss of control were predictive of becoming overweight or obese during the subsequent 1–2 years.

Although many studies have reported a strong cross-sectional association between binge eating and obesity (Field et al. 1999; French et al. 1999; Neumark-

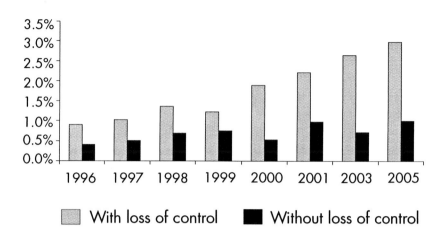

FIGURE 6–1. Prevalence of at least weekly overeating episodes among girls in the Growing Up Today Study (GUTS), 1996–2005.

Sztainer and Hannan 2000; Tanofsky-Kraff et al. 2004), few studies have examined the association prospectively. In the few longitudinal studies, binge eating was found to predict greater weight (Stice et al. 1999) or body fat gain (Tanofsky-Kraff et al. 2006), but we are unaware of any prospective studies investigating the association between development of overweight and overeating episodes with and without loss of control during the episode. The results of our study suggest that all overeating episodes (regardless of frequency or loss of control) are predictive of becoming overweight or obese.

In contrast, weekly binge eating was more strongly predictive than overeating episodes without a loss of control of starting to binge drink frequently, starting to use drugs, or developing high levels of depressive symptoms. The results suggest loss-of-control overeating may be predictive of a broader problem related to impulse control, which increases the risk of starting to use drugs or binge drink. In addition, weekly binge eating with a loss of control was strongly predictive of developing high levels of depressive symptoms. Some females may turn to drugs or alcohol to self-medicate depressive symptoms, which explains why loss-of-control overeating is related to all three adverse outcomes. More research is needed to better understand why loss-of-control overeating episodes are predictive of developing adverse substance use and mental health outcomes among some adolescent and young adult females.

One limitation of our study is that it does not represent a random sample of all U.S. female adolescents and young adults. The participants are daughters of nurses, and the sample is more than 90% white; thus we are unlikely to have children of

TABLE 6–2. Prospective association[a] of disordered eating predicting becoming overweight or obese in the subsequent 1–2 years among girls in the Growing Up Today Study

	Age-adjusted OR (95% CI)	*P*
Binge eating disorder[b]	1.7 (0.8–3.6)	0.1729
Subthreshold binge eating disorder[c]	2.3 (1.5–3.7)	0.0004
Bingeing ≥ weekly	1.9 (1.2–2.8)	0.0044
Overeating without loss of control ≥ weekly	2.1 (1.2–3.8)	0.0143
Bingeing ≥ monthly	2.0 (1.5–2.7)	< 0.0001
Overeating without loss of control ≥ monthly	1.5 (1.0–2.1)	0.0356

[a]Odds ratios and 95% confidence intervals from generalized estimating equation models of disordered eating predicting becoming overweight or obese by the subsequent follow-up assessment.
[b]Binge eating two or more times per week and not engaging in purging.
[c]Binge eating one or more times per week and not engaging in purging.

TABLE 6–3. Prospective association[a] of disordered eating predicting starting to binge drink frequently in the subsequent 1–2 years among girls in the Growing Up Today Study

	Age-adjusted OR (95% CI)	*P*
Binge eating disorder[b]	2.0 (1.2–3.3)	<0.0001
Subthreshold binge eating disorder[c]	2.1 (1.5–3.0)	<0.0001
Bingeing ≥ weekly	2.1 (1.5–2.8)	<0.0001
Overeating without loss of control ≥ weekly	1.2 (0.6–2.2)	0.6266
Bingeing ≥ monthly	1.8 (1.5–2.2)	<0.0001
Overeating without loss of control ≥ monthly	1.8 (1.4–2.3)	<0.0001

[a]Odds ratios and 95% confidence intervals from generalized estimating equation models of disordered eating predicting starting to binge drink by the subsequent follow-up assessment.
[b]Binge eating two or more times per week and not engaging in purging.
[c]Binge eating one or more times per week and not engaging in purging.

TABLE 6–4.   Prospective association[a] of disordered eating predicting starting to use drugs other than marijuana in the subsequent 2 years among girls in the Growing Up Today Study

	Age-adjusted OR (95% CI)	P
Binge eating disorder[b]	1.9 (0.6–6.2)	0.2780
Subthreshold binge eating disorder[c]	1.1 (0.4–3.0)	0.8675
Bingeing ≥ weekly	1.9 (1.1–3.3)	0.0196
Overeating without loss of control ≥ weekly	1.4 (0.5–4.0)	0.4943
Bingeing ≥ monthly	2.0 (1.4–2.9)	<0.0001
Overeating without loss of control ≥ monthly	1.4 (0.9–2.2)	0.1817

[a]Odds ratios and 95% confidence intervals from generalized estimating equation models of disordered eating predicting starting to use drugs other than marijuana by the subsequent follow-up assessment.
[b]Binge eating two or more times per week and not engaging in purging.
[c]Binge eating one or more times per week and not engaging in purging.

TABLE 6–5.   Prospective association[a] of disordered eating predicting developing high levels of depressive symptoms in the subsequent 2 years among girls in the Growing Up Today Study

	Age-adjusted OR (95% CI)	P
Binge eating disorder[b]	1.7 (0.5–6.0)	0.4103
Subthreshold binge eating disorder[c]	2.7 (1.3–5.7)	0.0064
Bingeing ≥ weekly	3.0 (1.7–5.3)	0.0001
Overeating without loss of control ≥ weekly	1.7 (0.8–3.9)	0.1948
Bingeing ≥ monthly	2.6 (1.8–3.7)	<0.0001
Overeating without loss of control ≥ monthly	1.5 (0.9–2.3)	0.0869

[a]Odds ratios and 95% confidence intervals from generalized estimating equations models of disordered eating predicting moving into the top quintile of depressive symptoms on the McKnight Risk Factor Survey IV six-item scale by the subsequent follow-up assessment.
[b]Binge eating two or more times per week and not engaging in purging.
[c]Binge eating one or more times per week and not engaging in purging.

lower socioeconomic status in the sample. As a result, it is unclear whether the results are generalizable to economically disadvantaged populations, nonwhite ethnic/racial groups, or males. However, there are many strengths in the current study that offset these limitations. The study is the largest study of disordered eating with repeated assessments of a wide range of outcomes and a long follow-up period. In addition, the study was sufficiently large to assess associations at different frequencies of overeating with becoming overweight, starting to binge drink or use drugs, or developing high levels of depressive symptoms.

Our results suggest that it would be prudent to retain the diagnostic criterion requiring that an individual experience a loss of control during an overeating episode. Although the frequency threshold for binge eating is being lowered from at least twice per week to at least once per week, our results demonstrate that even less frequent binge eating is predictive of starting to use drugs, binge drinking frequently, and developing high levels of depressive symptoms. Therefore, clinicians should be encouraged to screen for binge eating, and researchers focused on primary prevention interventions should aim to prevent both infrequent and clinically significant binge eating.

References

American Psychiatric Association: Diagnostic and Statistical Manual of Mental Disorders, 4th Edition. Washington, DC, American Psychiatric Association, 1994

Cole TJ, Bellizzi MC, Flegal KM, et al: Establishing a standard definition for child overweight and obesity worldwide: international survey. BMJ 320:1240–1243, 2000

Eddy KT, Celio Doyle A, Hoste RR, et al: Eating disorder not otherwise specified in adolescents. J Am Acad Child Adolesc Psychiatry 47:156–164, 2008

Field AE, Camargo CA Jr, Taylor CB, et al: Overweight, weight concerns, and bulimic behaviors among girls and boys. J Am Acad Child Adolesc Psychiatry 38:754–760, 1999

Field AE, Camargo CA Jr, Taylor CB, et al: Peer, parent, and media influences on the development of weight concerns and frequent dieting among preadolescent and adolescent girls and boys. Pediatrics 107:54–60, 2001

Field AE, Taylor CB, Celio A, et al: Comparison of self-report to interview assessment of bulimic behaviors among preadolescent and adolescent girls and boys. Int J Eat Disord 35:86–92, 2004

Field AE, Aneja P, Rosner B: The validity of self-reported weight change among adolescents and young adults. Obesity (Silver Spring) 15:2357–2364, 2007

Field AE, Javaras KM, Aneja P, et al: Family, peer, and media predictors of becoming eating disordered. Arch Pediatr Adolesc Med 162:574–579, 2008

French SA, Jeffery RW, Sherwood NE, et al: Prevalence and correlates of binge eating in a nonclinical sample of women enrolled in a weight gain prevention program. Int J Obes Relat Metab Disord 23:576–585, 1999

Herzog DB, Field AE, Keller MB, et al: Subtyping eating disorders: is it justified? J Am Acad Child Adolesc Psychiatry 35:928–936, 1996

Kann L, Warren CW, Harris WA, et al: Youth Risk Behavior Surveillance—United States, 1995. MMWR CDC Surveill Summ 45:1–84, 1996

le Grange D, Binford RB, Peterson CB, et al: DSM-IV threshold versus subthreshold bulimia nervosa. Int J Eat Disord 39:462–467, 2006

Mond J, Hay P, Rodgers B, et al: Use of extreme weight control behaviors with and without binge eating in a community sample: implications for the classification of bulimic-type eating disorders. Int J Eat Disord 39:294–302, 2006

Neumark-Sztainer D, Hannan PJ: Weight-related behaviors among adolescent girls and boys: results from a national survey. Arch Pediatr Adolesc Med 154:569–577, 2000

Patton GC, Coffey C, Carlin JB, et al: Prognosis of adolescent partial syndromes of eating disorder. Br J Psychiatry 192:294–299, 2008

Shisslak CM, Renger R, Sharpe T, et al: Development and evaluation of the McKnight Risk Factor Survey for assessing potential risk and protective factors for disordered eating in preadolescent and adolescent girls. Int J Eat Disord 25:195–214, 1999

Solomon CG, Willett WC, Carey VJ, et al: A prospective study of pregravid determinants of gestational diabetes mellitus. JAMA 278:1078–1083, 1997

Steiger H, Bruce KR: Phenotypes, endophenotypes, and genotypes in bulimia spectrum eating disorders. Can J Psychiatry 52:220–227, 2007

Stice E, Cameron RP, Killen JD, et al: Naturalistic weight-reduction efforts prospectively predict growth in relative weight and onset of obesity among female adolescents. J Consult Clin Psychol 67:967–974, 1999

Sullivan PF, Bulik CM, Kendler KS: The epidemiology and classification of bulimia nervosa. Psychol Med 28:599–610, 1998

Tanofsky-Kraff M, Yanovski SZ, Wilfley DE, et al: Eating-disordered behaviors, body fat, and psychopathology in overweight and normal-weight children. J Consult Clin Psychol 72:53–61, 2004

Tanofsky-Kraff M, Cohen ML, Yanovski SZ, et al: A prospective study of psychological predictors of body fat gain among children at high risk for adult obesity. Pediatrics 117:1203–1209, 2006

Wilfley DE, Bishop ME, Wilson GT, et al: Classification of eating disorders: toward DSM-V. Int J Eat Disord 40(suppl):S123–S129, 2007

Wonderlich SA, Joiner TE Jr, Keel PK, et al: Eating disorder diagnoses: empirical approaches to classification. Am Psychol 62:167–180, 2007

Zeger SL, Liang KY: Longitudinal data analysis for discrete and continuous outcomes. Biometrics 42:121–130, 1986

PART 2

EMPIRICAL APPROACHES TO CLASSIFICATION

Methodological Considerations and Research Findings

7

EMPIRICAL APPROACHES TO THE CLASSIFICATION OF EATING DISORDERS

Ross D. Crosby, Ph.D.
Stephanie Bauer, Ph.D.
Sonja A. Swanson, Sc.M.
Kathryn Gordon, Ph.D.
Stephen A. Wonderlich, Ph.D.
Thomas E. Joiner, Ph.D.

The standard diagnostic systems used in psychiatry and clinical psychology are ICD-10 (World Health Organization 1992) and DSM-IV (American Psychiatric Association 1994, 2000). Although their major purpose is to inform clinical practice, the diagnostic criteria specified in these systems are also often used in research. For example, researchers include or exclude participants in empirical studies based on the presence or absence of diagnostic criteria according to DSM-IV or ICD-10. They also use these criteria to evaluate the efficacy and effectiveness of therapeutic interventions.

The DSM-IV criteria for eating disorders represent conventions that have been widely accepted among clinicians and researchers. However, empirical studies increasingly point to the limitations of the current DSM-IV classification. Concerns have been raised, for example, regarding the validity of the anorexia nervosa, bulimia nervosa, and eating disorder not otherwise specified diagnoses as distinct diagnostic entities and the validity of the subtype distinctions for anorexia and bulimia nervosa (Wonderlich et al. 2007b, 2007c).

The system by which eating disorders are classified has important implications for clinical practice and research. Classification systems are challenged to demonstrate both their clinical utility and scientific validity (Wonderlich et al. 2007b). Any newly introduced system should prove superior in terms of these aspects compared with an existing approach. Thus, it has recently been recommended that alternative classification systems for eating disorders be tested against each other to empirically determine the best-supported system (Gordon et al. 2010).

The empirical approaches reviewed here provide several important tools in the study of eating disorder classification systems. First, these empirical approaches can be used to *confirm or validate* existing eating disorder classification systems (i.e., DSM or ICD). Results from several studies reported in this monograph (see Chapters 9 and 10, this volume) and elsewhere (Peterson et al., submitted) also provide strong empirical support for a new broad classification system of eating disorders proposed by Walsh and Sysco (2009). Observed differences in classification between empirical approaches and existing classification systems can help to inform modifications to those clinical systems. Second, empirical approaches to classification can be used to *evaluate specific diagnostic criteria.* This can be accomplished by comparing differences in empirically derived classification when a specific criterion (e.g., amenorrhea) is included or removed as an indicator variable in the statistical classification model. The finding that empirical classification does not change depending on the inclusion or exclusion of a specific criterion would suggest that this criterion does not contribute meaningfully to the classification system (e.g., see Crow et al., submitted). Finally, empirical approaches can be used to *discover or explore* new classification systems. For example, Wonderlich et al. (2005, 2007a) have used latent profile analysis to classify individuals with eating disorder on the basis of personality characteristics.

The review that follows provides an overview of current empirical approaches to the classification of eating disorders. First, cross-sectional approaches are distinguished that are either dimensional or categorical, or combine categorical and dimensional approaches. Next, two longitudinal approaches to eating disorder classification are considered. In closing, the implications of empirical approaches for future eating disorder research are considered.

Cross-Sectional Approaches to Eating Disorder Classification

Cross-sectional approaches to eating disorder classification can be divided into approaches that are dimensional, those that are categorical, and those that combine or compare dimensional and categorical approaches.

DIMENSIONAL APPROACHES

The primary analytic method for classifying individuals with eating disorder on the basis of dimensions is the *factor analytic* approach, which would include both exploratory and confirmatory applications. The primary research question addressed by this approach is: *Can individuals be meaningfully characterized in terms of their location(s) on one or more continuous dimensions?* This approach is reflected in the dimensional scales of many common eating disorder assessments. For example, the Eating Disorder Examination (Fairburn and Cooper 1993) generates continuous scales for all individuals on four dimensions: restraint, eating concerns, weight concerns, and shape concerns. Likewise, the Eating Disorder Inventory–2 (Garner 1991) includes three eating disorder dimensional subscales (i.e., drive for thinness, bulimia, and body dissatisfaction) and eight other related dimensional subscales.

A variety of statistical software is available for conducting factor analyses. General statistical packages such as PASW (SPSS 2009; formerly SPSS) and SAS (SAS Institute 2009) provide full-featured capabilities for performing exploratory factor analysis. There are also a number of software packages available for conducting confirmatory factor analysis, including Mplus (Muthén and Muthén 1998–2007), LISREL (Mels 2006), and EQS (Bentler 1995).

The dimensional approach assumes that 1) individuals can be characterized along one or more continua and that 2) the distances between individuals on these dimensions are meaningful. Thus, distinctions between individuals are considered to be primarily quantitative rather than qualitative. The utility of the dimensional approach is largely dependent upon the "true nature" of the construct(s) under consideration. If differences among individuals on the tested constructs reflect variations on continuously distributed traits without natural boundaries or qualitative distinctions among individuals, then the dimensional approach will be an appropriate method for identifying meaningful differences among individuals. However, a limitation of the dimensional approach is that no information is provided on the appropriateness of the dimensional approach in comparison with a categorical approach.

CATEGORICAL APPROACHES

One empirical approach to classifying individuals with eating disorder into distinct categories or classes can be subsumed under the rubric of *cluster analytic* techniques. This includes both *partitioning* approaches to clustering, such as the k-means approach, and *agglomerative* (i.e., hierarchical) approaches. The primary research question addressed by this approach is: *How can individuals be divided into meaningful subgroups?* A variety of studies have used cluster analytic techniques to identify subgroups of individuals with eating disorders or eating disturbances (Goldschmidt et al. 2008; Grilo 2004; Turner et al. 2009). Most statistical software packages, including PASW and SAS, provide a number of modules for conducting cluster analysis. Cluster analytic approaches assume that individuals can always be divided into subgroups. Unlike dimensional approaches, cluster analysis assumes that distinctions between individuals are primarily qualitative rather than quantitative. The primary utility of cluster analysis is that it provides an easy-to-use heuristic tool for dividing individuals into subgroups. However, objective methods for determining the appropriate number of clusters are only effective when symptom overlap between clusters is absent or minimal (Tonidandel and Overall 2004), which is a situation in eating disorder research that is likely to be quite uncommon. Furthermore, like factor analytic methods, cluster analysis cannot determine whether a categorical model better captures the structure of the data than a dimensional model (Beauchaine and Marsh 2006). Given these limitations, cluster analytic techniques are quite limited in terms of their utility in identifying meaningful classifications of eating disorder patients.

A second cross-sectional empirical approach to classifying individuals with eating disorders into distinct categories or classes can be subsumed under the rubric of *latent structure analyses*. These techniques, which are alternatively referred to as mixture models (McLachlan and Basford 1998), include both *latent class analysis* (LCA), which uses dichotomous indicators, and *latent profile analysis* (LPA), which can include categorical, ordinal, and continuous indicators (Lazarsfeld and Henry 1968). The primary research question addressed by this approach is: *Can individuals be divided into meaningful subgroups?* There are now a relatively large number of eating disorder studies that have used either LCA (Bulik et al. 2000; Keel et al. 2004; Myers et al. 2006; Pinheiro et al. 2008; Richardson et al. 2008; Striegel-Moore et al. 2005; Sullivan et al. 1998) or LPA (Duncan et al. 2007; Eddy et al. 2009, 2010; Jacobs et al. 2008; Mitchell et al. 2007; Steiger et al. 2009; Thomas et al. 2010; Wade et al. 2006; Wagner et al. 2006; Wonderlich et al. 2005, 2007a; see also Chapters 9, 10, and 14, this volume) to identify subgroups of individuals with eating disorders or eating disorder symptoms. There are a number of more specialized software packages, such as Mplus and Latent Gold (Statistical Innovations Inc. 2005), that provide features for conducting a variety of latent structure analyses. Like cluster analytic techniques, latent structure analysis is used to identify qualitatively distinct subgroups. However, unlike cluster analytic techniques, there is not an a priori assumption with latent structure analysis that individuals can be classified into subgroups. Instead, objective criteria (e.g., parsimony indices) are used to evaluate whether there is evidence to support the existence of latent classes. These criteria are used not only to evaluate the existence of latent classes but also to determine the optimal number and composition of the classes. This is one of the primary advantages of the latent structure approach in comparison with cluster analytic techniques. Another advantage of latent structure analysis is that groups are created in such a way as to maximize homogeneity within groups. Consequently, when latent structure analysis is used to study psychiatric conditions such as eating disorders, this may serve to create classes that are clinically homogeneous. However, a notable limitation of the latent structure analysis is the tendency in some situations to produce latent classes that represent different points along a continuum of severity (Uebersax 1999). Also, latent structure models are prone to identify spurious latent classes when only one group is contained within a population (Bauer and Curran 2004). Thus, it is not possible with latent structure analysis to determine whether the identified latent groups are truly discrete.

COMBINED APPROACHES

Two approaches that combine or compare dimensional and categorical approaches are considered. The first of these is taxometric analysis. *Taxometric analyses* are a set of interrelated procedures designed to address the question of whether two apparently discrete classes represent truly categorically distinct entities (i.e., taxa) or variations along an underlying continuum. The primary research question that is addressed is: *Are the classes of interest qualitatively distinct from each other or do they differ quantitatively along a continuum?* To date, four studies have used taxometric analysis to investigate the structure of eating disorders (Gleaves et al. 2000a, 2000b; Tylka and Subich 2003; Williamson et al. 2002). Three of the four studies have supported a categorical distinction between bulimia nervosa and normality. In addition, two of the studies suggest that the anorexia nervosa binge-purge subtype might fall within the same class as bulimia nervosa. Finally, the anorexia nervosa restricting subtype has been found to be qualitatively distinct (i.e., taxonic) from bulimia nervosa but not from normality. A suite of taxometric analysis software programs running under the R environment (R Development Core Team 2009) are available from Ruscio (2008). Taxometric analysis assumes that the sample, if categorically distinct, contains only two groups: a taxon and its complement; thus it is not appropriate when the sample contains more than two latent groups. One of the primary advantages of this approach is that it allows a direct comparison of dimensional and categorical models using a variety of tests. It is strongly advocated that multiple consistency tests be performed to replicate the conclusions using alternative taxometric procedures. Taxometric analysis assumes that 1) a true latent taxon should be detectable using multiple taxometric methods, and 2) agreement should be observed in estimates of distributional characteristics, both within and across taxometric methods. Some concerns have been raised about the tendency for taxometric analysis to identify spurious groups (Ruscio and Ruscio 2004); however, this tendency has been linked with sampling discrete subtypes (Beauchaine 2007), such has frequently been done in taxometric analysis studies of eating disorders (Gleaves et al. 2000a, 2000b; Williamson et al. 2002).

The second cross-sectional approach that combines dimensional and categorical components is *factor mixture modeling* (FMM; Lubke and Muthén 2005). FMM is a form of latent structure analysis that can compare purely dimensional models, purely categorical models, and models that combine dimensions and categories simultaneously. The primary research question addressed by this approach is: *Can the observed heterogeneity in a sample best be accounted for in terms of dimensions, categories, or a combination of both?* FMM has been used to investigate tobacco dependence (Muthén and Asparouhov 2006), substance use disorders (Muthén 2006), attention-deficit/hyperactivity disorder (Lubke et al. 2007), and performance-enhancing drug use (Hildebrandt et al. 2007). To date, only a single paper has used FMM to study heterogeneity in eating disorder symptoms. Keel et al. (submitted) evaluated the latent structure of bulimic syndrome using FMM, finding that a three-class solution with a single severity dimension best accounted for the heterogeneity in the data. FMM can be performed using Mplus software. FMM allows the direct comparison of models differing in combinations of dimensions and categories using objective fit indices. The advantage of FMM over taxometric analysis is that only the former is appropriate when the sample consists of multiple latent groups. One potential limitation of FMM is that to date, all published studies have found that a model combining categories and dimensions provides better fit than models including only dimensions or only categories. It is unclear whether there are circumstances in which this will not be the case.

Longitudinal Approaches to Eating Disorder Classification

There are currently two longitudinal empirical approaches to classification that have particular relevance to eating disorder classification. The first of these is *latent transition analysis* (LTA; Collins and Lanza 2010; Collins et al. 1994), which evaluates patterns of classification stability and transition among classes over time. The primary research question addressed by this approach is: *What is the probability of remaining in the same class versus transitioning to other classes over time?* LTA has been used to study patterns of transition in adolescent substance use (Chung and Martin 2005) and drinking patterns in young adults (Jackson et al. 2001). Two studies to date have utilized LTA to study patterns of transition in eating disorder symptoms. Peterson et al. (submitted) compared the stability of empirically derived classes with DSM-IV diagnoses over a 2-year period in 429 females with eating disorder symptoms. Empirically derived classes of eating disorder symptoms showed greater longitudinal stability compared with DSM-IV diagnoses, suggesting that modifying the criteria to be consistent with empirically based classification may reduce diagnostic crossover in eating disorders. Cain et al. (2010) used LCA and LTA to derive syndromes of concerns related to eating, weight and shape, and movement across these syndromes over 4 years in a sample of 1,498 college women. Five classes were identified, with membership in each class tending to be stable over time. A number of software packages can be used to conduct LTA, including Mplus and SAS

PROC LTA (Lanza and Collins 2008). LTA assumes that the same latent classes are applicable over time. Therefore, LTA is not appropriate when the latent structure changes over time. However, LTA does not require that transition probabilities remain constant over time. LTA is ideal for studying the stability of classification and how the inclusion/exclusion of specific indicators may influence stability patterns. The limitations of LCA and LPA as described earlier are also applicable to LTA (see subsection "Categorical Approaches" earlier in this chapter).

The second longitudinal approach applicable to the study of eating disorder classification is *latent growth mixture modeling* (LGMM; Muthén and Khoo 1998; Muthén and Muthén 2000). LGMM assumes that a sample is composed of a mixture of distinct subgroups, each defined by a prototypical growth curve or trajectory. LGMM is used to identify the optimal number of trajectories, the shape of these trajectories, and the composition of these trajectories. LGMM differs from LTA in that patterns of change over time are not between classes but rather continuous patterns of change over the observation interval. The primary research question of LGMM is: *Can prototypical patterns of change be identified in the sample?* Only two eating disorder studies to date have utilized LGMM. Crosby et al. (2009) used LGMM to identify daily mood patterns in bulimic women. Nine distinct daily patterns of negative affect were identified. The highest rates of binge eating and purging episodes were found to occur on days characterized by stable high negative affect or increasing negative affect over the course of the day. A second study (Lavender et al., in press) used semi-parametric growth mixture modeling to identify longitudinal trajectories for low body weight, binge eating, and purging in a more than 5-year period in 246 women seeking treatment for anorexia nervosa or bulimia nervosa. Four individual trajectories were identified for each of the eating disorder symptoms, with the shape of the trajectories similar across symptoms. LGMM can be performed using Mplus software. Like other forms of latent structure analysis, parsimony indices can be used to determine the optimal number of latent trajectories. In addition, the model provides information to determine the shape and composition of the trajectories. LGMM is ideal for identifying prototypical patterns of change in a given measured variable. LGMM assumes that the measurement properties of the construct (e.g., reliability) do not change over time. Like other latent structure analyses, however, LGMM does not provide information about whether the latent trajectories are qualitatively distinct.

Conclusion

Several empirical approaches to the classification of eating disorders are described in this chapter. Although the vast majority of the studies described have used only a single approach to classify eating disorder symptoms, these approaches are not necessarily mutually exclusive. At least one study has used multiple classification methods to study the latent structure of eating disorders. Keel et al. (Chapter 11, this volume) used LPA to identify five latent classes using data from 528 individuals recruited from the community for studies of bulimia nervosa and related eating disorders not otherwise specified. Taxometric analyses were then performed between pair-wise combinations of classes to determine whether they were qualitatively distinct from each other. Results generally supported qualitative distinctions among eating disorder classes and between eating disorder classes and normality.

A final consideration related to the classification of eating disorders is the importance of establishing the validity of the classification system. As observed by Wonderlich et al. (2007c): "It is relatively easy to devise conceptual models of eating disorder classification, but it is much harder to determine if these models are valid" (p. S40). They argued that for a classification system to be valid, 1) classes must differ on something other than the indicators that are used to derive these classes, and 2) these differences must be useful or important for some purpose. It will often be the case that different classification systems will be useful for different purposes. For example, one classification system may be useful for characterizing differences in response to treatment; another may have greater utility in predicting long-term outcome. Ultimately, the decision as to the "best" classification system may depend upon which validators are most important. Any classification system, regardless of whether it is clinically derived or empirically based, should be evaluated and compared with alternative systems in terms of utility and validity.

References

American Psychiatric Association: Diagnostic and Statistical Manual of Mental Disorders, 4th Edition. Washington, DC, American Psychiatric Association, 1994

American Psychiatric Association: Diagnostic and Statistical Manual of Mental Disorders, 4th Edition, Text Revision. Washington, DC, American Psychiatric Association, 2000

Bauer DJ, Curran PJ: The integration of continuous and discrete latent variable models: potential problems and promising opportunities. Psychol Methods 9:3–29, 2004

Beauchaine TP: A brief taxometrics primer. J Clin Child Adolesc Psychol 36:654–676, 2007

Beauchaine TP, Marsh P: Taxometric methods: enhancing early detection and prevention of psychopathology by identifying latent vulnerability traits, in Developmental Psychopathology, 2nd Edition. Edited by Cicchetti D, Cohen D. Hoboken, NJ, Wiley, 2006, pp 931–967

Bentler PM: EQS Structural Equations Program Manual. Encino, CA, Multivariate Software, 1995

Bulik CM, Sullivan PF, Kendler KS: An empirical study of the classification of eating disorders. Am J Psychiatry 157:886–895, 2000

Cain AS, Epler AJ, Steinley D, et al: Stability and change in patterns of concerns related to eating, weight, and shape in young adult women: a latent transition analysis. J Abnorm Psychol 119:255–267, 2010

Chung T, Martin CS: Classification and short-term course of DSM-IV cannabis, hallucinogen, cocaine, and opioid disorders in treated adolescents. J Consult Clin Psychol 73:995–1004, 2005

Collins LM, Lanza ST: Latent Class and Latent Transition Analysis: With Applications in the Social, Behavioral, and Health Sciences. New York, Wiley, 2010

Collins LM, Graham JW, Rousculp SS, et al: Latent transition analysis and how it can address prevention research questions. NIDA Res Monogr 142:81–111, 1994

Crosby RD, Wonderlich SA, Engel SG, et al: Daily mood patterns and bulimic behaviors in the natural environment. Behav Res Ther 47:181–188, 2009

Crow SJ, Swanson SA, Peterson CB, et al: Latent class analysis of eating disorders: relationship to mortality. Manuscript submitted for publication

Duncan AE, Bucholz KK, Neuman RJ, et al: Clustering of eating disorder symptoms in a general population female twin sample: a latent class analysis. Psychol Med 37:1097–1107, 2007

Eddy KT, Crosby RD, Keel PK, et al: Empirical identification and validation of eating disorder phenotypes in a multisite clinical sample. J Nerv Ment Dis 197:41–49, 2009

Eddy KT, le Grange D, Crosby RD, et al: Diagnostic classification of eating disorders in children and adolescents: how does DSM-IV-TR compare to empirically derived categories? J Am Acad Child Adolesc Psychiatry 49:277–287, quiz 293, 2010

Fairburn CG, Cooper Z: The Eating Disorder Examination (12th Edition), in Binge Eating: Nature, Assessment and Treatment. Edited by Fairburn CG, Wilson GT. New York, Guilford, 1993, pp 317–360

Garner D: Eating Disorder Inventory–2: Professional Manual. Odessa, FL, Psychological Assessment Resources, 1991

Gleaves DH, Lowe MR, Green BA, et al: Do anorexia and bulimia nervosa occur on a continuum? A taxometric analysis. Behav Ther 31:195–219, 2000a

Gleaves DH, Lowe MR, Snow AC, et al: Continuity and discontinuity models of bulimia nervosa: a taxometric investigation. J Abnorm Psychol 109:56–68, 2000b

Goldschmidt AB, Tanofsky-Kraff M, Goossens L, et al: Subtyping children and adolescents with loss of control eating by negative affect and dietary restraint. Behav Res Ther 46:777–787, 2008

Gordon KH, Holm-Denoma JM, Crosby RD, et al: The classification of eating disorders, in The Oxford Handbook of Eating Disorders. Edited by Agras WS. New York, Oxford University Press, 2010, pp 9–24

Grilo CM: Subtyping female adolescent psychiatric inpatients with features of eating disorders along dietary restraint and negative affect dimensions. Behav Res Ther 42:67–78, 2004

Hildebrandt T, Langenbucher JW, Carr SJ, et al: Modeling population heterogeneity in appearance- and performance-enhancing drug (APED) use: applications of mixture modeling in 400 regular APED users. J Abnorm Psychol 116:717–733, 2007

Jackson K, Sher K, Gotham HG, et al: Transitioning into and out of large-effect drinking in young adulthood. J Abnorm Psychol 110:378–391, 2001

Jacobs MJ, Roesch S, Wonderlich SA, et al: Anorexia nervosa trios: behavioral profiles of individuals with anorexia nervosa and their parents. Psychol Med 26:1–11, 2008

Keel PK, Fichter M, Quadflieg N, et al: Application of a latent class analysis to empirically define eating disorder phenotypes. Arch Gen Psychiatry 61:192–200, 2004

Keel PK, Crosby RD, Hildebrandt T, et al: Latent structure of eating disorders: a mixture modeling approach. Manuscript submitted for publication

Lanza ST, Collins LM: A new SAS procedure for latent transition analysis: transitions in dating and sexual behavior. Dev Psychol 42:446–456, 2008

Lavender JM, De Young KP, Franko DL, et al: An investigation of the joint longitudinal trajectories of low body weight, binge eating, and purging in women with anorexia nervosa and bulimia nervosa. Int J Eat Disord (in press)

Lazarsfeld PF, Henry NW: Latent Structure Analysis. Boston, MA, Houghton Mifflin, 1968

Lubke GH, Muthén B: Investigating population heterogeneity with factor mixture models. Psychol Methods 10:21–39, 2005

Lubke GH, Muthén B, Moilanen IK, et al: Subtypes versus severity differences in attention-deficit/hyperactivity disorder in the Northern Finnish Birth Cohort. J Am Acad Child Adolesc Psychiatry 46:1584–1593, 2007

McLachlan GJ, Basford KE: Mixture Models. New York, Marcel Dekker, 1998

Mels G: LISREL for Windows: Getting Started Guide. Lincolnwood, IL, Scientific Software International, 2006

Mitchell JE, Crosby RD, Wonderlich SA, et al: Latent profile analysis of a cohort of patients with eating disorder not otherwise specified. Int J Eat Disord 40:S95–S98, 2007

Muthén B: Should substance use disorders be considered as categorical or dimensional? Addiction 101(suppl):6–16, 2006

Muthén B, Asparouhov T: Item response mixture modeling: application to tobacco dependence criteria. Addict Behav 31:1050–1066, 2006

Muthén B, Khoo ST: Longitudinal studies of achievement growth using latent variable modeling. Learn Individ Differ 10:73–101, 1998

Muthén B, Muthén LK: Integrating person-centered and variable-centered analyses: growth mixture modeling with latent trajectory classes. Alcohol Clin Exp Res 24:882–891, 2000

Muthén LK, Muthén BO: Mplus User's Guide, 5th Edition. Los Angeles, CA, Muthén and Muthén, 1998–2007

Myers TC, Wonderlich SA, Crosby RD, et al: Is multi-impulsive bulimia a distinct type of bulimia nervosa: psychopathology and EMA findings. Int J Eat Disord 39:655–661, 2006

Peterson CB, Crow SJ, Swanson SA, et al: The longitudinal stability of eating disorders: comparing empirically derived and DSM-IV classifications. Manuscript submitted for publication

Pinheiro AP, Bulik CM, Sullivan PF, et al: An empirical study of the typology of bulimic symptoms in young Portuguese women. Int J Eat Disord 41:251–258, 2008

R Development Core Team: R: A Language and Environment for Statistical Computing. Reference Index Version 2.10.1. Vienna, Austria, R Foundation for Statistical Computing, 2009

Richardson J, Steiger H, Schmitz N, et al: Relevance of the 5-HTTLPR polymorphism and childhood abuse to increased psychiatric comorbidity in women with bulimia-spectrum disorders. J Clin Psychiatry 69:981–990, 2008

Ruscio J: Taxometric Programs for the R Computing Environment: User's Manual. Ewing, NJ, College of New Jersey, 2008

Ruscio J, Ruscio AM: Clarifying boundary issues in psychopathology: the role of taxometrics in a comprehensive program of structural research. J Abnorm Psychol 113:24–38, 2004

SAS Institute: SAS 9.2 Output Delivery System: User's Guide. Cary, NC, SAS Institute, 2009

SPSS: PASW Statistics for Windows, Release 18.0.0. Chicago, IL, SPSS, 2009

Statistical Innovations Inc: Latent GOLD, Version 4.5.0. Belmont, MA, Statistical Innovations Inc., 2005

Steiger H, Richardson J, Schmitz N, et al: Association of trait-defined eating disorder sub-phenotypes with (biallelic and triallelic) 5HTTLPR variations. J Psychiatr Res 43:1086–1094, 2009

Striegel-Moore RH, Franko DL, Thompson D, et al: An empirical study of the typology of bulimia nervosa and its spectrum variants. Psychol Med 35:1563–1572, 2005

Sullivan PF, Bulik CM, Kendler KS: The epidemiology and classification of bulimia nervosa. Psychol Med 28:599–610, 1998

Thomas JJ, Crosby RD, Wonderlich SA, et al: A latent profile analysis of the typology of bulimic symptoms in an indigenous Pacific population: evidence of cross-cultural variation in phenomenology. Psychol Med 29:1–12, March 2010 [Epub ahead of print]

Tonidandel S, Overall JE: Determining the number of clusters by sampling with replacement. Psychol Methods 9:238–249, 2004

Turner H, Bryant-Waugh R, Peveler R: An approach to sub-grouping the eating disorder population: adding attachment and coping style. Eur Eat Disord Rev 17:269–280, 2009

Tylka TL, Subich LM: Revisiting the latent structure of eating disorders: taxometric analyses with nonbehavioral indicators. J Couns Psychol 50:276–286, 2003

Uebersax JS: Probit latent class analysis with dichotomous or ordered category measures: conditional independence/dependence models. Appl Psychol Meas 23:283–297, 1999

Wade TD, Crosby RD, Martin NG: Use of latent profile analysis to identify eating disorder phenotypes in an adult Australian twin cohort. Arch Gen Psychiatry 63:1377–1384, 2006

Wagner A, Barbarich-Marsteller NC, Frank GK, et al: Personality traits after recovery from eating disorders: do subtypes differ? Int J Eat Disord 39:276–284, 2006

Walsh BT, Sysko R: Broad categories for the diagnosis of eating disorders (BCD-ED): an alternative system for classification. Int J Eat Disord 42:754–764, 2009

Williamson DA, Womble LG, Smeet MAM, et al: The latent structure of eating disorder symptoms: a factor analytic and taxometric investigation. Am J Psychiatry 159:412–418, 2002

Wonderlich SA, Crosby RD, Joiner T, et al: Personality subtyping and bulimia nervosa: psychopathological and genetic correlates. Psychol Med 35:649–657, 2005

Wonderlich SA, Crosby RD, Engel SG, et al: Personality-based clusters in bulimia nervosa: differences in clinical variables and ecological momentary assessment. J Pers Disord 21:340–357, 2007a

Wonderlich SA, Joiner TE, Keel PK, et al: Eating disorder diagnoses: empirical approaches to classification. Am Psychol 62:167–180, 2007b

Wonderlich SA, Crosby RD, Mitchell JE, et al: Testing the validity of eating disorders diagnoses. Int J Eat Disord 40(suppl):S40–S45, 2007c

World Health Organization: The ICD-10 Classification of Mental and Behavioural Disorders: Clinical Descriptions and Diagnostic Guidelines. Geneva, Switzerland, World Health Organization, 1992

8

LATENT STRUCTURE ANALYSES OF EATING DISORDER DIAGNOSES

Critical Review of Results and Methodological Issues

Scott J. Crow, M.D.
Sonja A. Swanson, Sc.M.
Carol B. Peterson, Ph.D.
Ross D. Crosby, Ph.D.
Stephen A. Wonderlich, Ph.D.
James E. Mitchell, M.D.

Currently, DSM-IV (American Psychiatric Association 1994, 2000) recognizes the diagnostic entities anorexia nervosa (AN), bulimia nervosa (BN), and eating disorder not otherwise specified (EDNOS) and also suggests binge eating disorder (BED) as a diagnostic criteria set for further study. For numerous reasons, these criteria are problematic. First, there are substantial similarities and high levels of crossover between these entities. Second, the existing diagnostic entities contain several severity specifiers (e.g., binge eating and purging frequency and duration) that,

Supported in part by P30 DK50456 and MH019901. The authors wish to acknowledge the valuable contributions of Karen Bandeen-Roche and Kung-Yee Liang.

for the most part, lack substantial empirical support. Finally, the criteria as currently applied lead to a preponderance of EDNOS diagnoses in most samples (Eddy et al. 2008; Fairburn and Bohn 2005; Turner et al. 2010). This appears to run counter to the intent of DSM, which states that "it is impossible for the diagnostic nomenclature to cover every possible situation" (p. 4): this suggests DSM categories would fail to capture a small percentage of affected individuals, when in fact they fail to capture the majority.

A variety of potential solutions have been proposed. These include the use of a single eating disorder diagnosis (Fairburn et al. 2003); the use of a dimensional as opposed to categorical eating disorder diagnosis (Williamson et al. 2005); and the use of broad diagnostic categories based on disordered eating behaviors (Walsh and Sysko 2009). In an attempt to better understand the current status of the eating disorder diagnostic system and to examine these potential solutions, a number of strategies have been used. One increasingly popular approach has been to derive diagnostic nomenclatures empirically, based on the assumption that meaningful underlying structures can be identified. This approach, often referred to broadly as latent structure analysis, has been used with increasing frequency in eating disorder research. This chapter reviews the results of the studies published to date and examines some specific methodological challenges in conducting and interpreting these analyses in eating disorders.

The general approach to latent structure analysis is reviewed in detail elsewhere in this volume. In brief, the method assumes that underlying structures can be detected through statistical analysis of data relating to a sample of subjects. The pattern detected by analysis of data utilizes measures thought to be operational measures of the underlying constructs; the measures are often referred to as *indicators* (other literature may refer to these as *manifest* or *response variables*). Once underlying structures have been identified, their usefulness is then examined by comparing the structures on clinically meaningful variables; these are often referred to as *validators*.

Of note, four studies to date (Gleaves et al. 2000a, 2000b; Tylka and Subich 2003; Williamson et al. 2002) have employed a somewhat different empirical classification strategy—taxometric analysis. Although this is a useful technique for determining whether a latent structure is best described by a continuum or continua versus by discrete classes/taxa, the present review focuses on latent structure analyses such as latent class analysis (LCA) or latent profile analysis (LPA).

Latent Structure Analyses of Eating Disorders

More than a dozen studies to date have been published that have employed empirical methods to examine diagnostic categories. As Table 8–1 reveals, the characteristics of the studies differ to some extent. Most importantly, some of the studies used epidemiological samples, either through community-based studies or through studies used to conduct twin research. Other studies have examined clinical samples of persons selected initially because they presented for eating disorder treatment or persons recruited for study because of their eating disorder diagnosis. Others have been restricted a priori to selected eating disorder subgroups (e.g., only subjects with an EDNOS diagnosis).

Among the community- and population-based studies, three investigations have examined the latent structure of eating disorders in full samples. Wade et al. (2006) completed an LPA in 1,002 twins using body mass index (BMI) and eating disorder symptoms as validators. A five-profile solution resulted in four largely unaffected profiles and a fifth that included disordered eating pathology. Duncan et al. (2007) examined latent structure in 3,723 twins using eating disorder symptoms as indicators. They also found five classes, but the classes distinguished included only one unaffected class and four distinct affected ones. Using bulimic symptoms, age, and BMI as indicators, Pinheiro et al. (2008) found a four-class solution for a sample of 2,028 female public school students, characterized by one unaffected class, one binge eating only class, one binge eating and purging class, and one purging only class.

Other studies that have used community samples have focused their models exclusively on the subset with eating disorder symptoms or diagnoses. Using a subsample of 474 women who had reported ever binge eating and/or self-induced vomiting from a population-based sample of 1,897 female twins, Sullivan et al. (1998) conducted LCA using nine bulimic symptoms as indicators. A four-class solution with two binge eating and two binge-purge classes was derived. Bulik et al. (2000) conducted LCA on a subsample of 1,071 twins who endorsed some degree of disordered eating symptoms from an initial twin sample of 2,163. LCA was conducted using eating disorder symptoms as indicators, and six classes were found, including three low-weight classes, one purging class, and one binge eating class. Keel et al. (2004) conducted LCA on 1,179 probands and affected relatives in genetic studies of eating disorders who entered because of a diagnosis of AN, BN, AN plus BN, or EDNOS. Eating disorder symptoms were used as indicators. A four-class solution was identified, with two low-weight and two purging classes. From an initial sample of 2,054, Striegel-Moore et al. (2005) employed latent class modeling with the 234 subjects who endorsed eating disorder symptoms. Using eating disorder symptoms as indicators, they found a three-class solution consisting of binge-purge, binge eating, and a purging class.

Four studies have examined broad eating disorder samples. Eddy et al. (2009) examined 687 individuals seeking treatment for eating disorders, using LPA with BMI and eating disorder symptoms as indicators, and found five profiles, including two low-weight profiles, two BN-like profiles, and one BED-like profile. Steiger et al. (2009, 2010) conducted LCA in 185 individuals with AN, BN, or EDNOS. Indicators included depression scale scores and personality trait measures, and a three-class solution based on temperament variables was derived. In another sample, Eddy

TABLE 8–1.　Characteristics of latent structure studies of eating disorders

Study	N	Sample	Method	Indicators	Validators	Results
Bulik et al. 2000	1,071	Female twins endorsing at least one eating disorder symptom (full sample $N=2,163$)	LCA	ED symptoms	Demographics, eating/weight variables, comorbidity, personality/attitudinal measures, co-twin risk/resemblance	6 classes
Duncan et al. 2007	3,723	Female adult twins	LCA	ED symptoms	Demographics, ED variables, comorbidity, suicidality	5 classes
Eddy et al. 2009	687	Patients seeking treatment with any ED	LPA	BMI, ED symptoms	Demographics, comorbidity, ED symptoms, medical symptoms, treatment utilization history	5 profiles
Eddy et al. 2010	401	Adolescents seeking ED treatment	LPA	Percent ideal body weight, ED symptoms	EDE subscales, BDI, self-esteem	3 profiles
Jacobs et al. 2009	433 trios	Proband-parent trios with AN proband	LPA	Personality and ED symptoms	ED and temperament plus state anxiety	3 profiles
Keel et al. 2004	1,179	547 probands with ED and 632 affected relatives in a family study	LCA	ED symptoms	Demographics, temperament, comorbidity	4 classes
Mitchell et al. 2007	403	Patients seeking treatment with EDNOS	LPA	BMI, ED symptoms	Demographics, EDE-Q subscales	5 profiles

TABLE 8–1. Characteristics of latent structure studies of eating disorders *(continued)*

Study	N	Sample	Method	Indicators	Validators	Results
Myers et al. 2006	125	BN	LCA	Impulsivity measures	Comorbidity, trauma history, demographics	2 classes
Pinheiro et al. 2008	2,028	Community	LCA	ED symptoms, BMI, age	EDE-Q subscales, SES	4 classes
Richardson et al. 2008	89	Women with full or subthreshold BN	LCA	Lifetime Axis I disorders	EDE, DAPP-BQ, 5-HTTLPR genotype, history of childhood abuse	2 classes
Steiger et al. 2009, 2010	185	AN/BN, EDNOS	LCA	DAPP, BIS, CES-D	Demographics, history of childhood abuse, BMI, 5-HTTLPR genotype, ED diagnosis and symptoms, psychiatric medication use	3 classes
Striegel-Moore et al. 2005	234	Subjects endorsing BN symptoms from a community sample (N=2,054)	LCA	BN symptoms	BMI, ED diagnosis, EDI subscales, demographics, Stunkard Figure Rating Scale, CES-D	3 classes

TABLE 8–1. Characteristics of latent structure studies of eating disorders *(continued)*

Study	N	Sample	Method	Indicators	Validators	Results
Sullivan et al. 1998	474	Subjects endorsing binge eating or self-induced vomiting from a population-based female twin sample (N=1,897)	LCA	BN symptoms	BMI, comorbid psychopathology, personality measures, demographics	4 classes
Wade et al. 2006	1,002	Twins	LPA	BMI, ED symptoms	MDD, EDE subscales, suicidality, first 16 years of life events	5 profiles
Wagner et al. 2006	55	Women recovered from AN or BN	LPA	Personality measures	Comorbid psychopathology, demographics	2 classes
Wonderlich et al. 2005	178	Women with full or sub-threshold BN	LPA	Psychiatric disorder and personality scales, 5-HTTLPR genotype	EDE-Q	3 classes
Wonderlich et al. 2007	131	Women with BN	LPA	DAPP	Comorbid psychopathology, treatment history, EMA measures	3 classes

Note. AN=anorexia nervosa; BDI=Beck Depression Inventory; BIS=Barratt Impulsivity Scale; BMI=body mass index; BN=bulimia nervosa; CES-D=Center for Epidemiologic Studies Depression Scale; DAPP=Dimensional Assessment of Personality Pathology; DAPP-BQ=Dimensional Assessment of Personality Pathology Basic Questionnaire; ED=eating disorder; EDE=Eating Disorders Examination; EDE-Q= Eating Disorders Examination Questionnaire; EDI=Eating Disorder Inventory; EDNOS=eating disorder not otherwise specified; EMA=ecological momentary assessment; LCA=latent class analysis; LPA=latent profile analysis; MDD=major depressive disorder; SES=socioeconomic status.

et al. (2010) studied a large group of treatment-seeking adolescents using LPA. Indicators were percent ideal body weight and eating disorder symptoms. Eating Disorder Examination subscale scores, depression ratings and self-esteem were used as validators. A three-profile solution resulted. One profile was marked by binge and purge behaviors; a second profile had high levels of exercise and high levels of eating disorder cognitions; and the third had low levels of each. Notably, both of the latter two profiles were heterogeneous in terms of weight status.

Finally, six studies have examined more diagnostically limited groups of individuals with eating disorders. In the first, Wonderlich et al. (2005) performed LPA on a sample of 178 women with full or subthreshold BN. Using one genetic and six psychiatric/personality indicators resulted in three classes characterized by their comorbidity and personality patterns. Myers et al. (2006) conducted LCA in 125 participants with BN who had taken part in an ecological momentary assessment study of BN, using impulsivity measures as indicators. Two classes were derived, one characterized by multi-impulsive bulimia behaviors and the other by their absence. In another study focused only on subjects with BN, Wonderlich et al. (2007) used personality measures as indicators on a sample of 131 females using LPA. Three BN-like classes that differed on temperament variables were derived. Richardson et al. (2008) conducted LCA on 89 women with BN spectrum disorders and used lifetime Axis I disorders as indicators. Two classes, defined by high and low comorbidity, were found. Whereas Wonderlich et al. (2005, 2007), Myers et al. (2006), and Richardson et al. (2008) focused only on subjects with BN or BN spectrum disorders, another analysis conducted by Mitchell et al. (2007) included 403 individuals with a diagnosis of EDNOS. Eating disorder symptoms and BMI served as indicators, and five profiles resulted, including a BED-like profile, profiles resembling subthreshold AN and subthreshold BN, and two more diverse profiles. Somewhat uniquely, Wagner et al. (2006) conducted LPA with a sample of 55 women who had recovered from AN or BN, using personality measures as indicators. The two classes that were derived were described as inhibited versus disinhibited in this small sample. With the exception of Mitchell et al. (2007), the latent structure analyses of these studies of special eating disorder subgroups tended to explore whether meaningful structures could be derived from other types of measures (e.g., personality) rather than using eating disorder symptoms as indicators.

One study using somewhat different methodology deserves comment. Jacobs et al. (2009) examined the latent structure in familial units. LPA was used in 433 AN trios—that is, constellations of an AN proband and two parents. A variety of attitudinal measures were used as indicators on these trios, and three different profiles resulted.

Table 8–2 summarizes the general latent structures found by these studies. Generally, most structures found classes that somewhat resemble AN, BN, BED, or, in the case of the community samples, an asymptomatic group, although rarely did these studies find all of these classes simultaneously. Of note, eight studies found

TABLE 8–2. Results of latent structure studies of eating disorders

Study	Asymptomatic class	Low weight or AN-like class	BN-like class	BED-like class	Other
Bulik et al. 2000	0	3: Low weight with binge eating; low weight without binge eating; anorexic	1: Bulimic	1: Binge eating	1: Shape/weight preoccupation
Duncan et al. 2007	1: Unaffected	0	0	0	4: Weight concerned; dieters; low weight gain; eating disorder
Eddy et al. 2009	0	2: Low weight with extreme versus minimal cognitive features	2: BN with vomiting versus multiple methods of purging	1: Binge eating	0
Eddy et al. 2010	0	2: Exercise/extreme cognitions; minimal behaviors/minimal cognitions	1: Binge-purge	0	0
Jacobs et al. 2009	0	0	0	0	3: Trio patterns

TABLE 8–2. Results of latent structure studies of eating disorders *(continued)*

Study	Asymptomatic class	Low weight or AN-like class	BN-like class	BED-like class	Other
Keel et al. 2004	0	2: RAN and RAN without body-related obsessive-compulsive features	2: Mixed AN/BN with multiple methods of purging; BN defined by vomiting	0	0
Mitchell et al. 2007	0	1: Sub-RAN	1: Sub-BN	1: Overweight resembling BED	2: Subsyndromal eating disorder; overweight with low pathology
Myers et al. 2006	0	0	2: High versus low impulsive BN		0
Pinheiro et al. 2008	1: Healthy	0	1: Binge eating and purging	1: Binge eating	1: Purging
Richardson et al. 2008	0	0	2: Low and high comorbidity	0	0
Steiger et al. 2009, 2010	0	0	0	0	3: Dissocial/impulsive; low psychopathology; inhibited/compulsive

TABLE 8–2. Results of latent structure studies of eating disorders *(continued)*

Study	Asymptomatic class	Low weight or AN-like class	BN-like class	BED-like class	Other
Striegel-Moore et al. 2005	0	0	1: Binge eating and purging	1: Binge eating	1: Purging
Sullivan et al. 1998	0	0	2: Both binge eating and vomiting differing by severity	2: Both binge eating with different cognitive features	0
Wade et al. 2006	3: Healthy weight; healthy/overweight; overweight/obese	1: Low weight	0	0	1: Eating disorder
Wagner et al. 2006	0	0	0	0	2: Inhibited; disinhibited
Wonderlich et al. 2005	0	0	3: Low comorbidity; affective-perfectionistic, and impulsive	0	0
Wonderlich et al. 2007	0	0	3: Interpersonal-emotional; stimulus-seeking hostile; low personality pathology	0	0

Note.   AN=anorexia nervosa; BED=binge eating disorder; BN=bulimia nervosa; RAN=restricting-type anorexia nervosa.

classes or profiles characterized by other features, including classes defined by purging in the absence of binge eating (Pinheiro et al. 2008; Striegel-Moore et al. 2005) or classes defined by more cognitive features (Steiger et al. 2010; Wagner et al. 2006). When classes did resemble DSM-IV disorders, they often did not align perfectly with DSM-IV criteria; for example, low-weight subjects who binged and purged were frequently in a BN-like class as opposed to being grouped with other low-weight subjects in an AN-like class (Keel et al. 2004; Mitchell et al. 2007), and subjects who endorsed bulimic behaviors at a subthreshold frequency for a BN diagnosis often were in the same class as subjects with the full diagnosis (e.g., Eddy et al. 2009). Additionally, many studies further subdivided their AN-, BN-, or BED-like constructs into multiple classes or profiles. One example of such a division is the findings supporting multiple BN-like classes divided by their choice of compensatory behaviors (e.g. Eddy et al. 2009; Keel et al. 2004); studies focusing on specific eating disorder subpopulations using indicators that are not eating disorder symptoms have found a variety of other distinctive divisions (e.g., comorbidity, personality).

Validity of Latent Structure Models in Eating Disorders

These studies have a wide array of sample characteristics, indicator choices, and resulting latent structures; they further differ on the validators used to justify their models. Many of these studies used demographic variables, including age, race/ethnicity, and sex, as validators. Other validators range from eating or weight variables, attitudinal or personality measures, genetics, and correlates of severity (e.g., comorbidity, suicidality, treatment utilization).

Depending on the sampling frame and indicator variables to some extent, studies also used eating and weight variables as validators. For example, the analyses of full community samples tended to use eating disorder diagnoses as validators, finding higher rates of diagnoses in their more pathological classes (Duncan et al. 2007; Pinheiro et al. 2008; Wade et al. 2006). Some of the eating disorder–specific samples that used eating disorder symptoms as indicators validated their models with subscales from widely used eating disorder measures, including the Eating Disorder Examination, Eating Disorder Examination Questionnaire, and Eating Disorder Inventory (Mitchell et al. 2007; Striegel-Moore et al. 2005). The use of eating disorder–related constructs as both indicators and validators raises some concern about circularity of findings. On the other hand, such studies have often used eating disorder behaviors as indicators and eating disorder cognition measures as validators, which might help to mitigate such concerns. Finally, most studies that did not include eating disorder symptoms in their indicators used an eating or weight measure to validate their findings (Richardson et al. 2008; Steiger et al. 2009, 2010; Wonderlich et al. 2005).

Some studies looked at personality or attitudinal measures to validate the classes or profiles derived. These validators were particularly common in community samples, where distinguishing between affected and unaffected classes was of interest. Bulik et al. (2000), Jacobs et al. (2009), Keel et al. (2004), and Sullivan et al. (1998) all utilized these measures as validators.

Three of the latent structure analyses of eating disorders considered genotypes, and two of these studies used genotypes as a validator (the third, Wonderlich et al. 2005, used it as an indicator). Both studies looked at whether the derived latent classes differed in terms of 5-HTTLPR. Both Steiger et al. (2009, 2010) and Richardson et al. (2008) found that distribution of the 5-HTTLPR polymorphisms differed across classes in their respective analyses, although the approaches to class creation and to the allele variable differed somewhat.

Perhaps the most clinically relevant set of validators utilized to date are those considered to be correlates of severity: psychiatric comorbidity (Bulik et al. 2002; Duncan et al. 2007; Eddy et al. 2009, 2010; Keel et al. 2004; Myers et al. 2006; Sullivan et al. 1998; Wagner et al. 2006; Wonderlich et al. 2005), other medical comorbidity (Eddy et al. 2009), suicidality (Wade et al. 2006), and treatment utilization (Eddy et al. 2009; Wonderlich et al. 2007). These validators were cross-sectional measures used to capture aspects of the clinical impact of disordered eating.

Finally, it is worth noting that although some of these studies used retrospective measures to validate their findings (e.g., history of child abuse [Myers et al. 2006; Richardson et al. 2008; Steiger et al. 2009, 2010]), none used a longitudinal outcome. Perhaps some of the most important questions to be addressed with latent structure analyses fall under this category (e.g., whether classes predict the course of the disorder, general health consequences, or even response to treatment). The justification of the clinical utility of the DSM categories is typically based on such validators.

Methodological Considerations and Challenges in Latent Structure Analyses of Eating Disorders

There are several methodological considerations to consider both when interpreting these studies and when conducting future studies. Some of these are universal to all latent structure analyses (e.g., use of information criteria), whereas others are particularly relevant to the eating disorder research field (e.g., local independence violations).

First, utilization of information criteria or other statistical "decision-makers" to determine the number of classes is not necessarily straightforward for this type of modeling. Unlike most regression analyses, generalized tests of significance such as likelihood ratio, score, or Wald's tests are not ideal, because assumptions underlying these theories are violated when comparing latent structures with different numbers of classes (Aitkin and Rubin 1985; Aitkin et al. 1981); nonetheless, these tests of significance were used in some of the earlier studies. Most studies use various information criteria to choose the optimal number of classes, including Akaike information criterion (AIC; Akaike 1973), Bayesian information criterion (BIC; Schwarz 1978), sample size adjusted Bayesian information criterion (ABIC; Sclove 1987), and consistent Akaike information criterion (CAIC; Bozdogan 1987). Although no single information criterion is definitively superior, it is important to understand that each approach has unique properties. Statistical simulation studies have tried to discern the circumstances under which these criteria perform optimally, and several aspects of study design (e.g., sample size) are known to influence the performance of these information criteria (Dayton and Macready 1988; Lin and Dayton 1997; Yang 2006). Moreover, these simulation studies have also looked for general trends in performance, including whether an information criterion tends to overestimate or underestimate the number of true classes. For example, AIC is considered "liberal" because it is most likely to overestimate the number of true classes, whereas BIC and CAIC are generally deemed "conservative" because of their tendency to underestimate the number of true classes. Whether a liberal or conservative information criterion is desirable is partially dependent on the short-term goals of latent structure analyses: although in the long term we of course want to identify the "correct" classes that underlie eating disorder pathology, over- or understratification has unique costs to genetics research, treatment outcome research, and so forth.

Prior to model selection, however, comes the choice of the model's indicators, and this choice can be particularly problematic in eating disorder latent structure analyses. Latent structure analyses assume local independence—that is, indicators are assumed to be independent of each other within classes (but not necessarily across classes). Local independence is one of the more attractive features of latent structure analyses, because it creates a model that has "clinically homogeneous" groups. However, this assumption needs to be tested, because violations of this assumption can greatly influence the accuracy of the results. Assuming local independence in settings that actually have local dependencies can lead to the identification of spurious classes (Suppes and Zanotti 1981) or biased solutions (Torrance-Rynard and Walter 1997; Vacek 1985). It is not clear that the local independence assumption has been tested in most of the published eating disorder LCAs and LPAs. Consider a hypothetical model that uses eating disorder symptoms as indicators, including both amenorrhea and BMI. If one considers two women who are known to belong to the same latent class in this model, and one has a BMI of 17 and the other has a BMI of 12, a clinician would assume that the woman with a BMI of 12 is more likely to have amenorrhea than the one with a BMI of 17; however, the model assumes that both women have the same probability because BMI is locally independent from amenorrhea within the latent class. There is evidence that this amenorrhea and BMI are dependent (Frisch and McArthur 1974), and it seems biologically implausible that this would be conditioned on class membership. As such, the use of both indicators would violate the local independence assumption and may lead to biased results or spurious classes in an LCA or LPA. As this hypothetical situation exemplifies, particular attention should be spent on testing the local independence assumptions in these models. Techniques can be used to address or relax this assumption when necessary.

Another practical issue that is especially relevant to eating disorder latent structure analyses is the implications of using sparse data. Sparseness is a characteristic of data matrices that have cells with zero or small counts. For example, suppose only two variables were used in the model, binge eating and vomiting frequencies, each measured with eight ordinal values (e.g., never, once per week, twice per week, etc.). The data matrix would then have $8 \times 8 = 64$ cells—that is, 64 different possible combinations of binge eating and vomiting frequencies. Of these 64 cells, one might expect the majority of observations near the diagonal of this matrix, where the frequencies of the binge episodes and vomiting behavior coincide. On the other hand, there might be relatively few or even no observations for high vomiting frequency coinciding with low binge eating frequencies. Such a pattern would then be considered sparse, because some of these 64 cells would be empty or have low counts. Of note, continuous variables are also affected by sparseness in some sense (one can picture this scenario by imagining trying to estimate the center and spread of a normal distribution of BMI for various levels of purging behaviors), but as fewer parameters are measured in an LPA with continuous variables compared with ordinal or categorical groups with several levels, the effect on model fitting may be less noteworthy. Many applications of latent variable modeling in eating disorder research rely on very sparse data; indeed, the latent class studies reviewed in this chapter range from having 16 to 32,768 possible cells, and their sample sizes range from 89 to 2,028. The studies using LPAs with ordinal or categorical indicators tend to have even more issues with sparseness. Thus it is important to keep in mind some of the consequences: it is not fully understood how sparseness influences replicability, in terms of both the latent structures found and even extraneous structures that may be identified only as a result of the particular data set's idiosyncrasies. Although these considerations raise concerns about analyzing very sparse data, it is also important to be reminded that it cannot be avoided for many scientific questions pertaining to eating disorder research. Even a simple model including indicators for binge eating, purging, and BMI can be problematic: if the sample size approaches infinity, for example, it is unlikely that the cell that crosses low levels of purging with a low BMI and high levels of binge eating will ever have more than a small count, but a model based on these three variables could be incredibly useful for discerning structures relating to anorexia nervosa, binge-purge type; BN; and BED. Analysts should take care to limit the number of indicators when they can, approach indicators from multiple coding methods (e.g., treating BMI as continuous versus two-, three- or four-level ordinal categories), consider testing the contribution of individual indicators to the model, and perhaps even explore the issue of replicability in these situations by cross-validating within their own dataset.

Another consideration in these types of modeling is the issue of class membership assignment. In latent structure modeling, subjects are not assumed to be perfectly classified into a class or profile; rather, the model finds underlying classes that represent the structure of the data and then subjects have a certain probability of belonging to each of the possible classes. To date, all latent structure analyses that have been conducted in the eating disorder field have assigned class membership to subjects based on the class that the subjects have the maximum posterior probability of belonging to, and they have used this assigned class membership in their validator comparisons. A problem with this approach is that it does not capture the uncertainty of latent class membership. By considering this membership fixed, the probabilistic structure of the latent class model is ignored and thus any post hoc comparison ignores possibly pertinent measurement error. Many alternatives to this approach have been proposed, including incorporating latent class probabilities into the validation analyses (Melton et al. 1994), using multiple imputations of class membership based on simulations of the estimated probabilities (Clogg 1995), and building the validator comparisons into a more complex latent variable regression framework directly (Bandeen-Roche et al. 1997; Dayton and Macready 1988). Although considering class membership as fixed may be preferable for clinical interpretation of these models, future analyses using latent structure models may benefit from exploration of these other approaches.

Finally, it is especially relevant to this type of modeling to remember that a model is just that: a model. The results of any latent structure analyses will be influenced by a variety of methodological factors, including sample size, missing data, base rates of symptom endorsement, measurement error, and many others. It is quite likely that the latent structure model derived from any one study will not exactly replicate the "true" population model in terms of the number or composition of classes. Investigators are cautioned to keep this fact in mind when interpreting findings from their studies. Replication is the hallmark of the scientific method, and its relevance for interpreting latent structure analyses in the eating disorder field should not be overlooked. Furthermore, different latent structure models may be important for different circumstances; for example, one latent structure may predict response to treatment, whereas another may be meaningful for genetic analyses.

Next Steps

Further work is needed in this area to replicate the results of studies conducted to date. Although the total number of latent structure analyses has become large, the sample design and modeling approaches are so highly variable that in some respects the actual N for the total number of studies is not 17 but more in the neighborhood of 2–4, depending on the particular scientific question. Thus, replication using both clinically derived and community samples is essential, especially using careful methodology that addresses issues of local independence, sparseness, and class membership assignment.

It would be extremely useful to expand the repertoire of validators from descriptive and concurrent variables to prospective ones. The goal of these latent structure analyses is to improve diagnosis (and in so doing, to guide the development of diagnostic algorithms such as DSM), and one major goal of diagnosis is to provide better clinical prediction of outcome and treatment response. Therefore, longitudinal outcome predictors and treatment response would be especially useful validators to examine.

References

Aitkin M, Rubin D: Estimation and hypothesis testing in finite mixture models. J R Stat Soc Ser B Methodol 47:67–75, 1985

Aitkin M, Andersen D, Hinde J: Statistical modeling of data on teaching styles. J R Stat Soc Ser A 144:419–461, 1981

Akaike H: Information theory and an extension of the maximum principle, in Second International Symposium on Information Theory. Edited by Petrov BN, Csaki BF. Budapest, Academai Kiado, 1973, pp 267–281

American Psychiatric Association: Diagnostic and Statistical Manual of Mental Disorders, 4th Edition. Washington, DC, American Psychiatric Association, 1994

American Psychiatric Association: Diagnostic and Statistical Manual of Mental Disorders, 4th Edition, Text Revision. Washington, DC, American Psychiatric Association, 2000

Bandeen-Roche K, Miglioretti D, Zeger S, et al: Latent variable regression for multiple discrete outcomes. J Am Stat Assoc 92:1375–1386, 1997

Bozdogan H: Model selection and Akaike's information criterion (AIC): the general theory and its analytical extensions. Psychometrika 52:345–370, 1987

Bulik CM, Sullivan PF, Kendler KS: An empirical study of the classification of eating disorders. Am J Psychiatry 157:886–895, 2000

Bulik CM, Sullivan PF, Kendler KS: Medical and psychiatric morbidity in obese women with and without binge eating. Int J Eat Disord 32:72–78, 2002

Clogg C: Latent class models, in Handbook of Statistical Modeling for the Social and Behavioral Sciences. Edited by Arminger G, Clogg C, Sobel ME. New York, Plenum, 1995, pp 311–359

Dayton CM, Macready GB: Concomitant-variable latent-class models. J Am Stat Assoc 83:173–178, 1988

Duncan AE, Bucholz KK, Neuman RJ, et al: Clustering of eating disorder symptoms in a general population female twin sample: a latent class analysis. Psychol Med 37:1097–1107, 2007

Eddy KT, Celio Doyle A, Hoste RR, et al: Eating disorder not otherwise specified in adolescents. J Am Acad Child Adolesc Psychiatry 47:156–164, 2008

Eddy KT, Crosby RD, Keel PK, et al: Empirical identification and validation of eating disorder phenotypes in a multisite clinical sample. J Nerv Ment Dis 197:41–49, 2009

Eddy KT, le Grange D, Crosby RD, et al: Diagnostic classification of eating disorders in children and adolescents: how does DSM-IV-TR compare to empirically derived categories? J Am Acad Child Adolesc Psychiatry 49:277–287, quiz 293, 2010

Fairburn CG, Bohn K: Eating disorder NOS (EDNOS): an example of the troublesome "not otherwise specified" (NOS) category in DSM-IV. Behav Res Ther 43:691–701, 2005

Fairburn CG, Cooper Z, Shafran R: Cognitive behaviour therapy for eating disorders: a "transdiagnostic" theory and treatment. Behav Res Ther 41:509–528, 2003

Frisch RE, McArthur JW: Menstrual cycles: fatness as a determinant of minimum weight for height necessary for their maintenance or onset. Science 185:949–951, 1974

Gleaves DH, Lowe MR, Green BA, et al: Do anorexia and bulimia nervosa occur on a continuum? A taxometric analysis. Behav Ther 31:195–219, 2000a

Gleaves DH, Lowe MR, Snow AC, et al: Continuity and discontinuity models of bulimia nervosa: a taxometric investigation. J Abnorm Psychol 109:56–68, 2000b

Jacobs MJ, Roesch S, Wonderlich SA, et al: Anorexia nervosa trios: behavioral profiles of individuals with anorexia nervosa and their parents. Psychol Med 39:451–461, 2009

Keel PK, Fichter M, Quadflieg N, et al: Application of a latent class analysis to empirically define eating disorder phenotypes. Arch Gen Psychiatry 61:192–200, 2004

Lin TH, Dayton CM: Model selection information criteria for non-nested latent class models. J Educ Behav Stat 22:249–264, 1997

Melton B, Liang KY, Pulver AE: Extended latent class approach to the study of familial/sporadic forms of a disease: its application to the study of the heterogeneity of schizophrenia. Genet Epidemiol 11:311–327, 1994

Mitchell JE, Crosby RD, Wonderlich SA, et al: Latent profile analysis of a cohort of patients with eating disorders not otherwise specified. Int J Eat Disord 40(suppl):S95–S98, 2007

Myers TC, Wonderlich SA, Crosby R, et al: Is multi-impulsive bulimia a distinct type of bulimia nervosa: psychopathology and EMA findings. Int J Eat Disord 39:655–661, 2006

Pinheiro AP, Bulik CM, Sullivan PF, et al: An empirical study of the typology of bulimic symptoms in young Portuguese women. Int J Eat Disord 41:251–258, 2008

Richardson J, Steiger H, Schmitz N, et al: Relevance of the 5-HTTLPR polymorphism and childhood abuse to increased psychiatric comorbidity in women with bulimia-spectrum disorders. J Clin Psychiatry 69:981–990, 2008

Schwarz G: Estimating the dimension of a model. Ann Stat 6:461–464, 1978

Sclove SL: Application of model-selection criteria to some problems in multivariate analysis. Psychometrika 52:333–343, 1987

Steiger H, Richardson J, Schmitz N, et al: Association of trait-defined, eating-disorder subphenotypes with (biallelic and triallelic) 5HTTLPR variations. J Psychiatr Res 43:1086–1094, 2009

Steiger H, Richardson J, Schmitz N, et al: Trait-defined eating-disorder subtypes and history of childhood abuse. Int J Eat Disord 43:428–432, 2010

Striegel-Moore RH, Franko DL, Thompson D, et al: An empirical study of the typology of bulimia nervosa and its spectrum variants. Psychol Med 35:1563–1572, 2005

Sullivan PF, Bulik CM, Kendler KS: The epidemiology and classification of bulimia nervosa. Psychol Med 28:599–610, 1998

Suppes P, Zanotti M: When are probabilistic explanations possible? Synthese 48:191–199, 1981

Torrance-Rynard VL, Walter SD: Effects of dependent errors in the assessment of diagnostic test performance. Stat Med 16:2157–2175, 1997

Turner H, Bryant-Waugh R, Peveler R: The clinical features of EDNOS: relationship to mood, health status and general functioning. Eat Behav 11:127–130, 2010

Tylka TL, Subich LM: Revisiting the latent structure of eating disorders: taxometric analyses with nonbehavioral indicators. J Couns Psychol 50:276–286, 2003

Vacek PM: The effect of conditional dependence on the evaluation of diagnostic tests. Biometrics 41:959–968, 1985

Wade TD, Crosby RD, Martin NG: Use of latent profile analysis to identify eating disorder phenotypes in an adult Australian twin cohort. Arch Gen Psychiatry 63:1377–1384, 2006

Wagner A, Greer P, Bailer UF, et al: Normal brain tissue volumes after long-term recovery in anorexia and bulimia nervosa. Biol Psychiatry 59:291–293, 2006

Walsh BT, Sysko R: Broad categories for the diagnosis of eating disorders (BCD-ED): an alternative system for classification. Int J Eat Disord 42:754–764, 2009

Williamson DA, Womble LG, Smeets MA, et al: Latent structure of eating disorder symptoms: a factor analytic and taxometric investigation. Am J Psychiatry 159:412–418, 2002

Williamson DA, Gleaves DH, Stewart TM: Categorical versus dimensional models of eating disorders: an examination of the evidence. Int J Eat Disord 37:1–10, 2005

Wonderlich SA, Crosby RD, Joiner T, et al: Personality subtyping and bulimia nervosa: psychopathological and genetic correlates. Psychol Med 35:649–657, 2005

Wonderlich SA, Crosby RD, Engel SG, et al: Personality-based clusters in bulimia nervosa: differences in clinical variables and ecological momentary assessment. J Pers Disord 21:340–357, 2007

Yang C: Evaluating latent class analysis models in qualitative phenotype identification. Comput Stat Data Anal 50:1090–1104, 2006

9

EMPIRICAL TAXONOMY OF PATIENTS WITH EATING DISORDERS

Marion P. Olmsted, Ph.D., C.Psych.
Stephen A. Wonderlich, Ph.D.
Traci McFarlane, Ph.D., C.Psych.
Ross D. Crosby, Ph.D.

The classification of eating disorders, at least as defined by DSM-IV (American Psychiatric Association 1994), has been plagued by an inordinate number of patients who do not meet criteria for anorexia nervosa (AN) or bulimia nervosa (BN) and consequently are classified in the default category of eating disorder not otherwise specified (EDNOS). This problem has been well documented (Fairburn and Bohn 2005), and numerous solutions have been discussed, including loosening the criteria for placement in AN or BN (Dalle Grave and Calugi 2007), creating broad categories that would have lower thresholds of acceptance than the current diagnostic categories (Walsh and Sysko 2009), and lumping all eating disorders together in one overarching diagnostic characterized by eating-related problems and concerns about shape and weight (Fairburn 2008). Despite these efforts to decrease the number of patients receiving an EDNOS diagnosis, there is very little empirical evidence characterizing the composition of the current EDNOS category. Two recent studies have taken large samples of EDNOS patients and either used a rational (Rockert et al. 2007) or empirical (Mitchell et al. 2007) means of identifying subgroups within EDNOS. Overall, it is clear that the EDNOS category seems to comprise diminutive forms of primary eating disorders as well as other potential classes such as night eating syndrome or purging disorder and various unique compilations of eating disorder symptomatology.

Paralleling the exploration of EDNOS, there has been a series of studies using empirical approaches to classify the full range of eating disorder possibilities. For example, eight studies (Bulik et al. 2000; Duncan et al. 2007; Eddy et al. 2009; Keel et al. 2004; Mitchell et al. 2007; Striegel-Moore et al. 2005; Sullivan et al. 1998; Wade et al. 2006) have used latent profile analysis (LPA) or latent class analysis to identify latent groupings of individuals with eating disorder. Although the number and composition of classes have been varied, several studies have identified classes resembling AN, BN, and binge eating disorder (BED), but the operationalization of these empirically derived classes is often different from that used in DSM-IV. With the exception of the study by Mitchell et al. (2007), these empirical approaches to taxonomy have not been used to characterize EDNOS specifically.

The present study had two primary aims. First, we intended to compare the latent structure of EDNOS with that of all eating disorders (EDNOS, AN, BN). Second, we sought to test the validity of identified latent classes across a wide variety of indicators, including demographic variables, clinical characteristics, and response to treatment.

Methods

SUBJECTS

Participants were females who sought treatment for their eating disorder and were referred to the Toronto General Hospital Eating Disorder Program between 1994 and 2006. The first contact consisted of a consultation interview conducted by an experienced psychiatrist or psychologist. The 1,617 patients who were diagnosed with an eating disorder at this interview, accepted a recommendation for day hospital or outpatient treatment, and attended a pretreatment assessment were included in the current study.

MEASURES

Patients completed a self-report questionnaire that requested information about demographic and clinical features. Symptom frequencies were initially assessed with a semistructured interview, the Eating Disorder Examination (EDE; Cooper and Fairburn 1987), and partway through the study, a switch was made to an abbreviated version of this interview.

STATISTICAL ANALYSIS

LPA (Lazarsfeld and Henry 1968) was conducted on the 688 patients with a diagnosis of EDNOS. LPA identifies the number and composition of latent (i.e., not directly observed) subgroups (or classes) from a heterogeneous sample by minimizing associations between measured indicators within these classes. The number of classes was determined by the Bayesian information criterion (BIC; Sclove 1987) parsimony index, the sample-size adjusted Bayesian information criterion (Yang 2006), and the consistent Akaike information criterion (Bozdogan 1987). Analysis was performed with Latent GOLD Version 4.5 software (Vermunt and Magidson 2000). Seven indicators of eating disorder pathology were selected from the EDE to represent the DSM-IV criteria sets for AN and BN. Indicators included body mass index (BMI; ≤17.5, >17.5 to <18.5, 18.5–24.9, 25–29.9, 30+), binge eating, vomiting and laxative use frequency in the previous month (none, one to three times, four to seven times, eight or more times), and fear of weight gain and loss of control (1 = never, to 6 = always). Missing values were estimated with full information maximum-likelihood estimation. LPA analysis was repeated with the full sample using the same procedures.

χ^2 analysis was used to compare empirical classification from the full-sample LPA with DSM-IV diagnoses, including subtypes of AN and BN, with BED separated from EDNOS. The identified classes from the full sample were compared on demographic and clinical features in order to characterize and validate these groups. Analysis of variance or χ^2 analyses on the full sample were then used to determine the proportion of variance in baseline validators that could be explained (via η^2 or ϕ^2) by the classes derived from LPA versus the DSM-IV diagnoses. Finally, separate analyses were conducted for patients treated in the day hospital ($n = 294$) and patients who participated in an outpatient psychoeducational group treatment ($n = 396$), with both empirical classes and DSM-IV diagnoses used to predict treatment outcome. These comparisons allowed a direct comparison of the DSM-based categories with the LPA-based classes.

Results

PATIENT CHARACTERISTICS

Table 9–1 presents demographic information and DSM-IV eating disorder diagnoses in the current sample. The vast majority of participants were female (96.9%), ranging in age from 17 to 70 years. The average duration of illness was more than 8.5 years. More than one-third of the sample (35.1%) met criteria for DSM-IV BN; almost one-quarter (22.4%) met criteria for AN; and the remainder of the sample (42.5%) met criteria for EDNOS, including 85 who met DSM-IV provisional criteria for BED.

LATENT PROFILE ANALYSIS

The LPA of EDNOS cases resulted in three classes, depicted in Figure 9–1. The y-axis represents standardized values on the indicators, with 0 representing the lowest

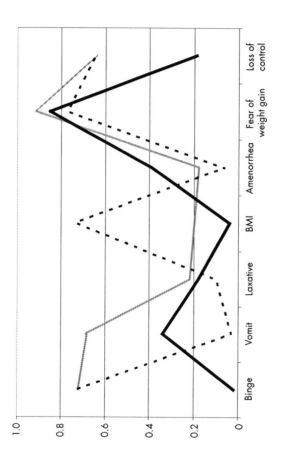

FIGURE 9–1. Latent profile analysis of eating disorder not otherwise specified sample (*N*=688).

Low weight restricting class: solid black line. Binge-purge class: solid gray line. Binge class: dashed black line. BMI=body mass index.

TABLE 9–1. Demographic and DSM-IV eating disorder diagnoses (*N*=1,617)

Female, *n* (%)	1,567 (96.9)
Age, mean ± SD (range)	28.7 ± 9.0 (17–70)
Body mass index, mean ± SD (range)	23.1 ± 7.3 (11.7–59.7)
Duration of illness in years, mean ± SD (range)	8.6 + 8.3 (0.1–57.0)
DSM-IV eating disorder diagnosis, *n* (%)	
Anorexia nervosa, restricting	161 (10.0)
Anorexia nervosa, binge-purge	201 (12.4)
Bulimia nervosa, purge	472 (29.2)
Bulimia nervosa, non-purge	95 (5.9)
Eating disorder not otherwise specified[a]	603 (37.3)
Binge eating disorder	85 (5.3)

[a]Excluding binge eating disorder.

and 1 the highest values and the lines representing the mean value for each class. The largest class (38.2%), depicted by the solid black line, is characterized by low BMI, absence of binge eating, and low levels of purging. This class was labeled "low weight restricting." The second class (37.4%), depicted by the solid gray line, is characterized by high levels of binge eating and purging, high fear of weight gain, and high loss of control. This class was labeled "binge-purge." The final class (24.4%), depicted by the dashed black line, is characterized by high levels of binge eating, absence of purging, and high BMI. This class was labeled "binge."

The results of LPA for the entire sample, which are shown in Figure 9–2, closely mirror those from the EDNOS sample. Again, three classes were identified, including a low weight restricting class (29.8%) shown by the solid black line, a binge-purge class (46.8%) shown by the solid gray line, and a binge class (23.4%) shown by the dashed black line.

ASSOCIATION BETWEEN EMPIRICAL CLASSIFICATION AND DSM-IV

Table 9–2 presents the cross-tabulation between empirical classes and DSM-IV diagnoses. There was a significant association between the empirical classes and DSM-IV diagnoses ($\chi^2_{10} = 1,489.7$; $P < 0.001$). The majority of patients with BN, purging subtype (94.1%) and AN, binge-purge subtype (69.7%) were classified in the binge-purge empirical class. Likewise, the majority of patients with AN, restricting subtype (93.8%) were assigned to the low weight restricting empirical class. All patients with BED or BN, nonpurging subtype were classified in the binge empirical class. Finally, patients with EDNOS were dispersed across the three empirical classes.

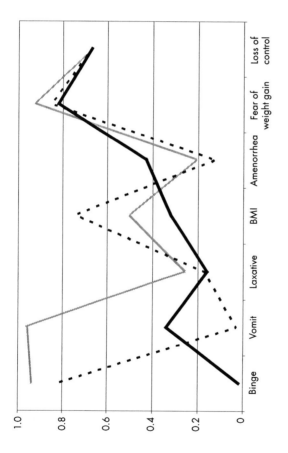

FIGURE 9–2.   Latent profile analysis of full sample (*N*=1,617).

Low-weight restricting class: solid black line. Binge-purge class: solid gray line. Binge class: dashed black line. BMI=body mass index.

TABLE 9–2. Empirical classification versus DSM-IV diagnosis

	Empirical class		
DSM-IV diagnosis	Binge-purge, *n* (%)	Low weight restricting, *n* (%)	Binge, *n* (%)
Anorexia nervosa, restricting	5 (3.1)	151 (93.8)	5 (3.1)
Anorexia nervosa, binge-purge	140 (69.7)	55 (27.4)	6 (3.0)
Bulimia nervosa, purge	444 (94.1)	1 (0.2)	27 (5.7)
Bulimia nervosa, non-purge	0 (0.0)	0 (0.0)	95 (100)
Eating disorder not otherwise specified[a]	168 (27.9)	275 (45.6)	160 (26.5)
Binge eating disorder	0 (0.0)	0 (0.0)	85 (100)

[a]Excluding binge eating disorder.

VALIDATION OF EMPIRICAL CLASSES

Comparisons between the three empirical classes on demographic and clinical characteristics are presented in Table 9–3. The binge-purge class was characterized by a higher number of previous eating disorder treatments and higher rates of alcohol abuse, drug abuse, and self-harm. As expected, the low weight restricting class was characterized by higher rates of hospitalization for treatment. Finally, the binge class was characterized by older age, a higher rate of male patients, and a longer duration of illness.

EMPIRICAL CLASSIFICATION VERSUS DSM-IV DIAGNOSES

Table 9–4 presents comparisons between empirical classification and DSM-IV diagnoses (with and without BED separated from EDNOS) in terms of the ability to account for differences in demographic and clinical characteristics at baseline. All three classification schemes were significantly associated with these validators. However, the empirical classification accounted for a higher proportion of the variance across all validators in comparison with either DSM-IV approach. This suggests that the empirical approach, which tends to group patients on the basis of similar binge-purge patterns, better distinguishes patients in terms of baseline demographic and clinical characteristics than the DSM-IV classification, which places more emphasis on weight.

TABLE 9–3. Comparison of latent classes on demographic and clinical characteristics

Characteristic	Binge-purge (n=757)	Low weight restricting (n=382)	Binge (n=378)	Significance
Age, mean ± SD	27.2 ± 7.5[a]	27.9 ± 9.1[a]	32.5 ± 10.4[b]	<0.001
Male, n (%)	17 (2.2)[a]	9 (2.4)[a]	20 (5.3)[b]	0.013
Duration of illness in years, mean ± SD	8.2 ± 7.4[a]	7.4 ± 8.5[a]	10.8 ± 9.7[b]	<0.001
Eating disorder treatments, mean ± SD	2.2 ± 2.5[a]	1.8 ± 2.7[ab]	1.6 ± 2.6[b]	0.020
Eating disorder hospitalizations, mean ± SD	0.5 ± 1.2[a]	0.8 ± 2.0[b]	0.3 ± 1.6[a]	<0.001
Alcohol abuse,[1] n (%)	176 (33.3)[a]	64 (22.5)[b]	62 (23.5)[b]	0.001
Drug abuse,[2] n (%)	107 (20.8)[a]	35 (12.5)[b]	46 (17.6)[ab]	0.013
Self-harm,[3] n (%)	246 (45.6)[a]	90 (30.6)[b]	94 (35.1)[b]	<0.001

Note. Cells without common superscripts are significantly different ($P<0.05$) based on Tukey's B or pairwise χ^2.
[1] $N=1,078$.
[2] $N=1,058$.
[3] $N=1,102$.

TABLE 9–4. Comparison of empirical and DSM-IV classifications on baseline validators

	Empirical	DSM-IV	
Baseline validator	BP, LWR, binge	AN, BN, EDNOS	AN, BN, BED, EDNOS
Age	0.059***	0.027***	0.047***
Gender	0.006**	0.005*	0.005*
Duration of illness	0.022***	0.016***	0.018***
Age at diagnosis	0.045***	0.023***	0.034***
Eating disorder treatments	0.016***	0.010*	0.011*
Eating disorder hospitalizations	0.015***	0.007*	0.008*

Note. Cell entries represent percent of variance accounted for based on η^2 or ϕ^2. AN = anorexia nervosa; BED = binge eating disorder; BN = bulimia nervosa; BP = binge-purge; EDNOS = eating disorder not otherwise specified; LWR = low weight restricting. *$P<0.05$; **$P<0.01$; ***$P<0.001$.

Comparisons between the empirical classification and DSM-IV diagnoses on treatment outcome revealed that no classification approach was significantly associated with outcome for either day hospital treatment or outpatient psychoeducational group treatment.

Discussion

The present LPA revealed a three-class latent structure for eating disorder patients, which included a binge-purge class, a low weight restricting class, and a binge eating class. These findings parallel several other recent studies (Peterson et al. 2009; see also Chapter 10, this volume). The binge class was discriminated from the other two classes by its propensity to contain older participants who were more likely to be male, with a longer duration of their disorder. The binge-purge class distinguished itself from the other classes with greater psychiatric comorbidity in the form of alcohol abuse, drug abuse, or self-harm. Those in the low weight restricting class were most likely to be hospitalized for an eating disorder.

Importantly, the three-class solution identified in the overall eating disorder sample was essentially replicated using only participants who were officially diagnosed as having EDNOS. The observation that the latent structure of EDNOS mirrors the latent structure of all eating disorders not only provides insight into the composition of EDNOS but also is consistent with recent evidence that subsyndromal eating disorder variants differ minimally from full-syndrome diagnoses across a wide range of validators (see Thomas et al. 2009). Moreover, the detection of three distinct classes in our LPA of EDNOS suggests there is meaningful variation within this broad diagnostic category, which is not consistent with transdiagnostic models of eating disorder classification (Fairburn 2008).

Finally, across a relatively broad range of demographic and clinical characteristics, the empirically based taxonomy accounted for more variance than the DSM-based taxonomy. The fundamental difference between the placement of participants in the DSM taxonomy versus the empirical taxonomy is the finding that low-weight individuals who binge eat and purge tend to be placed in the binge-purge class in empirical taxonomies but are placed in the AN category in the DSM taxonomy (i.e., AN, binge-purge type). Thus, at least on the validators examined in this study, the presence of binge eating and purging, regardless of weight, was a significant factor in discriminating classes on the demographic and clinical characteristics chosen as validators in the present study. It may be that various characteristics associated with binge-purge behavior (e.g., impulsive personality structure, psychiatric comorbidity) increase the predictive power of the empirical taxonomy by placing all such individuals in one class. However, as other studies have recently shown (see Chapter 10), when other validating variables are considered (e.g., mortality), empirically based taxonomies may perform less well.

The present study has several strengths, including use of a large eating disorder sample that represents a broad range of symptomatology. Also, the application of contemporary empirical taxonomy strategies and clinically meaningful validators enhances the usefulness of this study. However, the study is not without limitations. The sample was derived from a clinical population at one site and thus may be limited in terms of overall generalizability. Additionally, the validators are relatively limited in scope, and clinical utility would have been enhanced by inclusion of longitudinal variables. Finally, although LPA is a useful strategy for identifying naturally occurring groupings, it does not clarify whether the identified classes differ in nature as opposed to degree. Additional analyses, such as taxometrics, could help to clarify the nature of the boundary between the identified classes.

References

American Psychiatric Association: Diagnostic and Statistical Manual of Mental Disorders, 4th Edition. Washington, DC, American Psychiatric Association, 1994

Bozdogan H: Model selection and Akaike's information criterion (AIC): the general theory and its analytical extensions. Psychometrika 52:345–370, 1987

Bulik CM, Sullivan PD, Kendler KS: An empirical study of the classification of eating disorders. Am J Psychiatry 157:886–895, 2000

Cooper Z, Fairburn CG: The Eating Disorder Examination: a semi-structured interview for the assessment of the specific psychopathology of eating disorders. Int J Eat Disord 6:1–8, 1987

Dalle Grave R, Calugi S: Eating disorder not otherwise specified in an inpatient unit: the impact of altering the DSM-IV criteria for anorexia and bulimia nervosa. Eur Eat Disord Rev 115:340–349, 2007

Duncan AE, Bucholz KK, Neuman RJ, et al: Clustering of eating disorder symptoms in a general population female twin sample: a latent class analysis. Psychol Med 37:1097–1107, 2007

Eddy KT, Crosby RD, Keel PK, et al: Empirical identification and validation of eating disorder phenotypes in a multisite clinical sample. J Nerv Ment Dis 197:41–49, 2009

Fairburn CG: Cognitive Behavior Therapy and Eating Disorders. New York, Guilford, 2008

Fairburn CG, Bohn K: Eating disorder NOS (EDNOS): an example of the troublesome "not otherwise specified" (NOS) category in DSM-IV. Behav Res Ther 43:691–701, 2005

Keel PK, Fichter M, Quadflieg N, et al: Application of a latent class analysis to empirically define eating disorder phenotypes. Arch Gen Psychiatry 61:192–200, 2004

Lazarsfeld PF, Henry NW: Latent Structure Analysis. Boston, MA, Houghton Mifflin, 1968

Mitchell J, Crosby R, Wonderlich S, et al: Latent profile analysis of a cohort of patients with eating disorder not otherwise specified. Int J Eat Disord 40:S95–S98, 2007

Peterson CB, Crow SJ, Swanson S, et al: Longitudinal stability of empirically derived vs. DSM-IV classification of eating disorder symptoms. Presented at the Eating Disorders Research Society 15th annual meeting, Brooklyn, New York, September 2009

Rockert W, Kaplan AS, Olmsted MP: Eating disorder not otherwise specified: the view from a tertiary care treatment center. Int J Eat Disord 40:S99–S103, 2007

Sclove S: Application of model-selection criteria to some problems in multivariate analysis. Psychometrika 52:333–343, 1987

Striegel-Moore R, Franko DL, Thompson D, et al: An empirical study of the typology of bulimia nervosa and its spectrum variants. Psychol Med 35:1563–1572, 2005

Sullivan PF, Bulik CM, Kendler KS: The epidemiology and classification of bulimia nervosa. Psychol Med 28:599–610, 1998

Thomas J, Vartanian L, Brownell K: The relationship between eating disorder not otherwise specified (EDNOS) and officially recognized eating disorders: meta-analysis and implications for DSM. Psychol Bull 135:407–433, 2009

Vermunt JK, Magidson J: Latent GOLD User's Guide. Belmont, MA, Statistical Innovations Inc, 2000

Wade TD, Crosby RD, Martin NG: Use of latent profile analysis to identify eating disorder phenotypes in an adult Australian twin cohort. Arch Gen Psychiatry 63:1377–1384, 2006

Walsh BT, Sysko R: Broad categories for the diagnosis of eating disorders (BCD-ED): an alternative system for classification. Int J Eat Disord 42:754–764, 2009

Yang C: Evaluating latent class analyses in qualitative phenotype identification. Comput Stat Data Anal 50:1090–1104, 2006

10

VALIDATING EATING DISORDER CLASSIFICATION MODELS WITH MORTALITY AND RECOVERY DATA

Ross D. Crosby, Ph.D.
Manfred M. Fichter, M.D., Dipl.Psych.
Norbert Quadflieg, Dipl.Psych.
Stephen A. Wonderlich, Ph.D.

Classification systems of psychopathology are critical for both clinical and scientific purposes, but there have been increased concerns about the validity of many contemporary psychiatric disorders (Rounsaville et al. 2002). Similar concerns have been raised regarding the validity of eating disorder diagnoses in DSM-IV (American Psychiatric Association 1994), particularly regarding subtypes of anorexia nervosa (AN) and bulimia nervosa (BN), as well as potential new eating disorder diagnoses, such as purging disorder, binge eating disorder (BED), or night eating syndrome (Wonderlich et al. 2007b). In addition to concerns about the validity of eating disorder diagnoses, there has been a significant concern about the issue of diagnostic coverage of eating disorders given that the majority of individuals with eating disorder do not receive diagnoses of AN or BN but are placed in the default category of eating disorder not otherwise specified (EDNOS; Fairburn and Bohn 2005).

In an effort to address many of these concerns, researchers have proposed new models of eating disorder classifications (e.g., Fairburn 2008; Williamson et al.

2002). Also, researchers have increasingly studied eating disorder classification using empirical approaches to taxonomy such as latent class analysis (LCA), latent profile analysis (LPA), and taxometric analysis. To date, there have been at least eight studies that have used LCA or LPA to examine samples with eating disorder symptomatology (Bulik et al. 2000; Duncan et al. 2007; Eddy et al. 2009; Keel et al. 2004; Mitchell et al. 2007; Striegel-Moore et al. 2005; Sullivan et al. 1998; Wade et al. 2006). Several findings converge across these analyses, including evidence of classes resembling BN, AN, and BED; however, there has been little support for the subtypes of AN and BN as defined by DSM-IV.

Although these empirical approaches to taxonomy provide interesting new insights into the possible nomenclature of eating disorders, strong tests of the validity of these latent classes have not been conducted, particularly regarding clinically significant validators (Wonderlich et al. 2007a). These studies would be enhanced substantially by comparing empirically derived classes across clinically meaningful measures, such as longitudinal clinical course (including mortality) and response to treatment. Moreover, head-to-head comparisons between differing taxonomic systems would promote evidence-based classification. The present study utilized a large sample of eating disorder patients who were studied longitudinally to provide such clinically useful validation data. Importantly, this study also offers comparisons on eating disorder–related mortality that, to date, have not been published in empirical approaches to taxonomy.

Methods

SUBJECTS

Participants were from 635 consecutive admissions from September 1985 to June 1988 for inpatient treatment for eating disorders or obesity in Upper Bavaria, Germany. A total of 90 patients treated for obesity without any DSM-IV eating disorder diagnosis were excluded from the current analyses, leaving a sample of 545 patients. Details of the sample and assessment procedures are provided elsewhere (Fichter and Quadflieg 2004; Fichter et al. 2006, 2008).

MEASURES

The Structured Interview for Anorexia and Bulimia Nervosa Expert Rating (SIAB-EX; Fichter et al. 1991) was used to determine initial eating disorder diagnosis and eating disturbance, and the self-rating version of this instrument (Fichter and Quadflieg 2000) was used at the 12-year follow-up. Patients completed the Beck Depression Inventory (Beck et al. 1961) and the Hopkins Symptom Checklist–90 (Derogatis et al. 1974) at admission. The Psychiatric Status Rating Scale developed by Herzog et al. (1988) was used as a global eating disorder outcome scale, with scores ranging from 1 (usual self) to 6 (eating disorder diagnostic criteria fulfilled, severe). Mortality of all patients at 12-year follow-up was determined by the German Federal Health Monitoring System.

PROCEDURES

Patients were assessed at the beginning and end of intensive inpatient treatment and at 2-year, 6-year, and 12-year follow-up. At each follow-up, patients received a comprehensive questionnaire by mail. After the questionnaire was completed and returned, the patient was contacted for a detailed interview conducted by trained experts.

STATISTICAL ANALYSIS

LPA (Lazarsfeld and Henry 1968) was conducted using admission data from the 545 patients with an eating disorder diagnosis. Analysis was performed using Latent GOLD Version 4.5 software (Vermunt and Magidson 2000). Indicators included body mass index (BMI; ≤ 17.5, >17.5 to <18.5, 18.5–24.9, 25–29.9, 30+), binge eating, vomiting and laxative use at admission (none vs. any), and a body image rating (five ordered categories) from the SIAB-EX. Missing values were estimated with full-information maximum-likelihood estimation. The number of classes was determined using four parsimony indices: Bayesian information criterion (Sclove 1987), the sample-size adjusted Bayesian information criterion (Yang 2006), the Akaike information criterion (Akaike 1987), and the consistent Akaike information criterion (Bozdogan 1987).

χ^2 analysis was used to compare empirical classification from the LPA with admission DSM-IV eating disorder diagnoses. Empirical classes were compared on demographic and clinical characteristics at baseline using χ^2 or analysis of variance with Tukey honestly significant difference post hoc comparisons. Logistic regression analyses were performed using empirical classes or DSM-IV admission diagnoses to predict mortality and recovery (defined as absence of a DSM-IV eating disorder diagnosis) at 12-year follow-up (age at admission controlled for). Linear regression analysis was used to predict psychiatric status at 12-year follow-up (controlling for age at admission).

Results

PATIENT CHARACTERISTICS

Demographic and clinical characteristics at admission, along with DSM-IV eating disorder diagnoses, are presented in Table 10–1. The patient sample was predominantly female (95.8%), with a mean age of 26.4 years. More than one-third of the

TABLE 10–1.   Patient characteristics at admission ($N=545$)

Female, n (%)	522 (95.8)
Age, mean ± SD (range)	26.4 ± 7.1 (14.9–52.1)
Age at diagnosis, in years, mean ± SD	18.3 ± 6.3
Body mass index, mean ± SD (range)	20.9 ± 7.8 (10.4–57.2)
Body mass index ≤ 17.5, n (%)	209 (38.3)
Body mass index ≥ 30, n (%)	64 (11.7)
Treatment duration, in days, mean ± SD	93.6 ± 45.8
DSM-IV eating disorder diagnosis, n (%)	
Anorexia nervosa, restricting	30 (5.5)
Anorexia nervosa, binge-purge	74 (13.6)
Bulimia nervosa, purge	205 (37.6)
Bulimia nervosa, non-purge	15 (2.8)
Eating disorder not otherwise specified[a]	152 (27.9)
Binge eating disorder	69 (12.7)

[a]Excluding binge eating disorder.

sample had an admission BMI of less than 17.5 kg/m². Nearly 20% of the sample met criteria for DSM-IV AN, more than 40% met criteria for BN, and slightly more than 40% met criteria for EDNOS (including BED).

LATENT PROFILE ANALYSIS

LPAs produced a clear and unambiguous three-class solution, shown in Figure 10–1. The values in the graph represent standardized scores on the indicators, with 0 representing the lowest and 1 the highest values. The lines in the graph represent the mean value for each class on that indicator. The largest class (62.6%), depicted by the solid gray line, is characterized by high levels of binge eating and purging and high body image disturbance. This class was labeled "binge-purge." The second class (29.0%), depicted by the solid black line, is characterized by low levels of binge eating and purging and low weight. This class was labeled "low weight restricting." The final class (8.4%), depicted by the dashed black line, is characterized by high levels of binge eating, the absence of purging, high BMI, and high body image disturbance. This class was labeled "binge."

ASSOCIATION BETWEEN EMPIRICAL CLASSIFICATION AND DSM-IV

A significant association ($\chi^2_{10}=360.1$; $P<0.001$) was found between the empirical classes and DSM-IV diagnoses, as shown in Table 10–2. The majority (66.7%) of

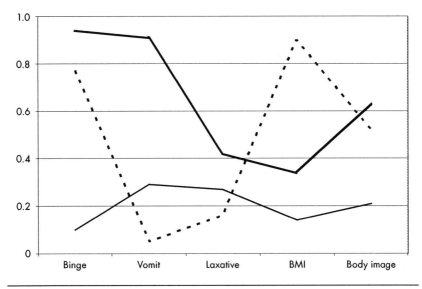

FIGURE 10–1.   Latent profile analysis (*N*=545).

Binge-purge class: solid gray line. Low weight restricting class: solid black line. Binge class: dashed black line.

BMI=body mass index.

patients with AN, restricting subtype were classified in the low weight restricting empirical class. Likewise, the majority of patients with BN, purging subtype (88.8%) or AN, binge-purge subtype (71.6%) were classified in the binge-purge empirical class. Finally, approximately half (50.7%) of the patients with BED and one-quarter (26.7%) of patients with BN, non-purge subtype were classified in the binge empirical class.

VALIDATION OF EMPIRICAL CLASSES

Table 10–3 presents a comparison of empirical classes on baseline demographic and clinical characteristics. The binge-purge class is characterized by the highest levels of depression and anxiety and the highest rates of a previous history of AN or BN. The low weight restricting class is characterized by the lowest BMI and the lowest levels of anxiety and depression. The binge class is characterized by the oldest age, highest BMI, and highest rates of a history of obesity.

EMPIRICAL CLASSIFICATION VERSUS DSM-IV DIAGNOSES

A total of 14 deaths (2.4%) were identified at 12-year follow-up in the sample. Figure 10–2 presents a comparison of the empirical classification and DSM-IV (with

TABLE 10–2. Empirical classification versus DSM-IV diagnosis

	Empirical class		
DSM-IV diagnosis	Binge-purge, n (%)	Low weight restricting, n (%)	Binge, n (%)
Anorexia nervosa, restricting	10 (33.3)	20 (66.7)	0 (0.0)
Anorexia nervosa, binge-purge	53 (71.6)	21 (28.4)	0 (0.0)
Bulimia nervosa, purge	182 (88.8)	17 (8.3)	6 (2.9)
Bulimia nervosa, non-purge	11 (73.3)	0 (0.0)	4 (26.7)
Eating disorder not otherwise specified[a]	53 (34.9)	98 (64.5)	1 (0.7)
Binge eating disorder	32 (46.4)	2 (2.9)	35 (50.7)

[a]Excluding binge eating disorder.

and without BED separated from EDNOS) in predicting 12-year mortality. Although both DSM-IV classifications significantly predicted mortality at 12 years, accounting for 7.2% and 8.2% of the criterion variance, the empirical classes did not significantly predict mortality. As expected, the highest rates of mortality were for those with AN.

Recovery data at 12 years were available for 342 patients. The number of patients with BED who were followed up was small ($n=8$), and therefore these patients were not separated from EDNOS patients assessed at 12-year follow-up. Rates of recovery at 12-year follow-up, defined as an absence of a DSM-IV eating disorder diagnosis, are presented for empirical and DSM-IV classifications in Figure 10–3. Again, DSM-IV diagnoses significantly predicted recovery, accounting for 2.8% of the criterion variance, whereas the empirical classification did not.

Psychiatric status at 12-year follow-up was available for 342 patients (Figure 10–4). Both the empirical classification and DSM-IV diagnoses significantly predicted psychiatric status at 12-year follow-up, with the empirical classification accounting for 1.9% of the criterion variance and DSM-IV diagnoses accounting for 2.4% of the variance.

Discussion

The present findings are consistent with an increasing number of studies suggesting that contemporary empirical approaches to classification produce three classes of individuals with ED: binge-purge, low weight restriction, and binge eating (Peterson et al. 2009; see also Olmsted et al., Chapter 9, "Empirical Taxonomy of

TABLE 10–3. Comparison of latent classes on demographic and clinical characteristics

Characteristic	Binge-purge (n=341)	Low weight restricting (n=158)	Binge (n=46)	Significance
Age, in years, mean ± SD	25.9 ± 6.6[a]	26.2 ± 7.0[a]	31.4 ± 8.6[b]	<0.001
Female, n (%)	326 (95.6)	152 (96.2)	44 (95.7)	0.952
Body mass index, mean ± SD	20.6 ± 6.1[a]	16.5 ± 3.5[b]	37.5 ± 7.7[c]	<0.001
Age at onset of eating disorder, in years, mean ± SD	17.7 ± 6.2	17.9 ± 9.2	15.8 ± 10.0	0.229
Beck Depression Inventory	23.3 ± 10.7[a]	15.3 ± 11.2[b]	22.2 ± 10.8[a]	<0.001
Symptom Checklist–90 Anxiety	1.4 ± 0.8[a]	0.9 ± 0.8[b]	1.3 ± 0.9[a]	<0.001
History of anorexia nervosa, n (%)	98 (28.7)[a]	41 (25.9)[a]	0 (0.0)[b]	<0.001
History of bulimia nervosa, n (%)	272 (79.8)[a]	42 (26.6)[b]	17 (37.0)[b]	<0.001
History of obesity, n (%)	40 (11.7)[a]	3 (1.9)[b]	41 (89.1)[c]	<0.001

Note. Cells without common superscripts are significantly different ($P<0.05$) based on Tukey's B or pairwise χ^2.

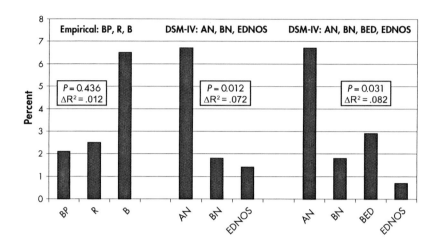

FIGURE 10–2.   Classification models and 12-year mortality ($N = 545$).

AN = anorexia nervosa; B = binge; BED = binge eating disorder; BN = bulimia nervosa; BP = binge-purge; EDNOS = eating disorder not otherwise specified; R = low weight restricting.

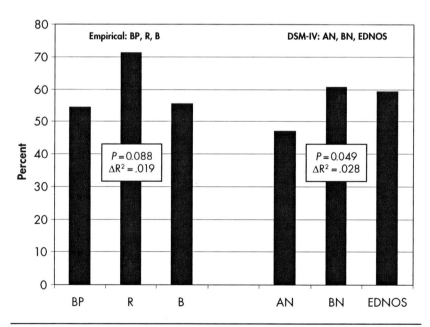

FIGURE 10–3.   Classification models and 12-year recovery ($N = 342$).

AN = anorexia nervosa; B = binge; BN = bulimia nervosa; BP = binge-purge; EDNOS = eating disorder not otherwise specified; R = low weight restricting.

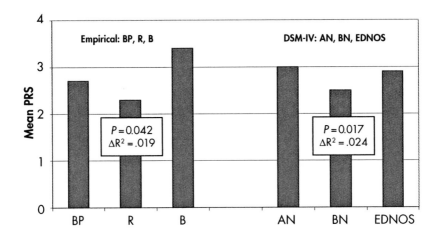

FIGURE 10–4. Classification models and 12-year psychiatric status (*N*=342).

AN = anorexia nervosa; B = binge; BN = bulimia nervosa; BP = binge-purge; EDNOS = eating disorder not otherwise specified; PRS = Psychiatric Rating Scale; R = low weight restricting.

Patients With Eating Disorders," this volume). These findings also provide empirical support for the recently developed broad categories model of eating disorders by Walsh and Sysko (2009). Although there is moderate correspondence between the empirical taxonomy and the DSM categories of AN, BN, and BED, empirical approaches tend to include low-weight individuals who binge eat and purge in the same class as normal-weight individuals who binge eat and purge (i.e., BN). This is in contrast to DSM-IV, in which low-weight individuals with binge-purge symptoms are considered to have a subtype of AN and to be qualitatively distinct from individuals with BN.

The present findings also suggest that a three-class empirical taxonomy displays meaningful external validity, with the low weight restricting class displaying lower levels of comorbid psychopathology than the other two classes, whereas the binge class tends to be older and more likely to have a history of obesity than the binge-purge and low weight restricting classes. As might be expected, the low weight restricting individuals tended to have the lowest BMIs and the individuals in the binge class displayed the highest BMIs. Thus, in terms of concurrent and historical demographic and clinical validators, the empirical taxonomy produces valid discriminations among classes.

However, validity tests on clinically relevant validators are most useful for testing models for clinical diagnostic purposes. The current findings regarding 12-year mortality and 12-year recovery are innovative and unique in empirical studies of eating disorder classification. In the mortality analysis, whether BED is broken out as a separate category or included in the EDNOS category, the DSM-IV classification scheme accounted for more variance in mortality than the empirical classification model. Similarly, the DSM classification model was superior to the empirical approach in accounting for diagnostic-related differences in 12-year recovery. Although differences between the DSM and empirical models were less pronounced in predicting 12-year psychiatric status, once again the DSM-IV model performed slightly better than the empirical taxonomy. These findings provide important validity data that have significant clinical utility. To the extent that a classification model should be useful in predicting course, the DSM model appears to have superior clinical utility in the present analysis. Such head-to-head comparisons on other validators have not consistently shown the DSM model to have greater validity or clinical utility than the empirical taxonomy. For example, the study by Olmsted et al. (see Chapter 9, "Empirical Taxonomy of Patients With Eating Disorders," this volume) suggested that the empirical taxonomy is more valid than the DSM-IV taxonomy in predicting concurrent clinical validators such as comorbidity and eating disorder history. Similarly, the study by Peterson et al. (2009) suggested that the empirical taxonomy is superior to the DSM-IV taxonomy in terms of diagnostic stability and reduction of diagnostic migration over time.

We speculate that the current findings are partially accounted for by the fact that the DSM-IV model separates all low-weight individuals from all other eating disorder patients and places them in one diagnostic class (i.e., AN). As noted previously, the empirical taxonomy tends to retain some low-weight individuals in the low weight restricting class, but other low-weight individuals are included in the binge-purge class. To the extent that low weight is a significant predictor of mortality and course, the separation of low-weight eating disorder patients into two different classes in the empirical taxonomy may reduce its predictive validity on clinically relevant validators that are correlated with weight, such as mortality and recovery.

The present study has several strengths, including a large eating disorder sample with substantial coverage of the domain of eating disorder symptomatology. Furthermore, the use of contemporary empirical taxonomy methodologies, such as LPA, with validators that are both longitudinal and clinically relevant make these findings quite unique in the empirical study of eating disorder classification. However, the study is limited by the fact that it was derived from a purely clinical population at one center, and thus it may not generalize to individuals with eating disorder who are not receiving clinical care or to those from other sites. Also, LPA is unable to determine whether the differentiations between classes are qualitative or quantitative, and alternative analyses, such as taxometric analysis, may be needed to clarify the nature of the boundary between empirical classes.

References

Akaike H: Factor analysis and AIC. Psychometrika 52:317–332, 1987

American Psychiatric Association: Diagnostic and Statistical Manual of Mental Disorders, 4th Edition. Washington, DC, American Psychiatric Association, 1994

Beck AT, Ward CH, Mendelson M, et al: An inventory for measuring depression. Arch Gen Psychiatry 4:561–571, 1961

Bozdogan H: Model selection and Akaike's information criterion (AIC): the general theory and its analytical extensions. Psychometrika 52:345–370, 1987

Bulik C, Sullivan P, Kendler K: An empirical study of the classification of eating disorders. Am J Psychiatry 157:886–895, 2000

Derogatis LR, Lipman RS, Rickels K, et al: The Hopkins Symptom Checklist (HSCL): a self-report symptom inventory. Behav Sci 19:1–15, 1974

Duncan A, Bucholz K, Neuman R, et al: Clustering of eating disorder symptoms in a general population female twin sample: a latent class analysis. Psychol Med 37:1097–1107, 2007

Eddy K, Crosby R, Keel P, et al: Empirical identification and validation of eating disorder phenotypes in a multisite clinical sample. J Nerv Ment Dis 197:41–49, 2009

Fairburn C: Cognitive Behavior Therapy and Eating Disorders. New York, Guilford, 2008

Fairburn C, Bohn K: Eating disorders NOS (EDNOS): an example of the troublesome "not otherwise specified" (NOS) category in DSM-IV. Behav Res Ther 43:691–701, 2005

Fichter MM, Quadflieg N: Comparing self- and expert rating: a self-report screening version (SIAB-S) of the Structured Interview for Anorexic and Bulimic Syndromes for DSM-IV and ICD-10 (SIAB-EX). Eur Arch Psychiatry Clin Neurosci 250:175–185, 2000

Fichter MM, Quadflieg N: Twelve-year course and outcome of bulimia nervosa. Psychol Med 34:1395–1406, 2004

Fichter MM, Elton M, Engel K, et al: Structured Interview for Anorexia and Bulimia Nervosa (SIAB): development of a new instrument for the assessment of eating disorders. Int J Eat Disord 10:571–592, 1991

Fichter MM, Quadflieg N, Hedlund S: Twelve-year course and outcome predictors of anorexia nervosa. Int J Eat Disord 39:87–100, 2006

Fichter MM, Quadflieg N, Hedlund S: Long-term course of binge eating disorder and bulimia nervosa: relevance for nosology and diagnostic criteria. Int J Eat Disord 41:577–586, 2008

Herzog DB, Keller MB, Lavori PW, et al: Short-term prospective study of recovery in bulimia nervosa. Psychiatry Res 23:45–55, 1988

Keel P, Fichter M, Quadflieg N, et al: Application of a latent class analysis to empirically define eating disorder phenotypes. Arch Gen Psychiatry 61:192–200, 2004

Lazarsfeld PF, Henry NW: Latent Structure Analysis. Boston, MA, Houghton Mifflin, 1968

Mitchell J, Crosby R, Wonderlich S, et al: Latent profile analysis of a cohort of patients with eating disorder not otherwise specified. Int J Eat Disord 40:S95–S98, 2007

Peterson CB, Crow SJ, Swanson S, et al: Longitudinal stability of empirically derived vs. DSM-IV classification of eating disorder symptoms. Presented at the Eating Disorders Research Society 15th annual meeting, Brooklyn, New York, October 2009

Rounsaville BJ, Alarcón RD, Andrews G, et al: Basic nomenclature issues for DSM-V, in A Research Agenda for DSM-V. Edited by Kupfer DJ, First MB, Regier DA. Washington, DC, American Psychiatric Association, 2002, pp 1–29

Sclove S: Application of model-selection criteria to some problems in multivariate analysis. Psychometrika 52:333–343, 1987

Striegel-Moore R, Franko D, Thompson D, et al: An empirical study of the typology of bulimia nervosa and its spectrum variants. Psychol Med 35:1563–1572, 2005

Sullivan P, Bulik C, Kendler K: The epidemiology and classification of bulimia nervosa. Psychol Med 28:599–610, 1998

Vermunt JK, Magidson J: Latent GOLD User's Guide. Belmont, MA, Statistical Innovations Inc, 2000

Wade T, Crosby R, Martin N: Use of latent profile analysis to identify eating disorder phenotypes in an adult Australian twin cohort. Arch Gen Psychiatry 63:1377–1384, 2006

Walsh BT, Sysko R: Broad categories for the diagnosis of eating disorders (BCD-ED): an alternative system for classification. Int J Eat Disord 42:754–764, 2009

Williamson DA, Womble LG, Smeets MA, et al: Latent structure of eating disorder symptoms: a factor-analytic and taxometric investigation. Am J Psychiatry 159:412–418, 2002

Wonderlich S, Crosby R, Mitchell J, et al: Testing the validity of eating disorder diagnoses. Int J Eat Disord 40:S40–S45, 2007a

Wonderlich S, Joiner T, Keel P, et al: Eating disorder diagnoses: empirical approaches to classification. Am Psychol 62:167–180, 2007b

Yang C: Evaluating latent class analyses in qualitative phenotype identification. Comput Stat Data Anal 50:1090–1104, 2006

11

LATENT STRUCTURE OF BULIMIC SYNDROMES

An Empirical Approach Utilizing Latent Profile Analyses and Taxometric Analyses

Pamela K. Keel, Ph.D.

Jill Holm-Denoma, Ph.D.

Ross D. Crosby, Ph.D.

Alissa A. Haedt, M.A.

Julie A. Gravener, M.A.

Thomas E. Joiner, Ph.D.

A key challenge facing the DSM-5 Eating Disorders Work Group is the need to "drain the swamp" that is the eating disorder not otherwise specified (EDNOS)

We would like to acknowledge the contributions of Drs. William Grove, John Ruscio, Tony Richey, and Kiara Timpano in the application and interpretation of taxometric analyses presented in this manuscript.

This work was supported by grants from the National Institute of Mental Health (R03 MH61320; R01 MH61836; R01 MH63758; PI: Pamela K. Keel). Portions of this work were presented at the 13th Annual Meeting of the Eating Disorders Research Society in Pittsburgh, PA and at a National Institute of Mental Health-sponsored meeting on classification of eating disorders in Washington, DC.

category, which currently contains any clinically significant disorder of eating that does not meet DSM-IV (American Psychiatric Association 1994) criteria for anorexia nervosa (AN) or bulimia nervosa (BN). Among the clinical presentations included in EDNOS are conditions that represent subthreshold versions of full-threshold disorders (e.g., all criteria met for BN except that the frequency of binge eating episodes and compensatory behaviors is less than twice/week). In addition, there are partial syndromes in which a key symptom required for a diagnosis is absent. For example, binge eating disorder (BED) resembles BN, with the exception that binge eating is not associated with the regular use of inappropriate compensatory behaviors. Similarly, purging disorder resembles BN, except that purging is not associated with binge eating episodes. In some circumstances, subthreshold EDNOS may reflect syndromes that differ only in severity from full-threshold syndromes. However, this is not clearly the case for partial EDNOS, because partial syndromes may include behavioral frequencies that exceed those required for a diagnosis. For example, an individual with purging disorder may endorse purging multiple times per day over years of her life, whereas an individual with BN may endorse binge eating and purging twice a week over the past 3 months. In such instances, it would be difficult to view the partial-syndrome EDNOS as a less severe variant of the full threshold disorder. Understanding whether partial-syndrome EDNOS that resemble BN represent variations on a dimension of severity or categorically distinct entities is crucial for understanding whether DSM-5 should add new categories or expand existing categories (so-called broad categories) to drain the EDNOS swamp.

Among various approaches used to examine the validity of alternative proposals for redefining eating disorders, latent class analysis (LCA), latent profile analysis (LPA), and taxometric analysis (TA) have been described as particularly useful for developing empirically based classifications (Wonderlich et al. 2007). These analytic approaches appear especially warranted for understanding the latent structure of bulimic syndromes, for which a single diagnosis or multiple diagnoses may be considered for the DSM-5.

Analytic Approaches to Determining Validity of Classification

LATENT CLASS AND LATENT PROFILE ANALYSES

Briefly, LCA and LPA examine associations among indicators to create homogeneous groups. Although a strength of LCA and LPA is their ability to determine the optimal number and composition of homogeneous groups, a noted weakness is a tendency to create spurious classes that represent different points along a continuum of severity (Uebersax 1999). Thus, differences in severity within one true category can create associations among observed symptoms/signs and produce additional classes that are not qualitatively distinct. This tendency may contribute to inconsistent results across LCA/LPA studies. Given mounting evidence that several mental disorders once thought to represent "true categories" may be better viewed as dimensions (Widiger and Samuel 2005), it is particularly important to evaluate whether thresholds for group membership identified in LCA and LPA actually represent boundaries between categorically distinct entities. If not, a single bulimic diagnosis may be warranted in which dimensional ratings of symptom frequencies are used to capture variation in illness severity.

TAXOMETRIC ANALYSIS

Briefly, TA examines associations among indicators to determine whether a true category (taxon) exists. A strength of TA is the ability to discriminate taxonic versus non-taxonic relationships for a superficially distinct condition. However, weaknesses are that TA tests for the presence of only one taxon at a time and requires the supposition of known groups for which indicators can be chosen to reveal the nature of associations in those groups. Thus, previous TA studies have relied on tests of syndromes as defined within DSM-IV rather than testing alternative, novel groups. Additionally, TA cannot render meaningful interpretations if multiple taxa are represented within the sample studied.

Current Study Methods

Given the distinct strengths and weaknesses of different statistical approaches, the current study used both LPA and TA to examine the latent structure of bulimic syndrome(s). Eating disorder symptoms were included in LPAs to empirically define groups. Resulting groups were then included in a series of TAs to determine whether latent groups represented true categories or profiles along a continuum of disordered eating. An advance over previous studies was the inclusion of large numbers of individuals who met DSM-IV criteria for BN (both purging and nonpurging subtypes) or BED; those who met research criteria for purging disorder (Keel et al. 2005, 2007); and individuals who reported an array of disordered eating features as well as those reporting no disordered eating. This enabled examination of potential distinctions between normality and bulimic syndrome(s) as well as potential distinctions among bulimic syndromes characterized by binge eating, purging, nonpurging compensatory behaviors, and various potential combinations of these features. Results of this examination are crucial for understanding whether cases currently residing in the EDNOS category can be best addressed by adding new categories to DSM-5 or by expanding thresholds for existing diagnoses within DSM-IV.

PARTICIPANTS

Participants (N=528; 4.7% male) were recruited from the community for studies of BN and related EDNOS conducted in the first author's (P.K.K.'s) lab between 1998 and 2007. These studies included assessment by the Structured Clinical Interview for DSM-IV Axis I Disorders (SCID-I; First et al. 1995), which was modified to omit skip rules in the eating disorders module (e.g., participants were asked about self-induced vomiting regardless of whether they endorsed binge eating). Mean age was 26.2 years, with a standard deviation of 7.3 years. Most participants (77.7%) were Caucasian, non-Hispanic; 9.7% were Asian, 5.9% were African American, 5.1% were Hispanic, and 1.7% were "other/mixed" or did not provide information on race/ethnicity.

PROCEDURES AND MEASURES

All participants completed written informed consent prior to participation, and procedures were approved by the Institutional Review Boards of Harvard University and the University of Iowa. The SCID-I was used to assess demographic information, treatment history, abuse history, current and lifetime mood, anxiety, substance use, eating, and impulse control disorders. Interrater reliability was good, ranging from κ=0.69 to κ=0.94 across disorders.

Based on SCID-I interviews, 137 participants (25.9%) had no lifetime history of an eating disorder, 70 (13%) had lifetime diagnoses of DSM-IV AN (62 with the binge-purge subtype); 168 (32%) had DSM-IV BN, purging subtype; 44 (8.3%) had DSM-IV BN, nonpurging subtype; 85 (16.1%) had DSM-IV BED; 59 (11.2%) had purging disorder (defined by purging through the use of self-induced vomiting, laxative use, or diuretic abuse at least twice per week, on average, over the previous 3 months; the absence of objectively large binge episodes; and the presence of undue influence of weight/shape on self-evaluation); and 24 (4.5%) had a nonpurging compensatory eating disorder defined by the use of excessive exercise or fasting at least twice per week, on average, over the previous 3 months, the absence of objectively large binge episodes, and the presence of undue influence of weight/shape on self-evaluation. These percentages exceed 100% because individuals could have more than one lifetime eating disorder diagnosis. For example, 38 participants (23%) with BN, purging subtype also had a lifetime history of AN.

ANALYSES

LPA was used to empirically define homogeneous groups of participants based on symptom profiles. The following symptoms of BN and AN were included in analyses: history of binge eating, compensatory behaviors, low weight, body image disturbance, and amenorrhea. Additional features of BED (e.g., binge eating episodes are associated with "eating alone because of being embarrassed by how much one is eating") were not included because they are conditionally dependent upon the presence of binge eating. In addition to these lifetime features, current body mass index was included. Height and weight were objectively measured in 336 participants (64%) and self-reported in 192 participants (36%). Numerous studies support the test-retest reliability and concurrent validity of self-reported height and weight with objectively measured height and weight in both clinical and nonclinical samples (Keel et al. 1999; Spencer et al. 2002; Stunkard and Albaum 1981). Features and coding ranges included in LPA are listed in the left-most column of Table 11–1. Analyses were conducted in LatentGOLD 3.0.6 (Statistical Innovations Inc. 2003) using the option of including cases with missing values. Unlike LCA, LPA does not produce a χ^2 test of fit. The optimal number of latent groups was based on the solution with the lowest Bayesian information criteria (BIC) because information-theoretic criteria are appropriate for model selection when comparing non-nested models (Markon and Krueger 2005).

Validation analyses were conducted to compare groups identified by LPA on demographic variables, Axis I disorders, clinical features, and treatment history, representing 16 independent comparisons made among groups. A Bonferroni-corrected P value of 0.0031 was used to control for family-wise error rate. When the omnibus test for a variable reached significance at $P<0.0031$, post hoc comparisons among groups were Bonferroni adjusted for the 10 possible pairwise comparisons to $P<0.005$.

Taxometric analyses were conducted with a suite of programs written in the R language (Ruscio 2008) to evaluate whether groups resulting from LPA represented categorically distinct entities or different loci on a continuum of disordered eating. For each pairwise comparison of latent groups identified with LPA, indicators were deemed suitable if they showed validities of 1.25 or greater and resulted in nuisance correlations less than 0.30 (Meehl 1995). Plots of observed data were coded independently by two raters ($\kappa=0.74$) with extensive training as taxonic, dimensional, or ambiguous. When raters disagreed, a third independent rater reviewed plots, and final ratings were based on the most common interpretation. A set of analyses was considered to indicate the presence of a taxon if they satisfied the following requirements: a) the ratio of independently rated taxonic to dimensional plots was greater than 1:1, and b) the comparison curve fit index (CCFI) was greater than 0.60. Analyses were considered to indicate dimensionality if a) the ratio of independently rated taxonic to dimensional plots was 1:1 or greater, and b) the CCFI was less than 0.40 (Beauchaine 2007; Ruscio 2007; Schmidt et al. 2005).

TABLE 11–1. Levels and distributions of eating disorder symptoms across latent groups (LGs) ($N=528$)

Symptom	LG1 ($n=135$), %	LG2 ($n=131$), %	LG3 ($n=110$), %	LG4 ($n=107$), %	LG5 ($n=45$), %
Binge eating					
0—None	96	0	19	7	2
1—Subthreshold loss of control	2	0	1	1	0
2—Loss of control/not large amount of food (SBEs), subthreshold frequency	3	0	7	8	0
3—SBEs, threshold (two or more times per week) frequency	0	12	10	21	0
4—Loss of control/large amount of food (OBEs), subthreshold frequency	0	3	21	7	9
5—OBEs, threshold (two or more times per week) frequency	0	85	41	58	89
Mean (SD)	0.1 (0.4)	4.7 (0.7)	3.4 (1.9)	3.9 (1.5)	4.8 (0.8)

TABLE 11–1. Levels and distributions of eating disorder symptoms across latent groups (LGs) (*N*=528) *(continued)*

Symptom	LG1 (*n*=135), %	LG2 (*n*=131), %	LG3 (*n*=110), %	LG4 (*n*=107), %	LG5 (*n*=45), %
Compensatory behaviors					
0—None	100	0	34	5	47
1—Nonpurging (e.g., fasting), subthreshold frequency	0	0	12	3	7
2—Nonpurging, threshold (two or more times per week frequency	0	13	17	12	19
3—Purging (e.g., vomiting), subthreshold frequency	0	2	11	7	7
4—Purging, threshold (two or more times per week) frequency	0	85	25	72	21
Mean (SD)	0 (0)	3.7 (0.7)	1.8 (1.6)	3.4 (1.1)	1.5 (1.6)
Refusal to maintain weight at minimally normal EBW					
0—None	93	81	85	9	87
1—Subthreshold (85% EBW < weight < 90% EBW)	6	8	10	18	7
2—Threshold (weight <85% EBW)	2	12	5	74	7
Mean (SD)	0.1 (0.3)	0.3 (0.7)	0.2 (0.5)	1.7 (0.6)	0.2 (0.5)

TABLE 11–1. Levels and distributions of eating disorder symptoms across latent groups (LGs) (*N*=528) *(continued)*

Symptom	LG1 (n=135), %	LG2 (n=131), %	LG3 (n=110), %	LG4 (n=107), %	LG5 (n=45), %
Body image disturbance					
0—No body image disturbance	84	0	11	0	3
1	3	0	1	0	0
2	13	0	65	3	9
3	0	2	11	2	0
4—Threshold fear of gaining weight and undue influence of weight/shape on self-evaluation	0	98	12	95	88
Mean (SD)	0.3 (0.7)	4.0 (0.1)	2.1 (1.0)	3.9 (0.4)	3.7 (0.9)
Amenorrhea					
0—None (0)	82	48	79	23	60
1—Subthreshold (no menstruation for less than 3 consecutive months)	7	3	9	8	0
2—Threshold (no menstruation for 3 or more consecutive months)	11	49	12	70	40
Mean (SD)	0.3 (0.6)	1.0 (1.0)	0.3 (0.7)	1.5 (0.8)	0.8 (1.0)
Current BMI (kg/m²), mean (SD)	22.2 (2.1)	23.5 (1.7)	22.5 (2.3)	20.6 (1.3)	37.4 (7.3)

Note. BMI = body mass index; EBW = expected body weight; OBE = objective bulimic episode; SBE = subjective bulimic episode.

Results

LATENT PROFILE ANALYSES

A single latent group solution provided a poor fit to data (log-likelihood [LL] = −4,180.99; BIC = 8,481.09) relative to solutions with additional groups, which improved model fit up to a five-group solution. The five-group solution reliably produced the lowest BIC value (LL = −3,450.40; BIC = 7,220.53; improvement in fit from four-group model: ΔBIC = 2.37; odds of the five-group model producing a better fit than the four-group model were 11:1) (Raftery 1995). Table 11–2 presents levels and distributions of eating disorder features across the latent groups.

LATENT GROUPS AND DSM-IV EATING DISORDERS

Significant associations between eating disorder diagnoses and latent group membership were found for lifetime DSM-IV AN ($\chi^2_8 = 281.92$; $P < 0.001$); BN, purging type ($\chi^2_8 = 195.18$; $P < 0.001$); BN, nonpurging type ($\chi^2_8 = 47.64$; $P < 0.001$); and BED ($\chi^2_8 = 189.51$; $P < 0.001$), and study diagnoses of purging disorder ($\chi^2_8 = 56.88$; $P < 0.001$) and compensatory eating disorder ($\chi^2_4 = 53.14$; $P < 0.001$). Figure 11–1 presents the distribution of lifetime eating disorder diagnoses across latent groups.

LPA supported a basic distinction between presence versus absence of eating disorders because the majority (95%) of individuals with no lifetime history of eating disorders were members of LG1 (see Figure 11–1). In support of the distinctions between the DSM-IV categories of AN and BN, most cases of AN occurred in LG4, whereas most cases of BN occurred in LG2. Cases of BED were most commonly observed in LG5. Cases of purging disorder were most commonly observed in LG4. Finally, cases of compensatory eating disorder were most commonly observed in LG3. However, the latter was the least frequent eating disorder and accounted for only 17% of cases in LG3. Whereas LG2, LG4, and LG5 were characterized by symptoms that defined the most common diagnosis in each group and high levels of body image disturbance, LG3 was characterized by a mix of behavioral features and moderate levels of body image disturbance (see Table 11–1). Specifically, 88%–98% of individuals in LG2, LG4, and LG5 endorsed both the undue influence of weight/shape on self-evaluation and an intense fear of gaining weight or becoming fat (weight phobia), whereas 65% of individuals in LG3 endorsed undue influence but denied weight phobia. We therefore provide the following descriptors to facilitate interpretation of validation analyses: LG1 = "healthy"; LG2 = "BN"; LG3 = an eating disorder with no weight phobia; LG4 = "AN"; LG5 = "BED."

TABLE 11–2. Validation analyses of latent groups (LGs) ($N=528$)

Axis I disorders	LG1 ($N=135$), n (%)	LG2 ($N=131$), n (%)	LG3 ($N=110$), n (%)	LG4 ($N=107$), n (%)	LG5 ($N=45$), n (%)	χ^2_4
Lifetime						
Mood	32 (24)[a]	98 (75)[b]	55 (51)[c]	83 (80)[b]	37 (84)[b]	112.96**
Anxiety	15 (11)[a]	53 (41)[b,c]	35 (33)[b]	46 (44)[b,c]	27 (63)[c]	52.81**
Substance use	20 (15)[a]	65 (50)[b]	28 (26)[a,c]	43 (42)[b,c]	25 (57)[b]	49.83**
Impulse-control	6 (5)[a]	39 (30)[b,c]	17 (16)[b]	36 (35)[c]	19 (43)[c]	49.96**
Current						
Mood	2 (2)[a]	39 (30)[b]	13 (12)[c]	25 (24)[b,c]	8 (19)[b,c]	43.63**
Anxiety	8 (6)[a]	35 (27)[b]	23 (21)[b]	33 (32)[b]	19 (44)[b]	37.81**
Substance use	0 (0)[a]	10 (8)[b]	3 (3)[a,b]	11 (11)[b]	0 (0)[a,b]	20.16**
Impulse-control	3 (2)[a]	24 (18)[b]	13 (12)[b]	21 (20)[b]	11 (25)[b]	25.00**
Clinical features						
Suicidality in mood episode[†]	18 (58)	28 (42)	25 (56)	17 (29)	9 (30)	12.67
Physical or sexual abuse/ assault	11 (8)[a]	33 (25)[b,c]	13 (12)[a,c]	19 (18)[a,c]	13 (29)[b,c]	20.20**
Global Assessment of Functioning score, mean (SE)	81.1 (0.8)[a]	58.1 (0.8)[b]	67.0 (1.0)[c]	57.2 (1.1)[b]	57.0 (1.7)[b]	$F_{4,485}=$ 120.10**

TABLE 11–2. Validation analyses of latent groups (LGs) (*N*=528) *(continued)*

Axis I disorders	LG1 (*N*=135), *n* (%)	LG2 (*N*=131), *n* (%)	LG3 (*N*=110), *n* (%)	LG4 (*N*=107), *n* (%)	LG5 (*N*=45), *n* (%)	χ^2_4
Treatment history						
Current treatment	2 (1)[a]	32 (25)[b,c]	19 (17)[b]	39 (37)[c]	15 (34)[b,c]	54.50**
Lifetime treatment	39 (29)[a]	102 (78)[b,c]	72 (65)[b]	97 (91)[c]	40 (89)[c]	131.10**
Hospitalization	0 (0)[a]	17 (13)[b,c]	4 (4)[a,c]	38 (36)[d]	11 (24)[b,d]	80.48**
Psychotropic medication use	3 (2)[a]	27 (21)[b,c]	12 (11)[b]	25 (24)[b,c]	18 (40)[c]	46.77**

Note. Lettered superscripts that differ represent significant differences between groups using a Bonferroni-corrected *P* value (*P*<0.005).
Race was self-reported by participants using categories presented by researchers for the purpose of tracking enrollment of racial and ethnic minorities for
National Institutes of Health–funded studies. http://grants.nih.gov/grants/funding/phs398/enrollmentreport.doc.
*P<0.0029; **P<0.001.
†Percentages are taken from among those with a lifetime history of a mood disorder (LG1, *n*=31; LG2, *n*=66; LG3, *n*=45; LG4, *n*=59; LG5, *n*=30).

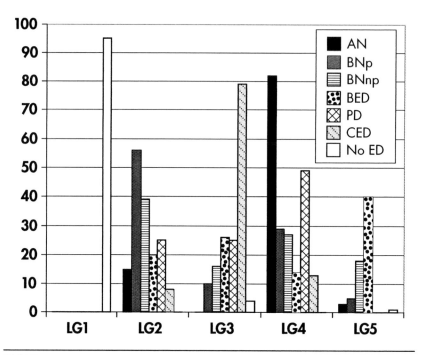

FIGURE 11–1.   Distribution of lifetime eating disorder diagnoses across latent groups (LGs).

AN = anorexia nervosa; BED = binge eating disorder; BNnp = bulimia nervosa, nonpurging subtype; BNp = bulimia nervosa, purging subtype; CED = nonpurging compensatory eating disorder; ED = eating disorder; PD = purging disorder.

VALIDATION ANALYSES

Table 11–2 presents results from validation analyses of Axis I disorders, clinical features, and treatment history. Significant differences were found for all Axis I disorders. The healthy group had lower lifetime prevalence for all Axis I disorders compared with the eating disorder groups, with the exception of not differing significantly on substance use disorders from the eating disorder group with no weight phobia. Similarly, the non-weight-phobic group reported lower lifetime prevalence of anxiety disorders compared with the BED group, lower prevalence of substance use disorders compared with the BN and BED groups, and lower prevalence of impulse-control disorders compared with the AN and BED groups. The AN, BN, and BED groups did not differ significantly on any lifetime Axis I disorder.

The healthy group reported fewer current comorbid Axis I disorders compared with the eating disorder groups, with the exception of not differing significantly on substance use disorders from the non-weight-phobic and BED groups. The eating disorder group with no weight phobia reported lower current prevalence of mood disorders compared with the AN, BN, and BED groups.

Significant differences were found for history of physical or sexual abuse/assault and interview-rated Global Assessment of Functioning (GAF) score. Both the BN and BED groups reported greater histories of abuse/assault compared with the healthy group, suggesting an association between traumatic history and disorders characterized by objectively large binge episodes. The AN, BN, and BED groups reported worse GAF scores compared with the non-weight-phobic and healthy groups, who also differed significantly from each other. Mean GAF scores were comparable among the AN, BN, and BED groups (range, 57.0–58.1), suggesting that these groups were characterized by similar illness severity and functional impairment.

The healthy group reported less treatment utilization compared with the eating disorder groups for almost all forms of treatment (rates of hospitalization for a mental disorder did not differ significantly between the healthy and non-weight-phobic groups). Compared with the group with eating disorders with no weight phobia, the AN group was more likely to be in current treatment; the AN and BED groups were more likely to have received some form of mental health treatment and to have been hospitalized during their lifetime; and the BED group was more likely to have been treated with psychotropic medicines. The AN group was more likely to have been hospitalized compared with the BN group.

TAXOMETRIC ANALYSES

Table 11–3 outlines indicators and taxometric methods used for each set of pairwise comparisons, CCFIs, rating of plots, and our final interpretation of the relationship (i.e., taxonic, dimensional, or ambiguous) between each pair of latent groups. Analyses generated 42 individual plots and 17 composite plots. For descriptive purposes, Figure 11–2 presents composite plots resulting in a taxonic interpretation (LG1 vs. LG4) and composite plots not resulting in a taxonic interpretation (LG2 vs. LG4).

Comparisons between the healthy group (LG1) and each of the eating disorder groups (LG2–LG5) supported that the eating disorder groups were categorically distinct from normality. Of note, the maximum eigenvalue (MAXEIG) CCFI value for comparing the healthy group with the BED group was below the suggested threshold for establishing taxonicity. However, resulting plots strongly supported taxonicity, as did findings using latent mode analysis, replicating previous findings comparing healthy and BED groups (Williamson et al. 2002).

The BN group presented some analytic difficulties. First, for all comparisons with other eating disorder groups, only two indicators were suitable for inclusion in TAs, restricting the methods that could be used. Second, results from mean above minus below a cut (MAMBAC) were inconsistent: CCFI for comparisons between BN and AN and between BN and BED supported a taxonic interpretation;

TABLE 11–3. Taxometric comparisons across latent groups

Latent groups[a]	Indicators	Suitable methods	CCFI	Plot ratings	Final interpretation
1 vs. 2	Binge eating Body image disturbance Compensatory behaviors	MAXEIG	0.683	3 of 3 taxonic	Taxonic
1 vs. 3	Binge eating Body image disturbance Compensatory behaviors	MAXEIG MAMBAC	0.601 0.684	3 of 3 taxonic 5 of 6 taxonic (1 dimensional)	Taxonic
1 vs. 4	Binge eating Body image disturbance Compensatory behaviors Refusal to maintain weight Amenorrhea	MAXEIG	0.721	5 of 5 taxonic	Taxonic
1 vs. 5	Binge eating Body image disturbance Compensatory behaviors BMI	MAXEIG L-Mode	0.512 0.764	3 of 4 taxonic (1 ambiguous) 1 of 1 taxonic	Likely taxonic
2 vs. 3	Body image disturbance Compensatory Behaviors	MAMBAC	0.536	1 of 2 taxonic (1 ambiguous)	Ambiguous

TABLE 11–3. Taxometric comparisons across latent groups *(continued)*

Latent groups[a]	Indicators	Suitable methods	CCFI	Plot ratings	Final interpretation
2 vs. 4	Refusal to maintain weight BMI	MAMBAC	0.606	0 of 2 taxonic (1 dimensional; 1 ambiguous)	Ambiguous
2 vs. 5	Compensatory behaviors BMI	MAMBAC	0.630	0 of 2 taxonic (2 ambiguous)	Ambiguous
3 vs. 4	Body image disturbance Refusal to maintain weight Amenorrhea	MAXEIG	0.598	2 of 3 taxonic	Likely taxonic
3 vs. 5	Body image disturbance BMI	MAMBAC	0.733	2 of 2 taxonic	Taxonic
4 vs. 5	Compensatory behaviors Refusal to maintain weight BMI	MAXEIG MAMBAC	0.520 0.748	2 of 3 taxonic (1 ambiguous) 4 of 6 taxonic (1 dimensional; 1 ambiguous)	Likely taxonic

Note. BMI = body mass index; CCFI = comparison curve fit index; L-Mode = latent mode analysis; MAMBAC = mean above minus below a cut; MAXEIG = maximum eigenvalue.

[a]1 = healthy; 2 = bulimia nervosa; 3 = mixed; 4 = anorexia nervosa; 5 = binge eating disorder.

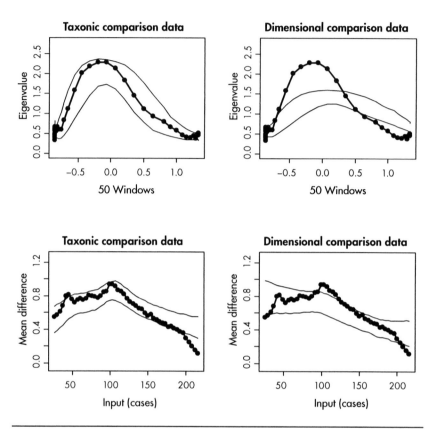

FIGURE 11–2. Composite plots for a comparison resulting in taxonic interpretation (latent group [LG]1 vs. LG4 using maximum eigenvalue, *top graphs*) and not resulting in taxonic interpretation (LG2 vs. LG4 using mean above minus below a cut, *bottom graphs*).

however, plots were rated as ambiguous. For comparison between the BN and non-weight-phobic groups, one MAMBAC plot supported taxonicity, but the CCFI fell within the ambiguous range.

The non-weight-phobic group appeared to have a taxonic relationship with the AN and BED groups. These results, when combined with the taxonic results of the healthy and non-weight-phobic groups, suggest that members of the latter group are qualitatively different from those without eating disorders and from those with eating disorders defined by the presence of weight phobia.

Finally, the relationship between the AN and BED groups appeared to be taxonic. The MAXEIG CCFI fell below the threshold for taxonicity; however, the MAMBAC CCFI and resulting plots from both methods supported a taxonic interpretation.

Discussion

The purpose of this study was to examine whether bulimic syndromes are best con-ceptualized as distinct categories or whether there is only one true bulimic disorder category. Results indicate that bulimic syndromes can be validly conceptualized as categorically distinct entities. Validation analyses indicated that the latent groups differed on comorbid disorders, abuse history, and treatment history. In several of these analyses, the eating disorder group with no weight phobia (LG3) had inter-mediate values between those reported for the healthy group (LG1) and the other eating disorder groups (LG2, LG4, and LG5), suggesting that this group could represent a midpoint on a continuum from being healthy to having an eating dis-order. However, TA indicated that the non-weight-phobic group was categorically distinct from both the healthy group and the other eating disorder groups, arguing against a dimensional interpretation. The single indicator that distinguished this latent group from the other eating disorder groups was level of body image distur-bance. Two previous LCA/LPA studies (Eddy et al. 2009; Keel et al. 2004) have produced latent groups characterized by lower body image disturbance. Given that body image disturbance is often measured as a continuous variable, these differ-ences have been interpreted as potentially reflecting spurious classifications that re-flect variation in illness severity within one true category. However, this is the first latent structure study to suggest body image disturbance may distinguish categor-ically distinct disorders of eating. Findings dovetail with recent results from a meta-analysis suggesting that AN without weight phobia may be qualitatively distinct from AN with weight phobia (Thomas et al. 2009).

Validation analyses for the LPA further suggested that it would be difficult to place the remaining latent eating disorder groups (LG2, LG4, and LG5) on a continuum of severity. Specifically, GAF scores were virtually indistinguishable among these three groups. Furthermore, depending upon the variable under consideration, the BN group (LG2), AN group (LG4), or BED group (LG5) appeared to be "most severe," implying that these latent groups may differ qualitatively rather than quantitatively. This interpretation was partially supported by TA. Specifically, comparisons of the AN and BED groups suggested a qualitative distinction, which represents a novel finding. Unfortunately, the latent eating disorder groups often differed on a small set of indicators, which restricted our ability to use TA for com-parisons with the BN group.

Replicating results from previous latent class (Eddy et al. 2009; Mitchell et al. 2007; Pinheiro et al. 2008; Striegel-Moore et al. 2005; Sullivan et al. 1998) and taxo-metric (Williamson et al. 2002) studies, BED emerged as a qualitatively distinct la-tent group, supporting its inclusion as an eating disorder category in DSM-5. The BED group was characterized by recurrent binge eating, obesity, and body image disturbance. Of these features, only one, recurrent binge eating, is included in the DSM-IV provisional criteria. Additional features proposed for a diagnosis of BED in DSM-IV (e.g., eating alone because of being embarrassed by the amount of food consumed) have demonstrated poor predictive value for making a diagnosis (Spitzer et al. 1993). Thus, it would be beneficial to include features that would add to the validity of the diagnosis. Based on our findings, body image disturbance could be included as a cognitive feature of BED, potentially as a diagnostic specifier (Grilo et al. 2008). Body image disturbance has reliably distinguished between obese individuals with and without BED (Devlin et al. 2003). Although results suggest that obesity was a defining feature of LG5, adding this as a sign of BED would be problematic for defining recovery. Several treatment studies have demonstrated that individuals with BED can make meaningful improvements in achieving symptom remission without achieving substantial weight loss (Wilson et al. 2007). If obesity were included in the definition of BED, such individuals might not be considered in remission, despite being indistinguishable from obese individuals with no eating disorder diagnosis.

Most cases of purging disorder were grouped in LG4 with AN. Conversely, most cases of compensatory eating disorder were found in LG3, which demonstrated a taxonic relationship to LG4. These results support recent findings suggesting that expanding the definition of purging disorder to include nonpurging inappropriate compensatory behaviors increases the heterogeneity and decreases its clinical significance (Haedt and Keel 2010). Purging disorder did not emerge as a distinct latent group, consistent with results from other studies in which BN and purging disorder fell into separate latent groups but the latter sorted with other syndromes characterized by purging, most notably AN (Eddy et al. 2009; Keel et al. 2004). Given similarities between them, almost all previous studies have sought to test the distinctiveness of purging disorder from BN (Binford and le Grange 2005; Keel et al. 2005, 2007; Wade 2007). However, our findings emphasize the need for more studies examining the distinctiveness of purging disorder from AN.

The current study's strengths include its large sample size, diversity of eating disorder presentations and severity, structured clinical interview assessments with high interrater reliability, and range of external validators. Despite these strengths, the study had certain weaknesses. First, we had a small number of compensatory eating disorder patients, and this may have limited our ability to detect whether this emerged as a distinct latent group. Second, coding of eating disorder features to produce independent indicators with adequate sensitivity for TA required combining some features as different levels in a single indicator (e.g., weight phobia and undue influence within a single body image disturbance indicator). These combinations reduced the number of indicators that could be included in TA. Finally, this study did not include an adequate number of individuals with restricting AN to address its relation to bulimic syndromes or normality.

Previous work (Williamson et al. 2002) posited the presence of only one taxonic feature, binge eating, that distinguished eating disorders from normality, suggesting that various bulimic syndromes may reside within a single category.

Our results provide convincing evidence that body image disturbance, compensatory behaviors, and body weight represent additional features that add to the qualitative distinctiveness of eating disorder syndromes. This has important implications for reconceptualizing EDNOS. Our analyses provide reasonably strong support for the validity of BED as being distinct from normality and related bulimic syndromes. However, more work is needed to understand syndromes characterized by purging and nonpurging compensatory behaviors in the absence of binge eating episodes. Beyond the immediate concerns of developing more informative diagnoses for DSM-5, identifying valid distinctions among eating disorder syndromes is central to answering questions related to their causes, consequences, treatment, and prevention.

References

American Psychiatric Association: Diagnostic and Statistical Manual of Mental Disorders, 4th Edition. Washington, DC, American Psychiatric Association, 1994

Beauchaine TP: A brief taxometrics primer. J Child Clin Adolesc Psychol 36:654–676, 2007

Binford RB, le Grange D: Adolescents with bulimia nervosa and eating disorder not otherwise specified–purging only. Int J Eat Disord 38:157–161, 2005

Devlin MJ, Goldfein JA, Dobrow I: What is this thing called BED? Current status of binge eating disorder nosology. Int J Eat Disord 34(suppl):S2–S18, 2003

Eddy KT, Crosby RD, Keel PK, et al: Application of latent profile analysis to empirically identify eating disorder phenotypes in a clinical sample. J Nerv Ment Dis 197:41–49, 2009

First M, Spitzer RL, Gibbon M, et al: Structured Clinical Interview for DSM-IV Axis I Disorders—Patient Edition (SCID/P). New York, Biometrics Research Department, New York State Psychiatric Institute, 1995

Grilo CM, Hrabosky JI, White MA, et al: Overvaluation of weight and shape in binge eating disorder and overweight controls: refinement of a diagnostic construct. J Abnorm Psychol 117:414–419, 2008

Haedt AA, Keel PK: Comparing definitions of purging disorder on point prevalence and associations with external validators. Int J Eat Disord 43:433–439, 2010

Keel PK, Mitchell JE, Miller KB, et al: Long-term outcome of bulimia nervosa. Arch Gen Psychiatry 56:63–69, 1999

Keel PK, Fichter M, Quadflieg N, et al: Application of a latent class analysis to empirically define eating disorder phenotypes. Arch Gen Psychiatry 61:192–200, 2004

Keel PK, Haedt A, Edler C: Purging disorder: an ominous variant of bulimia nervosa? Int J Eat Disord 38:191–199, 2005

Keel PK, Wolfe BE, Liddle RA, et al: Clinical features and physiological response to a test meal in purging disorder and bulimia nervosa. Arch Gen Psychiatry 64:1058–1066, 2007

Markon KE, Krueger RF: Categorical and continuous models of liability to externalizing disorders: a direct comparison in NESARC. Arch Gen Psychiatry 62:1352–1359, 2005

Meehl PE: Bootstraps taxometrics: solving the classification problem in psychopathology. Am Psychol 50:266–275, 1995

Mitchell JE, Crosby RD, Wonderlich SA, et al: Latent profile analysis of a cohort of patients with eating disorders not otherwise specified. Int J Eat Disord 40:S95–S98, 2007

Pinheiro AP, Bulik CM, Sullivan PF, et al: An empirical study of the typology of bulimic symptoms in young Portuguese women. Int J Eat Disord 41:251–258, 2008

Raftery AE: Bayesian model selection in social research (with discussion). Sociol Methodol 25:111–195, 1995

Ruscio J: Taxometric analysis: an empirically grounded approach to implementing the method. Crim Justice Behav 34:1588–1622, 2007

Ruscio J: Taxometric Programs for the R Computing Environment: User's Manual. Ewing, NJ, College of New Jersey, 2008

Schmidt NB, Kotov R, Joiner TE Jr: Taxometrics: Toward a New Diagnostic Scheme for Psychopathology. Washington, DC, American Psychological Association, 2005

Spencer EA, Appleby PN, Davey GK, et al: Validity of self-reported height and weight in 4808 EPIC-Oxford participants. Public Health Nutr 5:561–565, 2002

Spitzer RL, Yanovski S, Wadden T, et al: Binge eating disorder: its further validation in a multisite study. Int J Eat Disord 13:137–153, 1993

Statistical Innovations Inc: LatentGOLD Version 3.0.6 (computer program). Belmont, MA, Statistical Innovations Inc, 2003

Striegel-Moore RH, Franko DL, Thompson D, et al: An empirical study of the typology of bulimia nervosa and its spectrum variants. Psychol Med 35:1563–1572, 2005

Stunkard AJ, Albaum JM: The accuracy of self-reported weights. Am J Clin Nutr 34:1593–1599, 1981

Sullivan PF, Bulik CM, Kendler KS: The epidemiology and classification of bulimia nervosa. Psychol Med 28:599–610, 1998

Thomas JJ, Vartanian LR, Brownell KD: The relationship between eating disorder not otherwise specified (EDNOS) and officially recognized eating disorders: meta-analysis and implications for DSM. Psychol Bull 135:407–433, 2009

Uebersax JS: Probit latent class analysis with dichotomous or ordered category measures: conditional independence/dependence models. Appl Psychol Meas 23:283–297, 1999

Wade TD: A retrospective comparison of purging type disorders: eating disorder not otherwise specified and bulimia nervosa. Int J Eat Disord 40:1–6, 2007

Widiger TA, Samuel DB: Diagnostic categories or dimensions? A question for the Diagnostic and Statistical Manual of Mental Disorders—fifth edition. J Abnorm Psychol 114:494–504, 2005

Williamson DA, Womble LG, Smeets MA, et al: Latent structure of eating disorder symptoms: a factor analytic and taxometric investigation. Am J Psychiatry 159:412–418, 2002

Wilson GT, Grilo CM, Vitousek KM: Psychological treatment of eating disorders. Am Psychol 62:199–216, 2007

Wonderlich SA, Joiner TE Jr, Keel PK, et al: Eating disorder diagnoses: empirical approaches to classification. Am Psychol 62:167–180, 2007

PART 3

EATING AND FEEDING DISORDERS IN CHILDHOOD AND ADOLESCENCE

12

CLASSIFICATION OF EATING DISTURBANCE IN CHILDREN AND ADOLESCENTS

Proposed Changes for DSM-5

Workgroup for Classification of Eating Disorders in Children and Adolescents (WCEDCA)

Terrill D. Bravender, M.D., M.P.H.
Rachel Bryant-Waugh, M.Sc., D.Phil.
David B. Herzog, M.D.
Debra Katzman, M.D., FRCP(C)
Richard E. Kreipe, M.D.
Bryan Lask, M.D.
Daniel Le Grange, Ph.D.
James D. Lock, M.D., Ph.D.
Katharine L. Loeb, Ph.D.
Marsha D. Marcus, Ph.D.
Sloane Madden, M.B.B.S. (Hons.), FRANZP, CAPCert, FAED

This paper is dedicated to Mae Sokol-Burger, who passed away before getting to see her efforts on this work in this publication. We are grateful for her selfless contributions to the field.

Reprinted with permission from Bravender T, Bryant-Waugh R, Herzog D, et al; Workgroup for Classification of Eating Disorders in Children and Adolescents. *European Eating Disorders Review* 18(2):79–89, 2010. Copyright 2010, John Wiley and Sons.

Dasha Nicholls, M.B.B.S., MRCPsych, M.D.
Julie K. O'Toole, M.D., M.P.H.
Leora Pinhas, M.D.
Ellen Rome, M.D., M.P.H.
Mae Sokol-Burger, M.D.
Ulf Wallin, M.D., Ph.D.
Nancy Zucker, Ph.D.

Anorexia nervosa (AN), bulimia nervosa (BN), and related eating disorders are psychiatric syndromes that convey significant risk for medical problems, particularly among youth. AN has a point prevalence of 0.48%–0.7% among adolescent females (Ackard et al. 2007; Hoek 2006; Hoek and van Hoeken 2003). BN occurs in approximately 1%–2% of the adolescent population, whereas clinically significant bulimic behaviors occur in an additional 2%–3% (Hoek and van Hoeken 2003). Lewinsohn et al. (2001) indicated that although the hazard rates for a diagnosis of AN peak between the ages of 16 and 17 years, slopes begin increasing around the age of 10 years. For BN, a disorder that was previously reported to have a later age at onset than AN, the pattern is similar. The view put forward in this chapter is that the current diagnostic classification system requires greater sensitivity to the expression of disordered eating in children and adolescents (Cooper et al. 2002; Nicholls et al. 2000).

Disturbances in nutrition may be particularly harmful during vulnerable periods of brain development and physical growth. Adolescence is well recognized as a period of profound alteration in multiple influential domains: the physical changes of puberty, the social changes associated with increased peer influence, the increased opportunities to engage in both maladaptive and adaptive decisions—all against a backdrop of intensified emotional reactivity (Casey et al. 2000, 2008; Giedd et al. 1996, 1999). Many of these changes are instantiated at the neural level. Accumulating evidence supports the observation that extensive neural remodeling and synaptic pruning occur in the developing adolescent brain (Gogtay et al. 2004). Particularly, brain structures associated with motivated states and emotional experience have been reported to develop more rapidly than distributed neural circuitry associated with cognitive control, a developmental divergence that has been proposed to account, in part, for the increase in maladaptive decisions that occur during this developmental window as emotions hold more sway than rational cognition. Adaptive negotiation of this period leads to flexible, adaptive responding—in effect, the ability to use emotion to guide decisions, not dictate them (Ochsner and Gross 2005).

To be sure, these are challenges of *typical* adolescents. Any insult or trauma during this period of vulnerability greatly complicates these developmental challenges, whereas trauma or neglect prior to this period may cause divergence from a healthy developmental trajectory that becomes potentiated via the maturational processes of adolescence (Cook et al. 2009; De Bellis and Kuchibhatla 2006). Frank malnutrition and the threat of self-imposed malnutrition (whether or not it is actually realized) are traumatic experiences that threaten the well-being and physical status at any stage of development. It stands to reason that nutritional disturbance or deficit, defining features of eating disorders, during particularly vulnerable developmental periods can result in excessive and potentially permanent physical and psychological consequences (De Souza 2006). Because adequate nutrition is the necessary substrate for all biological growth, the fact that the malnutrition of eating disorders principally begins in adolescence and can also have its onset prior to adolescence necessitates flexibility in diagnostic boundaries based on developmental stage. Modifications to adult-defined boundaries of illness are needed to address the associated morbidity in the short term and to prevent more serious morbidity in the longer term (Eisler et al. 1997; Madden et al. 2009; Peebles et al. 2006). The failure to capture unique age-sensitive nuances of eating disturbance impedes case identification and the opportunity for early intervention. Furthermore, insensitivity to the developmental expression of nutrition inadequacy obscures differential diagnosis and inhibits identification and differentiation of related, clinically significant childhood nutritional presentations and disorders (Cooper et al. 2002; Nicholls et al. 2001; Watkins and Lask 2002). This chapter is intended to address these important issues by proposing changes to diagnostic criteria delineated in the current edition of DSM (DSM-IV; American Psychiatric Association 1994, 2000) to reflect pivotal developmental manifestations of symptom expression in children and adolescents. Although this opinion was framed while considering the criteria outlined in DSM-IV specifically, the issues addressed are also germane to current revisions being considered for revisions to the *International Statistical Classification of Diseases and Related Health Problems* (ICD-10; World Health Organization 2004).

Recommendations

A realistic goal for the current revision to DSM-IV is the creation of empirically validated amendments to existing criteria that characterize developmentally sensitive alterations in symptom expression seen in children and adolescents. There are important gaps in the current research literature pertaining to child and adolescent eating disorder diagnosis, as summarized by the following research questions. First, do eating disorders described in DSM-IV appear in childhood in a similar manner to adults? If so, an adult with AN and a child with AN would present with the same features. Second, do currently defined DSM-IV diagnoses appear in childhood and young adolescence, yet manifest in ways developmentally consistent with cognitive and emotional maturity? If so, a child can be diagnosed with AN, but given, as an example, maturational limitations in abstract reasoning, she might be unable to identify or articulate the fears of fatness associated with adult illness manifestations and would thus display a child-specific manifestation of AN. Nevertheless, her behavior might be entirely consistent with avoidance of any weight gain. Third, do children and adolescents manifest different eating disorders than described in older samples? For example, dietary restriction and weight loss without the stated fear of fatness may be a psychological entity entirely different from AN and might not be associated with concerted efforts to avoid gaining weight. The Work Group determined that the body of evidence was too limited to adequately adjudicate novel and separate diagnoses in children and adolescents (question 3) but considered this an area for future research. However, there is evidence that in some cases, eating disorders as expressed in childhood and adolescence differ from their adult-expressed counterparts (question 1). Thus, our goal in this chapter is to consider the current body of research in disordered eating in children and adolescents, to view the current diagnostic criteria in light of cognitive and developmental milestones of childhood and adolescence, and to integrate this body of evidence to arrive at proposed developmentally sensitive adaptations of existing criteria (question 2).

Recommended Changes to Existing Cognitive Criteria in Anorexia Nervosa and Bulimia Nervosa

Recommendation 1
Behavioral indicators should be permitted to substitute for internally referenced cognitive criteria.

Recommendation 2
Wording should be added that alerts health care professionals to developmental limitations that may preclude the ability to endorse a cognitive criterion.

Diagnostic criteria for eating disorders that require complex abstract reasoning may not be valid for children or adolescents. *Formal thought* is defined as the ability to integrate two or more lower-order, concrete processes to arrive at an intangible higher-order process (e.g., refusing food and exercising excessively to manage fears of being overweight) (Marini and Case 1994). In typically developing adolescents, formal thought emerges around 11–13 years old, whereas complex abstract reasoning continues to evolve into late adolescence (Rosso et al. 2004). Capacity for complex abstract reasoning is necessary to meet current criteria. For example, to determine the value of body weight and appearance in the determination of self-worth, an individual needs to rank several abstract constructs (such as trustworthiness, loyalty, attractiveness, and interpersonal competence) pertinent to self-evaluation. This capacity to describe internal experiences or compare and articulate multiple abstract concepts is not present in some children and adolescents.

The ability to perceive risk also continues to evolve throughout adolescence (Boyer 2006). Risk perception requires a child or adolescent to appreciate relative probabilities and to weigh these relative perceptions both immediately and in the future (Boyer 2006). For example, Criterion C for AN relates to denial of the seriousness of low body weight (Table 12–1). To perceive the seriousness of low body weight, a child must be able to consider the risk of his or her current weight relative to the risk of an alternative weight (such as being normal weight or overweight) and to project the long-term serious implications of this weight. Although research has been inconsistent, a conservative interpretation is that some preadolescents have difficulty perceiving the relative risk of alternative outcomes (Levin and Hart 2003), whereas both young and older adolescents may exhibit difficulties in appreciating distal negative consequences.

Behavioral indicators may serve as valid substitutes when internal experiences cannot be articulated in a manner consistent with adult presentations. Importantly, we cannot distinguish whether lack of endorsement of a cognition-based criterion is due to developmental insensitivity or to differences in symptom expression. However, given aforementioned limitations in cognitive development, behavioral indicators should be permitted to serve as substitutions for reliable descriptions of internal experiences. For example, severe and determined food restriction or selectivity that is designed to yield a low body weight (e.g., refusal to eat any fat or carbohydrates) could be considered as a proxy for expressed fear of weight gain. There are several precedents for this type of accommodation within the existing body of DSM-IV criteria (e.g., anxiety disorders). Moreover, parents or other caregivers can be enlisted as additional informants in assessing the presence and severity of behavioral indicators of the psychological features of AN and BN, a strategy utilized in measures of other forms of psychopathology in children and adolescents (e.g., depression) (Table 12–1).

TABLE 12–1.   Symptoms in current eating disorder diagnoses that reference cognitive events or experiences

Anorexia nervosa Criterion B: Intense fear of gaining weight, or becoming fat, even though underweight

Children may not verbally endorse fear of fatness, despite determined food refusal (of a quantitative and/or qualitative nature) that results in severe weight loss. This may either be a manifestation of anorexia nervosa in younger ages or reflect an alternative diagnosis. Specific fear of weight gain or compensatory behaviors may become apparent once weight restoration efforts commence. Behavioral indicators and/or parental report should serve as valid sources of information for this criterion.

Anorexia nervosa Criterion C: Disturbance in the way in which one's body weight or shape is experienced, undue influence of body weight and shape on self-evaluation, or denial of the seriousness of the current low body weight

Children and young adolescents may lack the capacity to appreciate abstract concepts such as self-worth or to describe the experience of their bodies in other than concrete or somatic terms. Children and both younger and older adolescents have a reduced capacity for general risk appraisal and thus may fail to appreciate the specific risk of extreme weight loss behaviors.

Bulimia nervosa Criterion D: Self-evaluation is unduly influenced by body shape and weight

Children and young adolescents may lack the capacity to appreciate abstract concepts such as self-worth or to describe the experience of their bodies in other than concrete or somatic terms.

Changes to Weight Loss Criterion in Anorexia Nervosa

Recommendation 3

Wording should be added to existing weight loss criteria that emphasizes the importance of an individual's previous growth and maturational trajectory in the determination of healthy weight status rather than a population-referenced cut point in the determination of clinical significance.

Although extreme weight loss or failure to make expected weight gain is a clinically significant symptom of AN (de Monléon et al. 1998), the sensitivity of current weight criteria in the detection of clinical severity has been questioned by numerous empirical investigations, professional organizations, and national treatment guidelines (Hebebrand et al. 2004; Nicholls and Stanhope 2000) (Table 12–2). Malnutrition has been convincingly demonstrated to negatively affect every system of the body both in individuals with AN and in those who are malnourished due to environmental or medical causes (de Monléon et al. 1998; Misra et al. 2004, 2005, 2006; Nicholls and Stanhope 2000). Of importance, however, is that severe weight loss may have more damaging effects at certain pivotal periods of development, and this may argue for more conservative definitions of weight loss during these sensitive periods (Nicholls et al. 2002). To illustrate, Peebles et al. (2006) compared children with AN, defined as 13 years of age or younger, with older adolescent patients. Children were reported to exhibit a lower percent ideal body weight, a shorter duration of illness, and a shorter temporal trajectory of weight loss (Peebles et al. 2006), highlighting the rapidity with which weight loss may confer potential harm. To be sure, a prepubescent child is likely to have lower fat stores than an adult (Nicholls et al. 2002). Thus, milder percentage weight loss may have more immediate negative impact, such as severe dehydration (Nicholls et al. 2002; Peebles et al. 2006). Of importance, whereas an adult needs to resolve symptoms to improve health, children and adolescents continue to grow and develop somatic processes with high-energy demands. Increased nutrition is necessary during this critical window to enable these processes to occur. To illustrate, malnourishment during adolescence is associated with low turnover of bone, with increased bone resorption without concomitant bone formation, a pattern different from that seen in menopausal women (Lennkh et al. 1999). Although weight restoration is an important determinant of bone mineral density, there appears to be a critical window during which such repair can occur (Brooks et al. 1998; Valla et al. 2000). To avoid the negative impact of malnourishment and to reflect the valid nutritional status of a child or adolescent adequately, developmentally sensitive definitions are required to ensure children are able to access appropriate treatment.

Accordingly, an alternative strategy to reliably define ideal weight for children and adolescents is to consider developmental trends in growth and physical maturity for that individual. To be sure, current weight criteria were never meant to be interpreted literally but rather to be used as a guide to determine when an individual's weight history warrants concern. In practice, however, these guidelines are far too often literally interpreted, with potentially deleterious consequences because individuals may be denied access to care by third-party payers due to failure to meet an arbitrary defined threshold. Thus, upcoming revisions have two challenges. First, weight criteria should be framed in a manner that is developmentally sensitive. Second, criteria must be framed so that they are clinically useful with no potential for misuse. Combined, such precautions would ensure that those who need care are not denied such treatment based on their weight loss history.

Current diagnostic complexity is due in part to the challenge of defining an optimal weight range for a growing child or adolescent. The degree of variation in phys-

TABLE 12–2. Weight criteria for the diagnosis of anorexia nervosa: critical issues for children and adolescents and corresponding proposed changes to DSM-IV

Anorexia nervosa Criterion A: Refusal to maintain body weight at or above a minimally normal weight for age and height (e.g., weight loss leading to maintenance of body weight less than 85% of that expected; or failure to make expected weight gain during period of growth, leading to body weight less than 85% of that expected)

In children and adolescents, consideration should be given to weight and height trends such as deviation from previous growth trajectories, percentage of weight loss, and/or body mass index centiles for age, rather than reliance on particular weight values in the determination of clinical threshold and severity.

In children and adolescents, the deleterious effects of weight loss may appear at a lower percentage weight lost relative to adults.

ical development at any one age during puberty is wide; for example, some children may be prepubertal, whereas others may have reached full adult maturity by the age of 12. With regard to eating disorders, this range can be widened further, because being underweight can result in pubertal delay or interruption. An average 16-year-old female, with the onset of menarche at 12.5 years of age, could therefore have reached full adult height and weight and thus her height and weight could be appropriately compared with centile charts or reported as standard deviations from population medians. However, if the eating disorder has an early onset, she may still have the height of an 11- or 12-year-old, making weight centiles more difficult to interpret. This is mainly an issue for premenarcheal-onset AN, because linear growth decelerates after menarche, with an average height gain averaging approximately 7 cm (2.8 inches) (Rosen 2004). Further complicating this issue is that although there are strong correlations between degree of emaciation and the frequency and severity of the medical sequelae of starvation, there is no "threshold" effect below which signs and symptoms of malnutrition occur (Swenne and Engström 2005).

Reporting nutritional status in terms of body mass index (BMI) standard deviation units or centiles (or percent BMI) provides an additional strategy to address problems with interpretation of weight, by adjusting weight for height, age, and sex. Many countries now have their own national reference centile charts for BMI for age. International BMI cutoffs for child overweight and obesity have been developed, and recently Cole et al. (2007) used similar methodology in order to improve international comparison of BMI in underweight growing children. Although these guidelines provide a laudable advance in increasing the consistency in the definition of thinness across the developmental spectrum, such reference BMI centiles only account for age and sex and do not take developmental maturity into account. Finally, as evidence of the potential for harm when criteria are interpreted literally, Madden et al. (2009) characterized the expression of early onset eating disorders in a nationally representative sample of 5- to 13-year-old Australian youth (Madden et al. 2009). Of importance, although only 51% met current weight criteria as defined by current diagnostic criteria, 61% had life-threatening complications of malnutrition (Madden et al. 2009). Accommodation for individual developmental trends is needed.

Changes to Amenorrhea Requirement in Anorexia Nervosa

Recommendation 4
Multiple physical systems should be evaluated for the clinical management of eating disturbance, but no single system should be required for diagnosis.

The requirement of amenorrhea in the diagnosis of AN is invalid for prepubescent children (Nicholls et al. 2000) and inappropriate for males (Abraham et al. 2005), and amenorrhea is not reliably reported by patients (Abraham et al. 2005; Swenne et al. 2005) (Table 12–3). The inadequacy of this criterion is widely accepted (National Institute for Clinical Excellence 2004; Society for Adolescent Medicine 2003), because research investigations with both adolescents and adults do not consistently require this feature in defining their clinical populations (Lock et al. 2006; Walsh et al. 2006). Furthermore, treatment recommendations from professional organizations advise clinicians that although medical signs, symptoms, and complications help characterize the clinical picture, they are not sufficient for diagnosis (National Institute for Clinical Excellence 2004). Thus, what is the role or necessity of menstrual dysfunction in the diagnosis of child and adolescent eating disorders? The principle here is that for eating disturbance to be clinically significant, there must be some evidence of physical risk or impairment. A review of the evidence suggests a middle ground: a recommendation that thorough diagnostic evaluation of children and adolescents take an expansive view of biological systems and consider a diverse array of biological abnormalities as contributing to the clinical picture of child and adolescent diagnosis, but not mandating specific abnormalities within a single system in the body for diagnosis.

The clinical profile of AN complicates sexual maturity rating. In females, the emaciated physical state and low estrogen associated with AN may reduce breast size and distort a health care professional's assessment of sexual maturity. In males,

---

TABLE 12–3.   Hypothalamic-pituitary axis dysfunction: critical issues for children and adolescents and corresponding proposed changes to DSM-IV

Anorexia nervosa Criterion D: In postmenarcheal females, amenorrhea (the absence of at least three consecutive cycles; a woman is considered to have amenorrhea if her periods occur only after hormone replacement, e.g., estrogen administration)

The effects of malnutrition evidence great variability. Clinicians should evaluate changes in multiple systems (e.g., cardiac, endocrine, gastrointestinal) for clinical management but refrain from using single physical sequelae as a diagnostic requirement (in children and adolescents).

---

similar regression may be witnessed in the effects of lowered testosterone on rating of Tanner stage (Tanner and Preece 1998).

Dysfunction in diverse physical systems may provide alternative or additional indicators of malnutrition resulting from disturbed eating in children and adolescents (Shamim et al. 2003). Several laboratories have supported the presence of significant medical abnormalities in diverse biological systems in both inpatient (Shamim et al. 2003) and outpatient (Misra et al. 2004) adolescents with eating disorders. Such variation demonstrates that there is not likely to be one specific metabolic profile in children, adolescents, or adults with AN. Rather, there may be an array of physiological signs in individuals with AN that aid in diagnosis.

Changes to Binge Eating Criteria in Bulimia Nervosa and Binge Eating Disorder

---

Recommendation 5
The experience of loss of control irrespective of the amount of calories consumed during an eating episode should be considered the hallmark of binge eating behavior in children.

Recommendation 6
Binge episodes should be a persistent symptom for diagnosis, but a lower frequency and duration are clinically significant in children. Episodes should occur at least once a month during the previous 3-month period for diagnosis.

Although adolescents with aberrant eating behaviors exhibit many features in common with adults, indicators of aberrant eating in children are age-specific and require assessment strategies sensitive to developmental context. In DSM-IV, *binge eating* is defined by consumption of an excessively large amount of food paired with the subjective experience of a loss of control over eating. Associated features of binge eating include the context in which eating occurs (e.g., in private), affective states that follow disturbed eating (e.g., shame and guilt), and the physiological state of the individual (e.g., feeling uncomfortably full following the episode). The assessment of these behaviors and experiences in children requires age-specific strategies (Table 12–4). Such strategies include the use of concrete examples and developmentally sensitive metaphors (e.g., a loss of control is similar to "a ball rolling down a hill") (Tanofsky-Kraff et al. 2004). When such strategies are employed, a subgroup of children endorses symptom profiles consistent with adult definitions of binge eating. However, an additional group endorses the subjective experience of loss of control without accompanying excessive food intake. As highlighted by Marcus and Kalarchian (2003), the clinical significance of *loss of control* relative to the quantity of calories consumed may provide a more developmentally valid index of aberrant eating. Indeed, in cross-sectional studies, any loss of control eating (i.e., one or more episodes) reported over the previous 4-week period is associated with greater adiposity (Neumark-Sztainer and Hannan 2000; Tanofsky-Kraff et al. 2004); elevations in psychiatric symptoms such as depression, anxiety, and body image disturbance (Glasofer et al. 2007; Tanofsky-Kraff et al. 2005); excessive weight gain (Tanofsky-Kraff et al. 2009b); and increased vulnerability to the abundant environmental triggers for dysregulated eating, such as excessive food availability (Tanofsky-Kraff et al. 2009a). Thus, consistent with the recommendations of Marcus and Kalarchian (2003) and supported by recent findings about the clinical implications of loss of control (Tanofsky-Kraff et al. 2009b), it may be that the experience of loss of control is an important consideration in the determination of clinical impairment, irrespective of the amount of food consumed.

Despite similar symptom presentations in children and adolescents relative to adults, lower symptom thresholds are recommended (Table 12–5). Research characterizing atypical eating patterns in adolescent BN and comparing threshold with subthreshold forms of this disorder indicates significant overlap in levels of impairment, patterns of psychiatric comorbidity (Binford and le Grange 2005; Eddy et al. 2008), and medical sequelae (le Grange et al. 2004), supporting the inadequacy of current diagnostic thresholds. Indeed, this finding is not unique to adolescents (le Grange et al. 2006). Current data suggest that the frequency and duration criteria for binge eating and purging in DSM-IV are not adequate (Crow et al. 2002; Sullivan and Kendler 1998). Furthermore, specific boundaries distinguishing subthreshold BN are extremely varied. Notwithstanding, in children there is added motivation to consider lower thresholds for diagnosis given the greater impact of similar medical sequelae at fragile developmental stages. Evidence to date supports the clinical significance of at least one episode of loss-of-control eating occurring

TABLE 12–4.   Binge eating: critical issues for children and adolescents and corresponding proposed changes to DSM-IV

Bulimia nervosa Criterion A: Recurrent episodes of binge eating. An episode of binge eating is characterized by both of the following: 1) eating, in a discrete period of time (e.g., within any 2-hour period), an amount of food that is definitely larger than most people would eat during a similar period of time and under similar circumstances; and 2) a sense of lack of control over eating during the episode (e.g., a feeling that one cannot stop eating or control what or how much one is eating).

In children and younger adolescents, the subjective experience of a loss of control may be a particularly robust indicator of aberrant eating behavior. However, care must be taken to ensure that children understand what is meant by "loss of control" through the use of developmentally appropriate assessment strategies, such as concrete examples or age-appropriate metaphors (e.g., the experience is "like a ball rolling down a hill" [Tanofsky-Kraff et al. 2004]). Behavioral indicators of loss-of-control eating, such as secretive eating, food seeking in response to negative affect, and food hoarding, should be considered in children younger than 12 years of age.

Given the prognostic significance of binge eating in children and young adolescents in relation to symptom severity and chronicity, a lower threshold for diagnosis should be considered.

for 3 months, a recommendation describing both a lower symptom frequency and a shorter duration of symptom expression. This practice is consistent with other childhood diagnoses (e.g., for dysthymic disorder the duration is 1 year instead of 2 years for adults). In sum, aberrant eating in children and adolescents overlaps significantly with adult manifestations, but behaviors do differ. The conservative strategy is to alert the health care community to divergent presentations and to consider a lower threshold of severity to protect children and adolescents from harmful sequelae of their disorders (Tanofsky-Kraff et al. 2008).

Changes to Criteria for Inappropriate Compensatory Mechanisms in Bulimia Nervosa

Recommendation 7
Lower thresholds of both symptom frequency and duration should be used to designate clinical levels of inappropriate compensatory mechanisms in children and adolescents.

TABLE 12–5. Compensatory behaviors: critical issues for children and adolescents and corresponding proposed changes to DSM-IV

Bulimia nervosa Criterion B: Recurrent inappropriate compensatory behavior in order to prevent weight gain, such as self-induced vomiting; misuse of laxatives, diuretics, enemas, or other medications; fasting; or excessive exercise

In children and younger adolescents, a lower threshold of symptom frequency and duration should be considered due to potential for acute medical sequelae in younger ages.

Given the potential severity of effects of extreme weight loss strategies on growth and development, lower thresholds of symptom severity are needed for children and adolescents. There is significant inter-individual variation in the response to extreme weight loss behaviors, variation that complicates the determination of a threshold of severity. For example, although some children may manifest electrolyte abnormalities with subthreshold levels of symptom frequency, for others laboratory results may fail to reveal significant medical sequelae until a chronic disease course has significantly progressed. Given the unpredictability of relating symptom frequency and duration to medical impairment, coupled with the severe cost of "missing" a serious disorder due to insensitive thresholds, the conservative strategy is the consideration of lower symptom thresholds for both symptom frequency and symptom duration. This strategy would alert clinicians to the serious nature of extreme weight loss behaviors, increasing the sensitivity of detection of severe clinical problems.

Subthreshold levels of extreme weight loss behaviors are clinically significant, predicting increased symptom severity as well as concurrent impairment in functioning. For example, in a representative community sample of 2,516 adolescents, Neumark-Sztainer et al. (2006) reported that subthreshold levels of extreme weight loss behavior predicted a one-point increase in BMI relative to adolescents not engaging in these behaviors. Furthermore, the presence of these behaviors at baseline resulted in a threefold increase in the likelihood of overweight at follow-up. Individuals who engaged in extreme weight loss behaviors were less likely to engage in health-promoting weight maintenance strategies such as fruit and vegetable consumption (Story et al. 1998). Several studies comparing the diagnosis of BN with subthreshold forms of this disorder found no difference in comorbid symptom severity or treatment response (Binford and le Grange 2005; le Grange et al. 2007; Schmidt et al. 2007). These results portend harm: adolescents engaging in even subthreshold levels of extreme weight loss strategies are positioned on a harmful trajectory predictive of unhealthy weight management and increased eating disturbance and appear to be as ill as those with threshold forms of BN.

Conclusion

The purpose of DSM "is to provide clear descriptions of diagnostic categories in order to enable clinicians and investigators to diagnose, communicate about, study, and treat people with various mental disorders" (American Psychiatric Association 1994, p. xxxvii). The goal of this consensus opinion is to improve the description of AN, BN, and eating disorders not otherwise specified as they pertain to children and adolescents to improve case identification, treatment, and research efforts in that segment of the population at highest risk for onset of these serious eating disorders. In the diagnosis of child and adolescent eating disorders, the data on proposed criteria modifications are convincing and their import is compelling, whereas the breadth of research is relatively small. This is due, in part, to the strategies that have been employed in the ascertainment of childhood eating disturbance—in effect, extrapolating from adult-defined symptoms. Although clinically significant but atypical presentations of eating disturbance also appear prominently in the adult population, developmental considerations increase the likelihood of such symptom constellations obscuring true AN or BN "caseness" among children and adolescents. The risks secondary to misdiagnosis during key periods of growth and development are grave. Advances in the diagnosis and research of eating disturbance in children and adolescents can only occur by adopting developmentally sensitive frameworks and methodologies. We recommend examining the topography and expression of symptoms of relevance for eating disorders through the lens of a developmental trajectory and defining child and adolescent eating pathology at the intersect of deviation from both healthy development and adult-defined diagnostic criteria.

References

Abraham SF, Pettigrew B, Boyd C, et al: Usefulness of amenorrhea in the diagnoses of eating disorder patients. J Psychosom Obst Gynecol 26:211–215, 2005

Ackard DM, Fulkerson JA, Neumark-Sztainer D: Prevalence and utility of DSM-IV eating disorder diagnostic criteria among youth. Int J Eat Disord 40:409–417, 2007

American Psychiatric Association: Diagnostic and Statistical Manual of Mental Disorders, 4th Edition. Washington, DC, American Psychiatric Association, 1994

American Psychiatric Association: Diagnostic and Statistical Manual of Mental Disorders, 4th Edition, Text Revision. Washington, DC, American Psychiatric Association, 2000

Binford RB, le Grange D: Adolescents with bulimia nervosa and eating disorder not otherwise specified–purging only. Int J Eat Disord 38:157–161, 2005

Boyer TW: The development of risk-taking: a multi-perspective review. Dev Rev 26:291–345, 2006

Brooks ER, Ogden BW, Cavalier DS: Compromised bone density 11.4 years after diagnosis of anorexia nervosa. J Womens Health 7:567–574, 1998

Casey BJ, Giedd JN, Thomas KM: Structural and functional brain development and its relation to cognitive development. Biol Psychol 54:241–257, 2000

Casey BJ, Getz S, Galvan A: The adolescent brain. Dev Rev 28:62–77, 2008

Cole TJ, Flegal KM, Nicholls D, et al: Body mass index cut offs to define thinness in children and adolescents: international survey. BMJ 335:194, 2007

Cook F, Ciorciari J, Varker T, et al: Changes in long term neural connectivity following psychological trauma. Clin Neurophysiol 120:309–314, 2009

Cooper PJ, Watkins B, Bryant-Waugh R, et al: The nosological status of early onset anorexia nervosa. Psychol Med 32:873–880, 2002

Crow SJ, Agras WS, Halmi K, et al: Full syndromal versus subthreshold anorexia nervosa, bulimia nervosa, and binge eating disorder: a multicenter study. Int J Eat Disord 32:309–318, 2002

De Bellis MD, Kuchibhatla M: Cerebellar volumes in pediatric maltreatment-related posttraumatic stress disorder. Biol Psychiatry 60:697–703, 2006

de Monléon JV, Simonin G, Giraud P, et al: Statural growth deficiency due to anorexia nervosa: a case in a patient with an unaffected identical twin [in French]. Ann Pediatr (Paris) 45:702–706, 1998

De Souza RG: Body size and growth: the significance of chronic malnutrition among the Casiguran Agta. Ann Hum Biol 33:604–619, 2006

Eddy K, Celio-Doyle A, Hoste R, et al: Eating disorder not otherwise specified in adolescents. J Am Acad Child Adolesc Psychiatry 47:156–164, 2008

Eisler I, Dare C, Russell GF, et al: Family and individual therapy in anorexia nervosa: a 5-year follow-up. Arch Gen Psychiatry 54:1025–1030, 1997

Giedd JN, Vaituzis A, Hamburger SD, et al: Quantitative MRI of the temporal lobe, amygdala, and hippocampus in normal human development: ages 4–18 years. J Comp Neurol 366:223–230, 1996

Giedd JN, Blumenthal J, Jeffries NO, et al: Brain development during childhood and adolescence: a longitudinal MRI study. Nat Neurosci 2:861–863, 1999

Glasofer DR, Tanofsky-Kraff M, Eddy KT, et al: Binge eating in overweight treatment-seeking adolescents. J Pediatr Psychol 32:95–105, 2007

Gogtay N, Giedd JN, Lusk L, et al: Dynamic mapping of human cortical development during childhood through early adulthood. Proc Natl Acad Sci U S A 101:8174–8179, 2004

Hebebrand J, Casper R, Treasure J, et al: The need to revise the diagnostic criteria for anorexia nervosa. J Neural Transm 111:827–840, 2004

Hoek HW: Incidence, prevalence and mortality of anorexia nervosa and other eating disorders. Curr Opin Psychiatry 19:389–394, 2006

Hoek HW, van Hoeken D: Review of the prevalence and incidence of eating disorders. Int J Eat Disord 34:383–396, 2003

le Grange D, Loeb K, Van Orman S, et al: Adolescent bulimia nervosa: a disorder in evolution? Arch Pediatr Adolesc Med 158:478–482, 2004

le Grange D, Binford RB, Peterson CB, et al: DSM-IV threshold versus subthreshold bulimia nervosa. Int J Eat Disord 39:462–467, 2006 le Grange D, Crosby R, Rathouz P, et al: A randomized controlled comparison of family based treatment and supportive psychotherapy for adolescent bulimia nervosa. Arch Gen Psychiatry 64:1049–1056, 2007

Lennkh C, de Zwaan M, Bailer U, et al: Osteopenia in anorexia nervosa: specific mechanisms of bone loss. J Psychiatr Res 33:349–356, 1999

Levin IP, Hart SS: Risk preferences in young children: early evidence of individual differences in reaction to potential gains and losses. J Behav Decis Mak 16:397–413, 2003

Lewinsohn PM, Striegel-Moore RH, Seeley JR: Epidemiology and natural course of eating disorders in young women from adolescence to young adulthood. J Am Acad Child Adolesc Psychiatry 39:1284–1292, 2001

Lock J, Couturier J, Agras WS: Comparison of long-term outcomes in adolescents with anorexia nervosa treated with family therapy. J Am Acad Child Adolesc Psychiatry 45:666–672, 2006

Madden S, Morris A, Zurynski YA, et al: Burden of eating disorders in 5–13-year-old children in Australia. Med J Aust 190:410–414, 2009

Marcus MD, Kalarchian MA: Binge eating in children and adolescents. Int J Eat Disord 349(suppl):S47–S57, 2003

Marini Z, Case R: The development of abstract reasoning about the physical and social world. Child Dev 65:147–159, 1994

Misra M, Aggarwal A, Miller KK, et al: Effects of anorexia nervosa on clinical, hematologic, biochemical, and bone density parameters in community-dwelling adolescent girls. Pediatrics 114:1574–1583, 2004

Misra M, Miller KK, Stewart V, et al: Ghrelin and bone metabolism in adolescent girls with anorexia nervosa and healthy adolescents. J Clin Endocrinol Metab 90:5082–5087, 2005

Misra M, Miller KK, Tsai P, et al: Elevated peptide YY levels in adolescent girls with anorexia nervosa. J Clin Endocrinol Metab 91:1027–1033, 2006

National Institute for Clinical Excellence: Core Interventions in the Treatment and Management of Anorexia Nervosa, Bulimia Nervosa, and Related Eating Disorders. London, National Institute for Clinical Excellence, 2004

Neumark-Sztainer D, Hannan PJ: Weight-related behaviors among adolescent girls and boys: results from a national survey. Arch Pediatr Adolesc Med 154:569–577, 2000

Neumark-Sztainer D, Wall M, Guo J, et al: Obesity, disordered eating, and eating disorders in a longitudinal study of adolescents: how do dieters fare 5 years later? J Am Diet Assoc 106:559–568, 2006

Nicholls D, Stanhope R: Medical complications of anorexia nervosa in children and young adolescents. Eur Eat Disord Rev 8:170–180, 2000

Nicholls D, Chater R, Lask B: Children into DSM don't go: a comparison of classification systems for eating disorders in childhood and early adolescence. Int J Eat Disord 28:317–324, 2000

Nicholls D, Christie D, Randall L, et al: Selective eating: symptom, disorder or normal variant. Clin Child Psychol Psychiatry 6:257–270, 2001

Nicholls D, Wells JC, Singhal A, et al: Body composition in early onset eating disorders. Eur J Clin Nutr 56:857–865, 2002

Ochsner KN, Gross JJ: The cognitive control of emotion. Trends Cogn Sci 9:242–249, 2005

Peebles R, Wilson JL, Lock JD: How do children with eating disorders differ from adolescents with eating disorders at initial evaluation? J Adolesc Health 39:800–805, 2006

Rosen DS: Physiologic growth and development during adolescence. Pediatr Rev 25:194–200, 2004

Rosso IM, Young AD, Femia LA, et al: Cognitive and emotional components of frontal lobe functioning in childhood and adolescence, in Adolescent Brain Development: Vulnerabilities and Opportunities. Edited by Dahl RE, Spear SE. New York, New York Academy of Sciences, 2004, pp 355–362

Schmidt U, Lee S, Beecham J, et al: A randomized controlled trial of family therapy and cognitive behavior therapy guided self-care for adolescents with bulimia nervosa and related disorders. Am J Psychiatry 164:591–598, 2007

Shamim T, Golden NH, Arden M, et al: Resolution of vital sign instability: an objective measure of medical stability in anorexia nervosa. J Adolesc Health 32:73–77, 2003

Society for Adolescent Medicine: Eating disorders in adolescents. J Adolesc Health 33:496–503, 2003

Story M, Neumark-Sztainer D, Sherwood N, et al: Dieting status and its relationship to eating and physical activity behaviors in a representative sample of US adolescents. J Am Diet Assoc 98:1127–1132, 1998

Sullivan PF, Kendler KS: Typology of common psychiatric syndromes: an empirical study. Br J Psychiatry 173:312–319, 1998

Swenne I, Engström I: Medical assessment of adolescent girls with eating disorders: an evaluation of symptoms and signs of starvation (see comment). Acta Paediatr 94:1363–1371, 2005

Swenne I, Belfrage E, Thurfjell B, et al: Accuracy of reported weight and menstrual status in teenage girls with eating disorders Int J Eat Disord 38:375–379, 2005

Tanner JM, Preece MA (eds): The Physiology of Human Growth (Society for the Study of Human Biology Symposium Series, Vol 29). Cambridge, UK, Cambridge University Press, 1998

Tanofsky-Kraff M, Yanovski SZ, Wilfley DE, et al: Eating-disordered behaviors, body fat, and psychopathology in overweight and normal-weight children. J Consult Clin Psychol 72:53–61, 2004

Tanofsky-Kraff M, Faden D, Yanovski SZ, et al: The perceived onset of dieting and loss of control eating behaviors in overweight children. Int J Eat Disord 38:112–122, 2005

Tanofsky-Kraff M, Marcus MD, Yanovski SZ, et al: Loss of control eating disorder in children age 12 years and younger: proposed research criteria. Eat Behav 9:360–365, 2008

Tanofsky-Kraff M, McDuffie JR, Yanovski SZ, et al: Laboratory assessment of the food intake of children and adolescents with loss of control eating. Am J Clin Nutr 89:738–745, 2009a

Tanofsky-Kraff M, Yanovski SZ, Schvey NA, et al: A prospective study of loss of control eating for body weight gain in children at high risk for adult obesity. Int J Eat Disord 42:26–30, 2009b

Valla A, Groenning IL, Syversen U, et al: Anorexia nervosa: slow regain of bone mass. Osteoporos Int 11:141–145, 2000

Walsh BT, Kaplan AS, Attia E, et al: Fluoxetine after weight restoration in anorexia nervosa: a randomized controlled trial. JAMA 295:2605–2612, 2006

Watkins B, Lask B: Eating disorders in school-aged children. Child Adolesc Psychiatr Clin N Am 11:185–199, 2002

World Health Organization: International Statistical Classification of Diseases and Related Health Problems, 10th Revision, 2nd Edition. Geneva, World Health Organization, 2004

13

VALIDATION OF A DIAGNOSTIC CLASSIFICATION OF FEEDING DISORDERS IN INFANTS AND YOUNG CHILDREN

Irene Chatoor, M.D.
Robert P. Hirsch, Ph.D.
Stephen A. Wonderlich, Ph.D.
Ross D. Crosby, Ph.D.

At present, DSM-IV (American Psychiatric Association 1994, 2000) lists feeding disorder of infancy and early childhood as the only diagnosis for a range of feeding difficulties in infants and young children. The diagnostic criteria are as follows:

The research for this work was supported by a grant from the National Institute of Mental Health (R01-MH58219) and a grant from the National Center for Research Resources awarded to the Children's Clinical Research Center (RR13297).

A special thanks to all the collaborators on the study: Jody Ganiban, Ph.D.; Benny Kerzner, M.D.; Miguel Macaoay, M.D.; Joyce Harrison, M.D.; Joan Pincus, M.D.; Laura McWade Paez, CPNP; Lori Stern, R.N.; Randi Simenson, M.S., OTR; Leila Becker, Ph.D.; Lauren Rhee, M.S., RD; Jacyln Shepard, M.A.; Laura Brinkmeier, B.A.; Amy Hahn, B.A.; Nicole Barber, B.A.

A. Feeding disturbance as manifested by persistent failure to eat adequately with significant failure to gain weight or significant loss of weight over at least 1 month.
B. The disturbance is not due to an associated gastrointestinal or other general medical condition (e.g., esophageal reflux).
C. The disturbance is not better accounted for by another mental disorder (e.g., rumination disorder) or by lack of available food.
D. The onset is before age 6 years.

These criteria have several limitations. The criterion "failure to eat adequately" does not address the different reasons why infants or young children may not eat adequately, which has implications for different etiologies of the feeding problems and need for different interventions. In addition, the criterion "failure to gain weight or loss of weight" does not address the feeding problems of a large number of young children who have a very limited diet but who eat adequate amounts of calories when given their favorite foods, and consequently gain adequate amounts of weight. The criteria in DSM-IV also exclude feeding problems associated with medical conditions.

As a result of the narrowness of the diagnostic criteria on the one hand and the lack of specificity on the other hand, different diagnostic labels have been used in the literature to describe overlapping symptomatology, and the same labels have been applied to describe different feeding problems (Chatoor and Ammaniti 2007). Many reports in the literature describe certain characteristics of a feeding disorder but fail to delineate how to differentiate this feeding disorder from other feeding disorders or from milder, transient forms of feeding difficulties.

To address the question of how to differentiate various feeding problems from one another and from transient or milder feeding difficulties, Chatoor (2002) first described a classification of six feeding disorders (feeding disorder of state regulation, feeding disorder associated with lack of parent-infant reciprocity, infantile anorexia, sensory food aversions, posttraumatic feeding disorder, feeding disorder associated with a concurrent medical condition). The initial criteria for these six feeding disorders were modified by the American Academy of Child and Adolescent Psychiatry's Task Force for Research Diagnostic Criteria: Infants and Preschool (Scheeringa et al. 2003) and were further developed with the help of a work group on diagnostic criteria in infants and young children that was supported by the American Psychiatric Association and whose findings were published in *Age and Gender Considerations in Psychiatric Diagnosis: A Research Agenda for DSM-V* (Narrow et al. 2007). These diagnostic criteria include clinical symptoms that are characteristic for each specific disorder and differentiate one feeding disorder from the other. In addition, each feeding disorder has measures of impairment that differentiate it from transient or milder forms of feeding difficulties. The impairment may be in the area of nutrition—for example, growth faltering, signs of malnutrition, specific dietary deficiencies in children with a limited diet, or inadequate food intake threatening the child's health and growth in posttraumatic feeding disorder. The impairment may also be in the child's oral motor, language, or social development, especially in children with sensory food aversions. On recommendation by the Task Force in 2003, impairment in the form of conflict in the parent-child relationship and parental stress was not included in the criteria (Scheeringa et al. 2003).

The first four feeding disorders arise most commonly during specific developmental periods. Feeding disorder of state regulation is commonly seen in the first few months of life; feeding disorder associated with lack of parent-infant reciprocity usually presents during the first year of life; both infantile anorexia and sensory food aversions become clinically evident most commonly between 6 months and 3 years, when young children are introduced to solid food and transitioned to self-feeding; and posttraumatic feeding disorder and feeding disorder associated with a medical condition can be observed in very young infants and in children of all ages.

In order to judge the validity of newly proposed diagnoses, Blashfield et al. (1990) suggested the following criteria:

1. There should be ample literature about the proposed syndrome.
2. The diagnostic criteria should be articulated clearly, and assessment instruments should exist that may be used for determining whether an individual meets criteria.
3. The proposed syndrome should be diagnosable with a high degree of reliability between two or more assessors.
4. Evidence should be available that the proposed syndrome can be differentiated from other (similar) syndromes.
5. Evidence should be provided regarding the coherence and validity of the syndrome.

The study described in this chapter was designed to determine whether these feeding disorders can be diagnosed with a high degree of reliability between three examiners, whether latent class analysis (LCA) can identify naturally occurring groups of feeding problems that agree with the clinical diagnoses, whether growth parameters differentiate between the four feeding disorders, and whether the four feeding disorders are associated with other psychopathology.

Method

The study was conducted by a multidisciplinary feeding disorders team at Children's National Medical Center in Washington, D.C., over a 5-year period. All children, ranging in age from 3 months to 6 years, who were referred to the clinic were invited to participate in the diagnostic study. No children with feeding disorder of state regulation or feeding disorder associated with lack of parent-infant reciprocity were referred to the clinic. These children were most likely admitted to the hospital's inpatient services, and their follow-up after admission is not known.

Chatoor (2002) proposed diagnostic criteria for the four feeding disorders presenting to the clinic and for oral motor feeding disorder, a nonpsychiatric diagnosis:

PROPOSED FEEDING DISORDERS

Infantile Anorexia

A. Refusal to eat adequate amounts of food for at least 1 month.
B. Onset of the food refusal often occurs during the transition to spoon- and self-feeding, typically between 6 months and 3 years of age.
C. Rarely communicates hunger, lacks interest in food and eating, and would rather play or talk than eat.
D. Shows faltering growth or signs of acute and/or chronic growth deficiency.
E. The food refusal did not follow a traumatic event to the oropharynx.
F. The food refusal is not due to an underlying medical illness.

Sensory Food Aversions

A. Consistently refuses to eat specific foods with specific tastes, textures, smells, temperatures, and/or appearances for at least 1 month.
B. Onset of the food refusal occurs during the introduction of a new type or taste of food.

Examples:

- May drink one type of milk but refuse another
- May eat smooth purees but gag and refuse baby food with lumps in it
- May eat crunchy snacks but refuse regular table foods

C. Aversive reactions to foods may range from grimacing and spitting out the food to gagging and vomiting.
D. After an aversive reaction, the child refuses to continue eating the food and frequently generalizes and refuses other foods with a similar color, appearance, or smell.
E. Is reluctant to try new foods but eats well when offered preferred foods.
F. Without supplementation, demonstrates specific dietary deficiencies (e.g., vitamins, iron, zinc, or protein) but usually does not show any growth deficiency and may even be overweight.
G. May show delayed oral motor and expressive speech development.
H. Starting during preschool years, may demonstrate anxiety around eating with others at school and avoid social situations that involve eating.
I. May have other sensory difficulties (e.g., sensitivity to touch, loud noises, bright lights).

J. Refusal to eat specific foods is not related to food allergies or any other medical illness.

Posttraumatic Feeding Disorder

A. Characterized by the acute onset of consistent food refusal.
B. Onset of the food refusal can occur at any age of the child, from infancy onward.
C. Food refusal follows a traumatic event or repeated traumatic insults to the oropharynx or gastrointestinal tract that trigger distress in the child (e.g., gagging, choking, vomiting, intubation, force feeding).
D. Food refusal may present in one of the following ways, depending on the feeding experience of the child in association with the traumatic event(s):

- Refuses bottle but may accept spoon
- Refuses solid food but may accept the bottle
- Refuses all oral feedings

E. Reminders of the traumatic event(s) cause distress, as manifested by one or more of the following:

- May show anticipatory distress when positioned for feeding
- Shows intense resistance when approached with bottle and/or food
- Shows intense resistance to swallow food that is placed in the infant's mouth

F. Food refusal poses an acute or long-term threat to the child's health, nutrition, and growth and threatens the progression of age-appropriate feeding development.

Feeding Disorder Associated With a Concurrent Medical Condition

A. Food refusal and inadequate food intake for at least 2 weeks.
B. The onset of the food refusal can occur at any age of the child and may wax and wane in intensity, depending on the underlying medical condition.
C. Readily initiates feeding, but over the course of feeding, shows distress and refuses to continue.
D. Has a concurrent medical condition that is believed to cause the distress.
E. Fails to gain age-appropriate weight or may even lose weight.
F. Medical management improves but may not fully alleviate the feeding problems.

Oral Motor Feeding Disorder (Nonpsychiatric Disorder)

A. Has difficulty sucking.
B. Has difficulty drinking milk from the cup.

C. Has difficulty chewing.
D. Has difficulty swallowing: may spit out food, may pocket food in cheeks, may gag or choke during feedings.

PARTICIPANTS

Approval for the study was obtained from the Institutional Review Board at Children's National Medical Center in Washington, D.C., and the written consent was explained to all parents. Over a 5-year period, 486 children were seen in the Multidisciplinary Feeding Disorders Clinic at Children's National Medical Center. The parents of 444 children consented to participate, whereas the parents of 42 children refused consent—primarily because they did not want to be videotaped during the feeding session. Complete data were obtained for 438 children and their parents.

The children ranged in age from 3 to 128 months. There were a few older children who were seen in the clinic because of their developmental delays. The median age was 24 months (mean, 29.1; standard deviation [SD], 19.4). Sixty-one percent were male and 39% were female. The ethnicities of the children, which were generally representative of the larger Washington metropolitan area, were 12% African American, 13% Asian American, 63% European American, 4% Hispanic, 5% mixed race, and 2% other. The parents were mostly college educated; the mean years (±SD) of education was 16.0 (±2.4) for the mothers and 16.3 (±2.4) for the fathers.

CLINICAL ASSESSMENTS

Medical Assessment

The children were first seen by a nurse practitioner or nurse, who, under the supervision of the chair of gastroenterology, took a medical and feeding history, performed a physical examination, and ordered medical tests as indicated.

Nutritional Assessment

The children were then seen by a nutritionist, who obtained measurements of weight, height, and head circumference and then calculated ideal body weight and ideal height. In addition, she reviewed a 3-day food record that the parents filled out before the visit, and she calculated the micronutrients (e.g., vitamins, iron, zinc, and protein) in the child's diet and compared them with the recommended daily allowances (RDAs) of these micronutrients.

Oral Motor Assessment

An occupational therapist or speech and language therapist assessed the child's oral motor and speech development and any other sensory difficulties the child might experience.

Psychiatric Assessment

One of two psychiatrists met with the parents; reviewed the feeding history and medical examination obtained by the nurse, the nutritional assessment, and the oral motor assessment; and then observed from behind a one-way mirror the mother and child during a lunch meal followed by 10 minutes of free play.

The mother was asked to feed the child foods that she usually fed him or her at home and to bring food for herself as well. She was instructed to feed her child in whatever manner she was used to feeding him or her at home. She was given a choice of a high chair or small chair for the child and was offered toys if she used them as distractions at home. After 20–30 minutes of feeding, the meal was terminated and the child was given a basket of age-appropriate toys in order to play with the mother.

The feeding was directly observed by the first psychiatrist and the nurse from behind the one-way mirror. At the same time, feeding and play were also videotaped for the independent assessment by the second psychiatrist and for the rating of mother-child interactions by blind observers. After the lunch meal, the first psychiatrist obtained additional information from the parents about the child's feeding behavior and family history as indicated.

After completion of their assessments, the psychiatrist and the nurse independently filled out a diagnostic form indicating which diagnoses they assigned to the child. At a later time, the second psychiatrist was given written reports of the feeding history, the medical assessment, the nutritional assessment, and the oral motor and sensory assessment, and also the videotape of mother and child during feeding and play. The second psychiatrist filled out the diagnostic form without having had direct contact with the child or the parents. The two psychiatrists alternated with the first and second evaluation.

OTHER MEASURES

The Child History Questionnaire

The Child History Questionnaire (Chatoor et al. 2001b) assesses race, religion, family structure, parental education, socioeconomic status, and a child's medical/developmental history since birth. It has been used by the principal investigator in several studies and was updated and revised by a group of psychiatrists at Children's National Medical Center in 2001. It is currently used in the department of psychiatry at Children's National Medical Center for research and clinical purposes.

Diagnostic Interview of Feeding Disorders in Infants and Young Children

The Diagnostic Interview of Feeding Disorders in Infants and Young Children (I. Chatoor, L. McWade, R. Simenson, et al. unpublished, 2000, 2001, 2002) was administered by the nurse on the team before her clinical assessment. The interview was first developed in 2000 but revised in 2001 and 2002 as we gathered more experience with it. It contains questions for the six feeding disorders classified by Chatoor (2002) as well as questions for two oral motor feeding disorders secondary to anatomical abnormalities or neurological impairment and questions about an oppositional feeding disorder. Each feeding disorder has two or three main questions that, if answered positively, lead to a set of additional questions to solidify the diagnosis.

Anthropometric Measures of Growth Deficiency

Children's growth status was assessed by weight, length/height, and head circumference using methods described by Gibson (1990). For the assessment of growth deficiency, we used criteria defined by Waterlow et al. (1977).

Acute malnutrition.   Weight for height reflects current or "acute" nutritional status. The reference "normal" is 50th percentile weight for height (Kuczmarski et al. 2000). The current weight divided by this number provides the percent of ideal body weight. Mild, moderate, and severe acute malnutrition correspond with 80%–89%, 70%–79%, and less than 70% of ideal weight, respectively.

Chronic malnutrition.   Chronic malnutrition is assessed by the child's height for age. The child's actual height is divided by the height that corresponds to the 50th percentile for age, or "ideal height." Mild, moderate, and severe chronic malnutrition correspond with 90%–95%, 85%–89%, and less than 85% of ideal height, respectively.

STATISTICAL ANALYSIS

Diagnostic agreement between the psychiatrist and nurse practitioner ($n=431$) and between the two psychiatrists ($n=438$) was assessed using kappa coefficients with 95% confidence intervals (CIs). LCA was performed on a subsample of 322 cases that had standard diagnostic data available. Because no children were seen in the clinic with feeding disorder of state regulation or feeding disorder associated with lack of parent-infant reciprocity, only dichotomous questions for the following five diagnoses were used for LCA:

- *Infantile anorexia:* Does not eat enough; not gaining weight; little interest in eating
- *Sensory food aversions:* Has a limited diet; consistently refuses certain foods
- *Feeding disorder associated with a medical condition:* Becomes uncomfortable during feeding; gets upset and stops eating; cannot calm himself or herself; tires quickly

- *Posttraumatic feeding disorder:* Refuses the bottle; refuses solid food; refuses all food; the food refusal started after traumatic events
- *Oral motor feeding disorder (nonpsychiatric diagnosis):* Has anatomical or neurological impairment; difficulty sucking; difficulty chewing; difficulty swallowing; difficulty drinking

Analyses were conducted with Latent GOLD Version 4.5 software (Statistical Innovations Inc. 2005). The number of latent classes was determined using several parsimony indices, including the Bayesian information criterion (Sclove 1987), the sample-size adjusted Bayesian information criterion (Yang 2006), the Akaike information criterion (Akaike 1987), and the consistent Akaike information criterion (Bozdogan 1987). The assumption of conditional independence was evaluated using bivariate residuals. Cross-tabulations were performed between empirical class membership (as determined by posterior probabilities) and feeding disorder diagnoses. Validation of the empirical latent classes was established by comparing the percent of cases within each class on acute malnutrition, chronic malnutrition, and head circumference less than 25%.

Results

INTERRATER AGREEMENT

Kappa coefficients (95% CI) between the psychiatrist and the nurse practitioner were 0.82 (0.77–0.88) for infantile anorexia, 0.77 (0.69–0.82) for sensory food aversions, 0.76 (0.68–0.74) for posttraumatic feeding disorder, and 0.58 (0.47–0.69) for feeding disorder associated with a medical condition. Kappa coefficients between the two psychiatrists were 0.71 (0.65–0.78) for infantile anorexia, 0.63 (0.55–0.70) for sensory food aversions, 0.62 (0.52–0.71) for posttraumatic feeding disorder, and 0.59 (0.48–0.69) for feeding disorder associated with a medical condition.

LATENT CLASS ANALYSIS

LCA was performed on a subsample of 322 cases (120 girls, 202 boys) with a mean age of 28.6 months (range, 3–120 months). Chatoor's (2002) proposed feeding disorder diagnoses were not mutually exclusive. A total of 148 children were diagnosed with infantile anorexia, 212 with sensory food aversion, 48 with posttraumatic feeding disorder, 47 with feeding disorder secondary to a medical condition, and 22 with oral motor feeding disorder. Table 13–1 shows the pattern of observed comorbid feeding disorder diagnoses. A total of 177 children (55.0%) had a single diagnosis, 135 (41.9%) had two feeding disorder diagnoses, and 10 (3.1%) had three diagnoses. The most common comorbidity by far was between infantile an-

TABLE 13–1.   Feeding disorder diagnostic comorbidity

Number of diagnoses	Diagnoses	Frequency
One (*n*=177)	SFA	94
	IA	52
	PTFD	13
	FDSM	13
	OMFD	5
Two (*n*=135)	IA + SFA	84
	PTFD + FDSM	14
	SFA + PTFD	11
	SFA + FDSM	7
	SFA + OMFD	7
	IA + FDSM	5
	FDSM + OMFD	3
	PTFD + OMFD	2
	IA + PTFD	1
	IA + OMFD	1
Three (*n*=10)	IA + SFA+ PTFD	3
	IA + SFA+ FDSM	2
	SFA + PTFD + OMFD	2
	Other	3

Note. FDSM=feeding disorder secondary to a medical condition; IA=infantile anorexia; OMFD=oral-motor feeding disorder; PTFD=posttraumatic feeding disorder; SFA=sensory food aversions.

orexia and sensory food aversions, either with or without another feeding disorder diagnosis.

LCA revealed a clear and unambiguous five-class solution. The results of the analyses are presented in Figure 13–1. The lines in the graph represent each of the five latent classes identified, the x-axis represents each of the dichotomous indicator variables organized by feeding disorder type, and the y-axis represents the proportion within each latent class endorsing that symptom. Class 1 (*n*=74; 23.0%) showed rates of endorsement exceeding 90% for each of the three symptoms of infantile anorexia and much lower rates of endorsement for all other symptoms. This class was labeled "infantile anorexia." Class 2 (*n*=84; 26.1%) showed high rates of endorsement for the two symptoms of sensory food aversions and low rates for all other symptoms. This class was labeled "sensory food aversions." Class 3 (*n*=25; 7.8%) showed rates of endorsement ranging from 0.4 to 0.8 on symptoms of oral-motor feeding disorder and rates of endorsement ranging from 0.4 to 0.6 on symptoms of infantile anorexia and sensory food aversions. Interpretation of this class must take into account the relative rates of endorsement in relation to other latent classes. Class 3 had much higher rates of endorsement on symptoms of oral-motor feeding disorder than any other class; in contrast, several other classes had higher rates of endorsement on symptoms of infantile anorexia and sensory food aversions in comparison to class 3. As such, class 3 was labeled "oral motor feeding disorder." Class 4 (*n*=105; 32.6%) showed high rates of endorsement on both infantile anorexia and sensory food aversions (the most frequently observed comorbidity) but low rates of endorsement on all other symptoms. This class was labeled "infantile anorexia plus sensory food aversions." Finally, class 5 (*n*=34; 10.6%) showed moderate rates of endorsement on most symptoms other than those from oral-motor feeding disorder. This class was labeled "mixture."

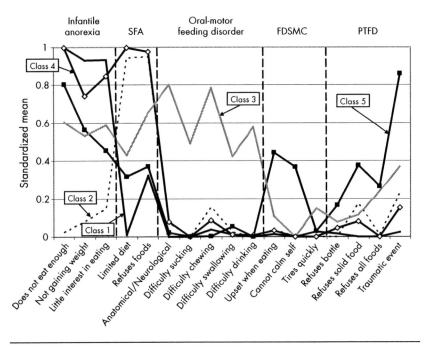

FIGURE 13–1. Latent class analysis of infants and children with feeding disorder diagnoses.

Standardized mean represents the proportion of cases in each class meeting the criteria. Class 1 is the *solid black line with no markers;* Class 2 is the *dashed black line;* Class 3 is the *solid gray line;* Class 4 is the *solid black line with open diamond markers;* Class 5 is the *solid black line with filled square markers.*

FDSMC = feeding disorder secondary to medical condition; PTFD = posttraumatic feeding disorder; SFA = sensory food aversions.

LATENT CLASS VERSUS FEEDING DISORDER DIAGNOSES

The relationship between latent class membership based upon posterior probabilities and feeding disorder diagnoses is presented in Table 13–2. A significant association was found between empirical and diagnostic classification (χ^2_{28}=349.29; P<0.001). Consistent with the interpretation of classes: 1) the majority (82.7%) of cases with a diagnosis of infantile anorexia only were assigned to class 1; 2) the majority (68.1%) of cases with a diagnosis of sensory food aversions only were assigned to class 2; 3) the majority (60.0%) of cases with a diagnosis of oral-motor feeding disorder only were assigned to class 3; 4) the majority (63.1%) of cases with a diagnosis of infantile anorexia and sensory food aversions without another diagnosis were assigned to class 4; and 5) class 5 included a mixture of cases with many different feeding disorder diagnoses.

VALIDATION OF EMPIRICAL CLASSES

Table 13–3 presents a comparison of latent classes on measures of malnutrition. Significant differences between latent classes in rates of acute malnutrition were observed (χ^2_4=68.35; P<0.001), with the highest rates found in class 1 (73.0%) and the lowest rates in class 2 (9.5%). A similar pattern of results was found for chronic malnutrition (χ^2_4=33.57; P<0.001), with the highest rates again found in class 1 (56.8%) and the lowest rates in class 2 (14.3%). Finally, head circumference also differed significantly by latent class (χ^2_4=44.40; P<0.001), with the highest rates of head circumference < 25% found in class 1 (54.1%) and the lowest rates in class 2 (7.1%).

Discussion

This study demonstrated that Chatoor's (2002) proposed diagnoses of infantile anorexia, sensory food aversions, and posttraumatic feeding disorder were diagnosed with high interrater agreement by two clinicians who had direct contact with the child and the parents (κ range, 0.76–0.82) and with good agreement by a third clinician, who determined the diagnoses from written reports and the observation of mother and child during feeding and play on videotape (κ range, 0.62–0.71). The diagnosis of feeding disorder associated with a medical condition had lower levels of agreement (κ=0.58 and 0.59, respectively). Whereas the majority of the children had a single diagnosis, 135 had two diagnoses, and 10 children carried three diagnoses. The most common feeding disorder was sensory food aversions (212 children), and the most common comorbidity was between infantile anorexia and sensory food aversions (84 children). Feeding disorder associated with a medical condition was often associated with other feeding disorders, especially with posttraumatic feeding disorder, which made the diagnosis more difficult.

The LCAs that examined the correspondence between the clinical feeding disorder diagnoses and empirical classes provided good empirical support for infantile

TABLE 13–2. Relationship between latent class membership and feeding disorder diagnoses

Feeding disorder diagnosis	n	Class 1: IA ($n=74$)	Class 2: SFA ($n=84$)	Class 3: OMFD ($n=25$)	Class 4: IA + SFA ($n=105$)	Class 5: Mixture ($n=34$)
				Latent class		
IA only	52	43 (82.7%)	0 (0%)	1 (1.9%)	7 (13.4%)	1 (1.9%)
SFA only	94	0 (0%)	64 (68.1%)	3 (3.2%)	24 (25.5%)	3 (3.2%)
OMFD only	5	0 (0%)	2 (40.0%)	3 (60.0%)	0 (0%)	0 (0%)
Feeding disorder secondary to medical condition only	13	4 (30.8%)	0 (0%)	3 (23.1%)	0 (0%)	6 (46.2%)
Posttraumatic feeding disorder only	13	0 (0%)	1 (7.7%)	1 (7.7%)	3 (23.1%)	8 (61.5%)
IA plus SFA	84	18 (21.4%)	7 (8.3%)	2 (2.4%)	53 (63.1%)	4 (4.8%)
Two other diagnoses	51	8 (15.7%)	5 (10.0%)	9 (17.6%)	14 (27.5%)	10 (19.6%)
Three other diagnoses	10	1 (10.0%)	0 (0%)	3 (30.0%)	4 (40.0%)	2 (20.0%)

Note. IA = infantile anorexia; OMFD = oral-motor feeding disorder; SFA = sensory food aversions.

TABLE 13–3.   Validation of latent classes on measures of malnutrition

Validator	Latent class				
	Class 1: IA ($n=74$)	Class 2: SFA ($n=84$)	Class 3: OMFD ($n=25$)	Class 4: IA+SFA ($n=105$)	Class 5: Mixture ($n=34$)
Acute malnutrition	54 (73.0%)	8 (9.5%)	8 (32.0%)	51 (48.6%)	15 (44.1%)
Chronic malnutrition	42 (56.8%)	12 (14.3%)	12 (48.0%)	46 (43.8%)	12 (35.3%)
Less than 25% head circumference	40 (54.1%)	6 (7.1%)	13 (52.0%)	38 (36.2%)	11 (32.4%)

Note.   IA=infantile anorexia; OMFD=oral-motor feeding disorder; SFA=sensory food aversions.

anorexia, sensory food aversions, comorbid infantile anorexia and sensory food aversions, and oral motor feeding disorder as distinct classes. A clear class of both posttraumatic feeding disorder and feeding disorder associated with a medical condition did not emerge, likely because of the low number of children presenting with the two disorders, the frequent comorbidity between posttraumatic feeding disorder and feeding disorder associated with a medical condition, and the comorbidity with other feeding disorders. However, the empirical support for the two feeding disorders seen most commonly in the clinic and for their frequent comorbidity was encouraging.

Further support for the difference between infantile anorexia and sensory food aversions came from the growth data, which included measurements of weight, height, and head circumference and review of the children's growth charts. About 15% of children with infantile anorexia showed faltering growth on their growth charts but were still within the normal range, whereas the majority of these children were found to have some form of acute, chronic, or combined forms of malnutrition. In contrast, 75% of the children with sensory food aversions had normal growth parameters. Interestingly, the growth patterns of children with both feeding disorders were very similar to those of children with infantile anorexia only; the sensory food aversions did not seem to contribute to their growth problems.

Children with posttraumatic feeding disorder, those with feeding disorder associated with a medical condition, children who had a combination of these two feeding disorders, and children with three feeding disorders showed a mixed picture, including normal growth parameters and various degrees of acute, chronic, or combined forms of malnutrition. This may be explained by the different times in the course of their illness when the children were referred and by the fact that some were given tube feedings to safeguard their nutrition.

Head circumference measurements, which were taken at the time of evaluation, also showed some differences between the groups. Whereas only a small percentage of children with sensory food aversions and less than 20% of those with infantile anorexia showed a small head circumference (less than the fifth percentile for age), about 40% of children with feeding disorder associated with a medical condition and those with three feeding disorders were found to have a small head circumference. This finding speaks to the seriousness of the feeding difficulties in children who have medical conditions and in those who have several feeding disorders at the same time.

The findings add to previous validity studies of Chatoor's (2002, 2009) proposed diagnoses. An early study by Chatoor et al. (1997a, 1997b) demonstrated that when rated by blind observers and compared with healthy mother-infant pairs, mothers and infants with feeding disorder of state regulation (then called feeding disorder of homeostasis) and those with feeding disorder associated with lack of parent-infant reciprocity (then called feeding disorder of attachment) were characterized by low dyadic reciprocity. Additionally, the latter group demonstrated high maternal noncontingency. In contrast, mothers and toddlers with infantile anorexia showed only somewhat less reciprocity than control subjects but demonstrated high scores on dyadic conflict, struggle for control, talk, and distraction. The next study by Chatoor et al. (1998) examined mother-toddler interactions of toddlers with infantile anorexia, toddlers with sensory food aversions (then called picky eaters), and healthy control children. The same pattern emerged; the mothers and toddlers with infantile anorexia showed significant problems in all interactional domains, but their feeding interactions were primarily characterized by intense dyadic conflict, struggle for control, talk, and distraction. Interestingly, the mothers and toddlers with sensory food aversions showed similar interactional problems but not to the same degree of severity as those with infantile anorexia. An additional study by Chatoor et al. (2001a) compared the interactions of mothers and toddlers with infantile anorexia with those of mothers and toddlers with posttraumatic feeding disorder and with mothers and toddlers who were healthy eaters. Although the interactions of the mothers and toddlers with posttraumatic feeding disorder were also characterized by high conflict similar to those with infantile anorexia, these toddlers demonstrated intense feeding resistance when positioned for feeding and approached with food, and resistance to swallowing food, which differentiated them from the healthy eaters and from those with infantile anorexia.

Conclusion

Infantile anorexia, sensory food aversions, and posttraumatic feeding disorder can be diagnosed with high interrater agreement and involve different growth patterns and different mother-infant/toddler interactions during feeding. The clinical diagnoses of infantile anorexia and sensory food aversions and the comorbidity of these two feeding disorders in some children could be confirmed empirically through LCA. The smaller number of children with posttraumatic feeding disorder and with feeding disorder associated with a medical condition, and the frequent comorbidity of these feeding disorders with other feeding disorders, did not bring the same clear results of distinct latent classes. However, clinically these feeding disorders can be well differentiated, and accurate diagnosis is essential for successful intervention. A few studies have demonstrated that treatment that may be helpful for one feeding disorder may be ineffective or contraindicated for the other. A randomized, controlled study showed the effectiveness of a behavioral intervention and the ineffectiveness of regulating meals and appetite in the treatment of posttraumatic feeding disorder (Benoit et al. 2000). However, the pilot study by Chatoor et al. (1997a, 1997b) and a recent randomized, controlled treatment study of infantile anorexia demonstrated that facilitating internal regulation of eating through the awareness of hunger and fullness is an effective treatment for this feeding disorder (Chatoor et al. 2009). Although these are only a few studies that testify to the effectiveness of specific interventions for specific feeding disorders, the price of not diagnosing and not treating these feeding disorders when the children are young is too high, as we are beginning to learn from a longitudinal study of infantile anorexia in Rome, Italy, by Lucarelli et al. (2007). The children not only continue to show feeding and growth problems but also develop serious symptoms of anxiety disorders as well as attention and behavioral problems.

References

Akaike H: Factor analysis and AIC. Psychometrika 52:317–332, 1987

American Psychiatric Association: Diagnostic and Statistical Manual of Mental Disorders, 4th Edition. Washington, DC, American Psychiatric Association, 1994

American Psychiatric Association: Diagnostic and Statistical Manual of Mental Disorders, 4th Edition, Text Revision. Washington, DC, American Psychiatric Association, 2000

Benoit D, Wang EE, Zlotkin SH: Discontinuation of enterostomy tube feeding by behavioral treatment in early childhood: a randomized controlled trial. J Pediatr 137:498–503, 2000

Blashfield RK, Sprock J, Fuller AK: Suggested guidelines for including or excluding categories in the DSM-IV. Compr Psychiatry 31:15–19, 1990

Bozdogan H: Model selection and Akaike's information criterion: the general theory and its analytical extensions. Psychometrika 52:345–370, 1987

Chatoor I: Feeding disorders in infants and toddlers: diagnosis and treatment. Child Adolesc Psychiatr Clin N Am 11:163–183, 2002

Chatoor I: Diagnosis and Treatment of Feeding Disorders in Infants, Toddlers, and Young Children. Washington, DC, Zero to Three: National Center for Infants, Toddlers, and Families, 2009

Chatoor I, Ammaniti M: Classifying feeding disorders of infancy and early childhood, in Age and Gender Considerations in Psychiatric Diagnosis: A Research Agenda for DSM-V. Edited by Narrow W, First M, Regier D, et al. Washington, DC, American Psychiatric Association, 2007, pp 227–242

Chatoor I, Getson P, Menvielle E, et al: A feeding scale for research and clinical practice to assess mother-infant interactions in the first three years of life. Infant Ment Health J 18:76–91, 1997a

Chatoor I, Hirsch R, Persinger M: Facilitating internal regulation of eating: a treatment model for infantile anorexia. Infants Young Child 9:12–22, 1997b

Chatoor I, Hirsch R, Ganiban J, et al: Diagnosing infantile anorexia: the observation of mother infant interactions. J Am Acad Child Adolesc Psychiatry 37:959–967, 1998

Chatoor I, Ganiban J, Harrison J, et al: Observation of feeding in the diagnosis of posttraumatic feeding disorder of infancy. J Am Acad Child Adolesc Psychiatry 40:595–602, 2001a

Chatoor I, Thomas J, Warren S, et al: The Child's History Questionnaire. Washington, DC, Children's National Medical Center, 2001b

Chatoor I, Hirsch R, Ganiban J, et al: Facilitating internal regulation: a treatment model for infantile anorexia, in Eating Disorders Research Society: Scientific Program and Abstracts. Brooklyn, NY, 2009, p 76

Gibson RS: Principles of Nutritional Assessment. New York, Oxford University Press, 1990

Kuczmarski RJ, Ogden CL, Grummer-Strawn LM, et al: CDC growth charts: United States. Adv Data 314:1–27, 2000

Lucarelli L, Cimino S, Petrocchi M, et al: Infantile anorexia: a longitudinal study on maternal and child psychopathology, in Eating Disorders Research Society: Scientific Program and Abstracts. Pittsburgh, PA, 2007, p 148

Narrow WE, First MB, Sirovatka PJ, et al: Age and Gender Considerations in Psychiatric Diagnosis: A Research Agenda for DSM-V. Washington, DC, American Psychiatric Association, 2007

Scheeringa M, Anders T, Boris N, et al: Research diagnostic criteria for infants and preschool children: the process and empirical support. J Am Acad Child Adolesc Psychiatry 42:1504–1512, 2003

Sclove S: Application of model-selection criteria to some problems in multivariate analysis. Psychometrika 52:333–343, 1987

Statistical Innovations Inc: Latent GOLD, Version 4.5.0. Belmont, MA, Statistical Innovations Inc, 2005

Waterlow JC, Buzina R, Keller W, et al: The presentation and use of height and weight data for comparing the nutritional status of groups of children under the age of 10 years. Bull World Health Organ 55:489–498, 1977

Yang C: Evaluating latent class analyses in qualitative phenotype identification. Comput Stat Data Anal 50:1090–1104, 2006

14

EATING DISORDERS IN CHILDREN AND ADOLESCENTS

Diagnostic Differences and Clinical Challenges

Julie K. O'Toole, M.D., M.P.H.
Janiece E. DeSocio, Ph.D., R.N., PMHNP-BC
Daniel J. Munoz, Ph.D.
Ross D. Crosby, Ph.D.

The scheduled publication of DSM-5 is of great interest to researchers and clinicians in the field of childhood-onset eating disorders. The appropriateness of existing diagnostic criteria for children has long been debated, and consensus is growing regarding the need for developmentally sensitive criteria that promote earlier identification and treatment (Bravender et al. 2010).

This chapter describes Kartini Clinic's contribution of research data and clinical observations to the March 2009 Eating Disorders Classification and Diagnostic Conference. The systematic use of a semistructured diagnostic interview

We are honored to contribute our voice to the voices of this international forum of colleagues dedicated to the recognition and treatment of eating disorders in children and adolescents.

(the Rating of Eating Disorder Severity for Children [REDS-C]) allowed us to quantify the severity of 16 eating disorder symptoms for a sample of 323 children and adolescents evaluated and treated at Kartini Clinic.

Historically, taxonomists, and more recently geneticists, have focused on identifying recognizable patterns in human disease (Jones and Smith 2005). Many human diseases, such as meningitis, tuberculosis, rheumatoid arthritis, lupus, diabetes, and so on, have recognizable patterns of symptoms but are known to present differently in children than in adults. We approached our study with these questions in mind: How relevant and robust are the DSM-IV (American Psychiatric Association 1994, 2000) criteria in describing eating disorder symptom patterns in a pediatric sample? Are there recognizable symptom patterns unique to children and adolescents with eating disorders? In this chapter, we draw from our research findings and clinical observations to present rationale for changes in DSM diagnostic criteria for eating disorders as they apply to children and adolescents.

Methods

DESCRIPTION OF SETTING

Kartini Clinic is a regional center for evaluation and treatment of children and adolescents with eating disorders located in the Pacific Northwest. The clinic was founded in 1999 and is recognized for family-based treatment of children and adolescents with severe and persistent eating disorder symptoms. The name "Kartini" was chosen in honor of a Javanese princess who was born in 1879 and was identified throughout Southeast Asia as an icon for women's rights and education. The clinic's interdisciplinary treatment approach encompasses pediatric medicine, adolescent medicine, child psychiatry, psychology, social work, physical therapy, and various allied health professions. Therapeutic modalities include medical care, psychopharmacology, family therapy, individual therapy, milieu therapy, art therapy, movement therapy, and yoga. Educational tutoring is incorporated to ameliorate the effects of school absence while children are in the day treatment program. Treatment is offered on a continuum of inpatient hospitalization, day treatment, and outpatient treatment. Approximately 90 patients per year are admitted to the inpatient service for medical stabilization, and a much smaller number of patients who do not meet hospitalization criteria are admitted directly to the day treatment programs. Two day treatment programs are offered: one for college-age youth and one for children and adolescents. Patients treated for anorexia nervosa (AN) and related syndromes range in age from 6 to 22 years. New patients who are age 21 or older are referred elsewhere for adult eating disorder services.

Children and families from within and outside the United States have sought evaluation and treatment at Kartini Clinic, resulting in the aggregation of a large repository of clinical data from patients with childhood-onset eating disorders. Additionally, parents' routine completion of extensive family history questionnaires provides information for construction of genograms that often display a multigenerational spectrum of related disorders. The collection of these data has supported research collaboration with colleagues from the University of Rochester; Pacific University; Vanderbilt University; research centers in Ulleval, Norway, and the United Kingdom; and the Neuropsychiatric Research Institute in Fargo, North Dakota.

SAMPLE

Data from a sample of 323 patients, ages 6–18 years, were extracted from archived clinical records. All patients were admitted to Kartini Clinic between 1999 and 2008 and completed baseline assessments, including the REDS-C as the basis for quantifying eating disorder symptom severity. Other admission data coded for this analysis included patients' height, weight, vital signs (lying and standing), temperature, Tanner stage sexual maturity rating, and menstrual status. Eating disorder diagnoses were determined by history taking, review of the family history questionnaire, physical examination and physical parameters, laboratory test values, and data from the REDS-C diagnostic interview. Distribution of clinical diagnoses by gender, age, and intake body mass index (BMI) is displayed in Table 14–1.

MEASURES

Item scores from the 16 symptoms assessed with the REDS-C were used to quantify the eating disorder symptoms of patients in this analysis. An adult version of the REDS was developed by Elliot Goldner at the University of British Columbia in 1998. Julie O'Toole adapted the REDS for use with children in 1999, with Dr. Goldner's permission (personal communications, 1999). The REDS-C is developmentally appropriate for children and adolescents and can be used with children as young as 6 years of age, with parent input. Each item is scored on a scale from 0 to 4 or 0 to 5, with higher scores indicating greater symptom severity. An item score of 2 or above is considered clinically meaningful. The clinician administers the REDS-C to the child, beginning with question prompts listed with each item and expanding or individualizing the interview as necessary to derive the most accurate symptom ratings. Administration time is approximately 20–30 minutes. Input is elicited from parents to clarify information acquired from the child as necessary, and item scores may be adjusted based on parental input. Items evaluated by the REDS-C include inadequate food intake, diminished food range, binge quantity, objective binge frequency, purge frequency, purge methods, frequency of compulsive or compensatory exercise, BMI adjusted for age, severity of the child's weight loss goals, cognitive drive for thinness, body image disturbance, denial of the seriousness of weight loss, social impact, and physical impact. Factor analysis of the REDS-C yielded three underlying factors/subscales: severity of malnutrition, severity of binge-purge symptoms, and severity of cognitive distortions. Items measuring restricting symptoms are included in the malnutrition subscale. The cognitive distortions subscale includes items measuring the severity of weight loss goals, cognitive drive for thinness, body image disturbance, and denial of the seriousness of weight loss. Cronbach α for the three subscales ranges from 0.79 to 0.88. Interrater reliability was computed based on the item and total scores of three independent raters, with a single-item reliability of 97% and an average interrater reliability of 99%. Research on the REDS-C was approved by the Legacy Health Systems Institutional Review Board (DeSocio et al., in review).

Measures used to collect patient biometrics included standard instruments and procedures for measuring blood pressure (lying and standing), pulse (lying and standing), and height and weight. BMI was calculated using the standard formula ([weight in pounds × 703] divided by [height in inches squared]). BMIs were graphed and coded for severity based on pediatric BMI percentile charts for age. Breast and pubic Tanner staging were used to measure pubertal status. Female menstrual status was recorded as primary amenorrhea or date of last menstrual period for postmenarcheal females and was derived from patient and parent reports. Data from the family history questionnaire, completed by parents at intake, were used to code patient history of child sexual abuse and/or history of self-injurious behaviors.

STATISTICAL ANALYSIS

Data retrieval and coding forms were created to systematize data extraction from paper charts and electronically scanned archives. Data were entered into SPSS Version 15.0 for analysis. Descriptive statistics were computed for the sample as a whole and for subgroups by diagnosis and age.

Latent profile analyses (LPAs) were performed with Latent GOLD Version 4.5 software (Vermunt and Magidson 2000). Six indicators of eating disorder symptoms were used for LPA analysis: 1) BMI percentile (3rd, 5th, 10th, 25th, 50th, 75th, 85th, 90th, 95th, 97th); 2) binge eating frequency (0 = none, 1 = < twice/week, 2 = > twice/week, 3 = daily); 3) purging frequency (0 = none, 1 = < twice/week, 2 = > twice/week, 3 = daily); 4) drive for thinness (0 = least, 5 = most); 5) preoccupation with weight and shape (0 = least, 5 = most); and 6) body image disturbance (0 = least, 5 = most). Model fit was evaluated using several parsimony indices, including the Bayesian information criterion (Sclove 1987), the sample-size adjusted Bayesian information criterion (Yang 2006), the Akaike information criterion (Akaike 1987), and the consistent Akaike information criterion (Bozdogan 1987). LPA classes were compared on baseline demographic and clinical characteristics using analysis of variance with Tukey honestly significant difference post hoc compar-

TABLE 14–1. Baseline demographics and clinical characteristics of the Kartini sample

Intake diagnosis	Sample, n (%)	Gender, n		Mean intake age, years (SD)	Mean intake body mass index (SD)
		Male	Female		
Anorexia nervosa, restricting subtype	173 (54)	22	151	13.5 (2.32) Range, 7.1–18.5	16.9 (2.66) Range, 10.5–27.8
Anorexia nervosa, binge-purge subtype	68 (21)	7	61	15.6 (1.52) Range, 13.0–18.8	19.0 (1.97) Range, 14.1–23.8
Eating disorders not otherwise specified	32 (10)	4	28	12.2 (2.87) Range, 7.3–18.5	16.8 (3.36) Range, 11.5–27.4
Bulimia	20 (6)	0	20	16.1 (1.55) Range, 13.2–18.5	23.1 (2.73) Range, 19.5–28.2
Food phobia	14 (4)	5	9	10.9 (1.48) Range, 8.5–13.8	15.2 (2.07) Range, 12.2–19.7
Selective eating	8 (2.5)	4	4	10.0 (3.08) Range, 6.1–15.3	16.2 (2.78) Range, 14.1–22.6
Binge eating	3 (1)	0	3	11.7 (1.02) Range, 10.5–12.5	23.7 (3.53) Range, 20.3–27.4
Other	5 (1.5)	0	5	10.8 (2.05) Range, 8.2–12.9	20.0 (2.92) Range, 16.7–23.9
Total sample	**N=323**	**42 (13%)**	**281 (87%)**	**13.7 (2.61) Range, 6.1–18.8**	**17.7 (3.15) Range, 10.5–28.2**

isons for continuous measure, and χ^2 with follow-up pairwise post hoc comparisons for categorical measures. Significance levels were set at 0.05 throughout.

Results

Table 14–1 provides a description of the clinical sample. The average age of patients in the sample was 13.7 years, the majority were female (87%), and three-quarters were diagnosed with one of the AN subtypes. The mean BMI at intake was 17.7 (range, 10.5–28.2), indicating a predominantly underweight population.

Table 14–2 displays age-adjusted BMI percentiles for patients by diagnostic group, as measured at intake. The meaning of a child's BMI is relative to his or her age and is more appropriately represented in relationship to BMI percentiles of children of the same age and gender. Although in some ways a problematic biometric, BMI percentiles adjusted for age serve as another parameter of medical compromise and can be useful in evaluating severity of illness.

Table 14–3 displays the mean scores on selected items of the REDS-C by diagnostic subgroup. Severity scores of 2.0 or higher on symptom items are considered clinically meaningful. Patterns of high symptom scores distinguish patients within different diagnostic groups. For example, patients with selective eating (as opposed to AN) are distinguished by relatively low scores on inadequate food intake and relatively high scores on diminished food range. Patients in both subtypes of AN have relatively high scores on inadequate food intake and physical impact compared with patients with bulimia nervosa (BN), who score lower on these two symptom dimensions but score as high as patients with AN on drive for thinness and preoccupation with body weight and shape. Children with food phobia (also referred to as functional dysphagia) score high on inadequate amount of food but show no clinically significant endorsement of cognitive symptoms.

Table 14–4 identifies selected items on the REDS-C that serve as a reasonable match for the existing DSM-IV diagnostic criteria for AN. All patients included in Table 14–4 were recognized by Kartini clinicians as having childhood-onset AN. The table is informative in displaying the proportion of these patients who would not have met existing DSM-IV criteria for a diagnosis of AN, and thus would have been relegated to the diagnostic classification of eating disorder not otherwise specified (EDNOS).

TABLE 14–2. Age-adjusted body mass index percentiles by diagnosis at intake

Intake diagnosis	<3rd percentile	3rd–9th percentile	10th–24th percentile	25th–49th percentile	≥50th percentile
Anorexia nervosa, restricting subtype ($n=173$)	54 (31.2%)	26 (15.0%)	37 (21.4%)	25 (14.5%)	31 (17.9%)
Anorexia nervosa, binge-purge subtype ($n=68$)	7 (10.3%)	8 (11.8%)	17 (25.0%)	15 (22.1%)	21 (30.9%)
Eating disorder not otherwise specified ($n=32$)	9 (28.1%)	4 (12.5%)	6 (18.8%)	4 (12.5%)	9 (28.1%)
Bulimia ($n=20$)	0 (0%)	0 (0%)	0 (0%)	1 (5.0%)	19 (95.0%)
Food phobia ($n=14$)	5 (35.7%)	2 (14.3%)	2 (14.3%)	2 (14.3%)	3 (21.4%)
Selective eating ($n=8$)	0 (0%)	2 (25.0%)	2 (25.0%)	2 (25.0%)	2 (25.0%)
Binge eating ($n=3$)	0 (0%)	0 (0%)	0 (0%)	0 (0%)	3 (100%)
Other ($n=5$)	0 (0%)	0 (0%)	1 (20.0%)	0 (0%)	4 (80.0%)
Total sample ($N=323$)	75 (23.2%)	42 (13.0%)	65 (20.1%)	49 (15.2%)	92 (28.5%)

TABLE 14–3. Summary of mean (SD) scores on selected Rating of Eating Disorder Severity for Children items by diagnosis

	Intake diagnosis				
	AN-R (n=173)	AN-BP (n=68)	BN (n=20)	Food phobia (n=14)	Selective eating (n=8)
Inadequate food	3.4 (1.1)	3.3 (1.2)	0.9 (1.0)	2.8 (1.7)	1.6 (1.1)
Diminished food range	2.8 (1.4)	3.0 (1.5)	1.1 (1.0)	0.9 (1.5)	3.1 (1.0)
Objective binge frequency	0.2 (0.6)	1.3 (1.2)	2.0 (1.0)	0.2 (0.6)	0.4 (0.7)
Purge frequency	0.1 (0.4)	2.6 (1.4)	2.5 (1.2)	0.0 (0.0)	0.0 (0.0)
Compensatory exercise	2.1 (1.6)	2.6 (1.4)	1.5 (1.4)	0.0 (0.0)	0.1 (0.4)
Drive for thinness	2.2 (1.8)	2.6 (1.8)	3.0 (2.1)	0.0 (0.0)	0.1 (0.4)
Preoccupation with weight/shape	2.9 (1.7)	3.8 (1.4)	3.8 (1.5)	0.8 (1.0)	0.5 (1.1)
Body image disturbance	1.5 (1.4)	2.4 (1.5)	2.5 (1.3)	0.1 (0.3)	0.1 (0.4)
Physical impact	3.0 (1.4)	3.1 (1.2)	1.6 (1.3)	1.8 (1.6)	0.4 (0.5)

Note.   AN-BP=anorexia nervosa, binge-purge subtype; AN-R=anorexia nervosa, restricting subtype; BN=bulimia nervosa.

TABLE 14–4. DSM-IV criteria represented by Rating of Eating Disorder Severity for Children item scores in patients diagnosed with anorexia nervosa, divided by age

Age group, years	Criterion A: Refuse body weight ≥85%[a]	Criterion B: Intense fear of weight gain[b]	Criterion C: Body image disturbance[c]	Binge-purge subtype criterion: Purge to avoid weight gain[d]
Ages 7–11 (*n*=43)	18 (42%)	25 (58%)	22 (51%)	0 (0%)
Ages 12 and 13 (*n*=80)	40 (50%)	49 (61%)	42 (53%)	15 (19%)
Ages 14 and 15 (*n*=64)	38 (59%)	36 (56%)	43 (67%)	29 (45%)
Ages 16–18 (*n*=54)	31 (57%)	28 (52%)	27 (50%)	24 (44%)
Subtotal anorexia nervosa subtypes (*n*=241)	127 (53%)	138 (57%)	134 (56%)	68 (28%)

[a]REDS-C score ≥ 2 on item 10, "Severity of Weight Loss Goal."
[b]REDS-C score ≥ 2 on item 11, "Cognitive Drive for Thinness."
[c]REDS-C Score ≥ 2 on item 13, "Body Image Disturbance."
[d]REDS-C Score ≥ 1 (ever purged) on item 7, "Purge Frequency."

LPA revealed a clear and unambiguous four-class solution. Figure 14–1 presents the standardized means for each of the four latent classes on each indicator, with 0 representing the lowest value in the sample and 1 the highest, and with the value of the line representing the mean for each class. The largest class (38.1%) is characterized by low BMI percentile, the absence of binge eating and purging, and low levels of cognitive eating disturbance. This class was labeled "low weight/low cognitive disturbance" and is depicted by the dashed black line. The second largest class (27.6%) is characterized by low BMI percentile, the absence of binge eating and purging, and moderate levels of cognitive eating disturbance. This class was labeled "low weight/moderate cognitive disturbance" and is depicted by the solid black line. The third class (23.5%) is characterized by higher BMI percentile, more frequent binge eating and purging, and moderate levels of cognitive eating disturbance. This class was labeled "binge-purge/moderate cognitive disturbance" and is depicted by the dashed gray line. The smallest class (10.8%) is characterized by higher BMI percentile, more frequent binge eating and purging, and the highest levels of cognitive eating disturbance. This class was labeled "binge-purge/high cognitive disturbance" and is depicted by the solid gray line.

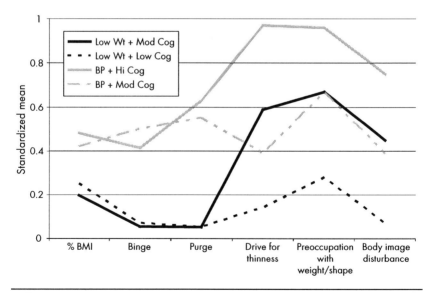

FIGURE 14–1.　Standardized means of symptom indicators in four latent classes.

The standardized mean is the value of the indicator, standardized on a 0 (lowest) to 1 (highest) scale.

BMI=body mass index; BP=binge-purge; Hi Cog=high cognitive disturbance; Low Cog=low cognitive disturbance; Low Wt=low weight; Mod Cog=moderate cognitive disturbance.

Table 14–5 presents cross-tabulations between the empirical classes derived from LPA and clinical intake diagnosis. Almost 90% of AN/restricting patients were classified in one of the two low weight classes, whereas slightly more than 90% of AN/binge-purge patients and 95% of BN patients were classified in one of the two binge-purge classes. This finding is consistent with other studies in this volume (see Chapters 8 and 9) in which low-weight patients were assigned to different empirical classes depending upon the presence or absence of binge eating and purging. In addition, more than 80% of patients with EDNOS and all patients with food phobia or selective eating were classified in the low weight/low cognitive eating disturbance class.

Comparisons between classes on baseline demographic and clinical characteristics are presented in Table 14–6. Patients in the binge-purge classes were older, had a higher BMI percentile, were more developed in terms of pubertal staging, and were more likely to have a history of self-injurious behavior.

Discussion

Characteristics of our sample are consistent with literature describing an atypical presentation for children and adolescents with eating disorders (Bryant-Waugh et al. 1992, 1996; Nicholls et al. 2000; Rosen 2003). Our data clearly show that not all children whom we recognize as having childhood-onset AN either subscribe to or acknowledge intense fears of weight gain or body image disturbance (Table 14–4). More than 40% of these patients, across all age groups, said they were willing to accept a weight at or above 85% of their expected body weight but were simply not able to get there. We remain curious regarding the reasons for this, although some authors have postulated it is a reflection of cognitive immaturity in reasoning and insight (Becker et al. 2009a, 2009b; Boyer 2006; Rosso et al. 2004).

By current DSM-IV criteria, children and adolescents with restricting symptoms who do not report fear of weight gain or cognitive distortions are, by default, diagnosed with EDNOS. As can be seen in Table 14–4, adherence to the DSM-IV criteria of refusal to gain weight to 85% of expected body weight would have forced almost half of our sample into the diagnostic category of EDNOS. At Kartini Clinic, we recognize that childhood-onset illnesses, including AN, may display a range of symptoms different than those seen in adults. We believe that diagnosing these children and adolescents with EDNOS instead of AN can have far-reaching negative consequences. Misconceptions about EDNOS are falsely reassuring, given the high mortality rate for these disorders (Crow et al. 2009). A diagnosis of EDNOS can mask the severity of a child's illness, allowing clinicians and parents to minimize the urgency of treatment ("let's wait and see"), patients to minimize the seriousness of their symptoms ("I'm not as bad as they are"), and insurance companies to deny benefits because "the patient doesn't meet criteria."

TABLE 14–5. Empirical classification by clinical intake diagnosis

	Empirical class, n (%)			
Clinical intake diagnosis	Low weight/ Low cognition	Low weight/ Moderate cognition	Binge-purge/ Moderate cognition	Binge-purge/ High cognition
Anorexia nervosa, restricting subtype	67 (38.7)	87 (50.3)	12 (6.9)	7 (4.0)
Anorexia nervosa, binge-purge subtype	4 (5.9)	2 (2.9)	44 (64.7)	18 (26.5)
Eating disorder not otherwise specified	26 (81.3)	0 (0.0)	6 (18.8)	0 (0.0)
Bulimia	1 (5.0)	0 (0.0)	9 (45.0)	10 (50.0)
Food phobia	14 (100)	0 (0.0)	0 (0.0)	0 (0.0)
Selective eating	8 (100)	0 (0.0)	0 (0.0)	0 (0.0)
Binge eating disorder	1 (33.3)	0 (0.0)	2 (66.7)	0 (0.0)
Other	2 (40.0)	0 (0.0)	3 (60.0)	0 (0.0)

TABLE 14–6. Latent profile analysis baseline comparisons

Baseline characteristic	Empirical class				Significance
	Low weight/ Low cognition	Low weight/ Moderate cognition	Binge-purge/ Moderate cognition	Binge-purge/ High cognition	
Age in years, mean (SD)	12.6 (2.6)[a]	13.3 (2.4)[a]	15.2 (2.2)[b]	15.5 (1.6)[b]	<0.001
Female, n (%)	102 (82.9)	75 (84.3)	70 (92.1)	34 (97.1)	0.062
Body mass index percentile	27.0 (27.0)[a]	20.5 (22.5)[a]	43.2 (28.9)[b]	47.5 (29.3)[b]	<0.001
Standing pulse, mean (SD)	86.8 (17.7)	83.1 (20.3)	81.1 (15.5)	83.9 (13.7)	0.171
Standing systolic blood pressure, mean (SD)	94.9 (13.1)	92.9 (10.5)	98.5 (12.7)	96.9 (11.9)	0.047
Standing diastolic blood pressure, mean (SD)	66.2 (11.0)	66.1 (9.4)	69.0 (9.5)	64.1 (11.1)	0.098
Tanner breast stage, mean (SD)	2.7 (1.4)[a]	2.9 (1.4)[a]	3.9 (0.8)[b]	4.1 (0.6)[b]	<0.001
Tanner pubic stage, mean (SD)	2.8 (1.4)[a]	3.0 (1.3)[a]	3.9 (0.8)[b]	4.1 (0.5)[b]	<0.001
History of child sexual abuse, n (%)	4 (3.9)	10 (13.9)	5 (7.7)	1 (3.1)	0.069
History of self-injury, n (%)	7 (9.5)[a]	11 (18.6)[ab]	15 (33.3)[b]	9 (39.1)[b]	0.002

Note. Cell entries without common superscripts are different ($P<0.05$) based upon Tukey honestly significant difference or pairwise χ^2.

LPA yielded four distinct, empirically derived classifications in our sample: 1) low weight/low cognitive disturbance, 2) low weight/moderate cognitive disturbance, 3) binge-purge/moderate cognitive disturbance, and 4) binge-purge/high cognitive disturbance (see Tables 14–5 and 14–6 and Figure 14–1). The finding of four distinct classes in the Kartini sample is similar to findings from other studies (Eddy et al. 2010; see also Chapters 8 and 11, this volume). Similar to Eddy et al. (2010), a significant main effect of age on purging symptoms was detected in our sample (Table 14–6). Table 14–4 shows that purging symptoms associated with AN were absent in the Kartini sample prior to age 12 years and increased after age 14 years.

Unexpected findings of the LPA included 19 patients diagnosed by Kartini clinicians with AN, restricting subtype but classified in LPA binge-purge categories (Table 14–5). Further examination of REDS-C item scores for these 19 patients revealed the following: 15 reported binge episodes but did not purge, and of those with only binge symptoms, 10 reported episodes of binge eating that were "just large enough" to be considered an objective binge and 4 were scored as "subjective" binge episodes only. Thus, a portion of children and adolescents with AN report binge eating but do not purge. These children predominantly engage in restrictive eating punctuated by occasional episodes of eating larger amounts of food, which are usually followed by feelings of guilt and a return to restricting. Also of interest was one 10-year-old girl in our sample who was diagnosed with AN, restricting subtype but classified within a binge-purge category due to symptoms of spitting. Although this symptom is rare in our experience, we have treated other young patients with AN who display frequent spitting because of refusal to swallow their own saliva. Another rare symptom observed in this population is rumination.

On the basis of these findings and our clinical experiences, we believe eating disorders can be conceptualized as recognizable patterns of brain (mal)functioning, with behavioral variations in younger patients that may be accounted for within the framework of developmental neurobiology. Similar to conclusions drawn by Beumont and Touyz (2003), we believe current diagnostic criteria do not allow clinicians to recognize the neurobiological manifestations of AN in its early stages, when treatment has greater potential to be effective and disabling effects are more likely to be prevented. Waiting for extreme emaciation and delusional cognitions to substantiate a diagnosis of AN may contribute to the chronicity of this disorder and the failure of heroic treatment efforts to bring patients to full symptom remission. As proposed by Insel and Wang (2010), the cognitive and behavioral symptoms associated with mental illness may be better understood as late-stage manifestations of underlying neurodevelopmental disorders. This shift in conceptualization of mental disorders, such as AN, would refocus treatment efforts from late-stage amelioration of symptoms to early detection, prevention, and preemptive interventions.

Conclusion

Our findings support arguments made by Bravender et al. (2010) for more developmentally relevant and flexible criteria for diagnosing eating disorders in children and adolescents. We recommend consideration of the following criteria, which we believe more accurately capture the presentation of AN in children and adolescents: 1) inability or refusal to eat adequately despite having done so in the past; 2) restricting calories globally or specifically (e.g., fats), resulting in weight loss regardless of starting point; *or* 3) failure to gain adequate weight in a child whose Tanner stage/age would predict weight gain (i.e., "crossing growth lines" in a downward direction); *and* 4) the absence of other medical diagnoses, such as hyperthyroidism, exogenous deprivation, brain tumor, and so on, that could otherwise account for these symptoms. Additional recommendations for the recognition and treatment of childhood-onset AN are listed in Table 14–7.

TABLE 14–7.   Recommendations for recognizing and treating childhood-onset anorexia nervosa

---

1. Premorbid weight is more important than "ideal" or "average" weight.
2. No arbitrary weight loss cut point should be necessary for diagnosis (e.g., 85%): Catch it early!
3. Amenorrhea is not necessary for diagnosis.
4. Intense fear of fat or fear of becoming fat may not be present, or if present, may not be acknowledged.
5. Body perception disturbance may be missing or not admitted to.
6. Children may be aware of the seriousness of their weight loss but be unable to change their behaviors related to food and exercise.
7. Relentless fidgeting, refusal to sit, and motor agitation are part of a common recognizable pattern of anorexia nervosa in pediatric patients.
8. A rare but recognizable pattern in some children is food restriction based on fear of abdominal pain or nausea as reasons given for not eating.
9. Extinction of eating disorder behaviors and complete weight restoration are essential to return a child or adolescent to health and reestablish normal growth and development.
10. Once symptoms abate and children are weight restored (state), they still have the underlying neurobiological vulnerabilities (traits) associated with the disease and thus require ongoing vigilance by parents and health care providers.

References

Akaike H: Factor analysis and AIC. Psychometrika 52:317–332, 1987

American Psychiatric Association: Diagnostic and Statistical Manual of Mental Disorders, 4th Edition. Washington, DC, American Psychiatric Association, 1994

American Psychiatric Association: Diagnostic and Statistical Manual of Mental Disorders, 4th Edition, Text Revision. Washington, DC, American Psychiatric Association, 2000

Becker AE, Eddy KT, Perloe A: Clarifying criteria for cognitive signs and symptoms for eating disorders in DSM-V. Int J Eat Disord 42:611–619, 2009a

Becker AE, Thomas JJ, Pike KM: Should non-fat-phobic anorexia nervosa be included in DSM-V? Int J Eat Disord 42:620–635, 2009b

Beumont PJ, Touyz SW: What kind of illness is anorexia nervosa? Eur Child Adolesc Psychiatry 12:20–24, 2003

Boyer TW: The development of risk-taking: a multiperspective review. Dev Rev 26:291–345, 2006

Bozdogan H: Model selection and Akaike's information criterion: the general theory and its analytical extensions. Psychometrika 52:345–370, 1987

Bravender T, Bryant-Waugh R, Herzog D, et al: Classification of eating disturbance in children and adolescents: proposed changes for DSM-V. Eur Eat Disord Rev 18:79–89, 2010

Bryant-Waugh R, Lask B, Shafran R: Do doctors recognize eating disorders in children? Arch Dis Child 67:103–105, 1992

Bryant-Waugh R, Hankins M, Shafran R: Prospective follow-up of children with anorexia nervosa. J Youth Adolesc 25:431–437, 1996

Crow SJ, Peterson CB, Swanson SA: Increased mortality in bulimia nervosa and other eating disorders. Am J Psychiatry 166:1342–1346, 2009

DeSocio J, O'Toole J, He H, et al: REDS-C rating of eating disorder severity interview for children and adolescents: psychometric properties and comparison with the modified EDI-2. Manuscript in review

Eddy KT, le Grange D, Crosby RD, et al: Diagnostic classification of eating disorders in children and adolescents: how does DSM-IV-TR compare to empirically derived categories? J Am Acad Child Adolesc Psychiatry 49:277–288, 2010

Insel TR, Wang PS: Rethinking mental illness. JAMA 303:1970–1971, 2010

Jones KL, Smith DW: Smith's Recognizable Patterns of Human Malformations, 6th Edition. New York, Elsevier Saunders, 2005

Nicholls D, Chater R, Lask B: Children into DSM don't go: a comparison of classification systems for eating disorders in children and early adolescents. Int J Eat Disord 28:317–324, 2000

Rosen D: Eating disorders in children and young adolescents: etiology, classification, clinical features and treatment. Adolesc Med 14:49–59, 2003

Rosso IM, Young AD, Femia LA, et al: Cognitive and emotional components of frontal lobe functioning in childhood and adolescence, in Adolescent Brain Development: Vulnerabilities and Opportunities. Edited by Dahl RE, Spear SE. New York, New York Academy of Sciences, 2004, pp 355–362

Sclove S: Application of model-selection criteria to some problems in multivariate analysis. Psychometrika 52:333–343, 1987

Vermunt JK, Magidson J: Latent GOLD User's Guide. Belmont, MA, Statistical Innovations Inc, 2000

Yang C: Evaluating latent class analyses in qualitative phenotype identification. Comput Stat Data Anal 50:1090–1104, 2006

15

LOSS OF CONTROL OVER EATING IN CHILDREN AND ADOLESCENTS

Marian Tanofsky-Kraff, Ph.D.
Susan Z. Yanovski, M.D.
Jack A. Yanovski, M.D., Ph.D.

With the possible inclusion of binge eating disorder (BED) in the upcoming DSM-5 and the alarming rates of adult (Flegal et al. 2010) and pediatric (Ogden et al. 2010) obesity observed in the United States, identifying and illuminating developmental precursors to both conditions is imperative. This chapter focuses on one specific behavior pattern—loss-of-control (LOC) eating in youth—and considers the evidence for LOC as an important risk factor for excessive weight gain and exacerbated disordered eating.

Research support: Intramural Research Program, National Institutes of Health, grant Z01-HD-00641 (to J.A.Y.) from the National Institute of Child Health and Human Development, supplemental funding from National Center on Minority Health and Health Disparities and Office of Behavioral and Social Sciences Research (to J.A.Y.), National Institute of Diabetes and Digestive and Kidney Diseases grant 1R01DK080906-01A1 (to M.T.K.), and Uniformed Services University of the Health Sciences grant R072IC (to M.T.K.). Dr. Yanovski is a commissioned officer in the U.S. Public Health Service. Disclaimer: The opinions and assertions expressed herein are those of the authors and are not to be construed as reflecting the views of the U.S. Public Health Service, Uniformed Services University of the Health Sciences, or the U.S. Department of Defense.

In contrast to classic binge episodes that require the consumption of a large amount of food in addition to a lack of control over what or how much is being consumed, *LOC eating* refers to the sense of being unable to stop eating regardless of the episode size. In this chapter, we address five key questions: 1) When in life does binge eating first begin? For this section, we include only those studies that examined classic binge episodes that involve a reportedly large amount of food accompanied by a sense of LOC over eating. The observed cross-sectional psychological and physiological correlates of binge eating are also reviewed. 2) Do canonical binge eating episodes independently predict the development of adverse physiological and/or psychological outcomes? We then consider the potential impact of LOC eating episodes, using this term to encompass both classic binge eating episodes and episodes in which LOC is experienced without consumption of an objectively large amount of food, to investigate the three final questions: 3) Does the size of LOC eating episodes matter? 4) Does LOC eating with or without consumption of a large amount of food predict an adverse physiological and psychological outcome? 5) What is the impact of binge and LOC eating on body weight and body composition in youth, over both the short term and the longer term? Finally, we consider a sixth question, namely, should there be a child-specific conceptualization of LOC eating?

Question 1: When Does Binge Eating First Begin?

Retrospective studies of adults with BED have suggested that the initiation of binge eating episodes occurs well before adulthood. The recalled average age of first binge episode ranges from 10.6 to 16 years across studies (Abbott et al. 1998; Binford et al. 2004; Grilo and Masheb 2000; Marcus et al. 1995; Mussell et al. 1995; Spurrell et al. 1997), with one study reporting that nearly 6% of adults recollected first binge eating by age 5 years (Spurrell et al. 1997). Such findings have prompted a number of researchers to investigate binge eating behaviors in children and adolescents.

The prevalence of BED, defined according to the DSM-IV (American Psychiatric Association 1994, 2000) criteria, among youth is low. Rates range from approximately 1% in adolescent community samples (e.g., Stice et al. 2009) to more than 6% among obese teenagers seeking weight loss therapy (e.g., Glasofer et al. 2007). Although few children and adolescents meet all symptom criteria for BED, it appears that episodes of binge eating may emerge as early as 6 years of age (Lamerz et al. 2005; Morgan et al. 2002; Tanofsky-Kraff et al. 2004). Most studies used questionnaire methods to assess binge eating; these studies tend to find greater prevalence of binge eating than do structured interview methods. The prevalence rates for binge eating in the absence of the full syndrome are estimated to range from approximately 6% to 57%, with the highest percentages among weight loss treatment–seeking (versus community) samples and higher prevalence among adolescents (versus children; e.g., Goossens et al. 2007, 2009b; Tanofsky-Kraff 2008). Furthermore, binge eating has been found to occur with greater frequency (e.g., 2:1) among girls compared with boys in survey-based assessments (Ackard et al. 2003).

The emergence and considerable prevalence of binge eating in childhood are of concern because of its links to high body weight and poor psychosocial adjustment. Cross-sectional data point to a relationship between the presence of binge eating episodes in children and overweight or obesity in children and adolescents. For instance, among young children (6 years of age), parental reports of children's binge eating were correlated with children's overweight status (Lamerz et al. 2005). In a large survey-based study of boys and girls (9–14 years), children's self-report of binge eating in the past month was associated with higher body weight (Field et al. 1999). A consistent relationship between binge eating and body weight also has been found among older children. In a school-based sample, overweight adolescents were more likely to report binge eating than their normal-weight peers (Neumark-Sztainer et al. 1997). Similar findings have been reported in other adolescent community samples using survey methods (Ackard et al. 2003; Field et al. 1997). Because of selection by participants' body weight, most studies of weight loss treatment–seeking overweight children and adolescents find that those reporting binge eating, whether based on questionnaire or interview methods, have a body mass index (BMI, kg/m^2) similar to that of children and adolescents who do not endorse binge eating (Glasofer et al. 2007; Goldschmidt et al. 2008; Mirch et al. 2006). However, regardless of whether youth are presenting for weight loss therapy or are not seeking treatment, children and adolescents with binge eating can be distinguished by greater psychological symptoms (e.g., depression and disordered eating attitudes) compared with their counterparts without binge eating (e.g., Goossens et al. 2007, 2009b; Tanofsky-Kraff 2008). The relationship between binge eating and psychological distress may be physiologically important, because there are data linking depressive symptoms to insulin resistance in youth (Shomaker et al. 2009b).

Further evidence for the importance of binge eating behaviors among children comes from laboratory data suggesting that youth who self-report binge eating are distinguishable by observable eating patterns likely to promote excessive weight gain. Mirch et al. (2006) studied a sample of 60 obese (BMI > 95th percentile for age and sex) boys and girls (6–12 years of age) seeking medication weight loss treatment. Ten youth endorsed at least one episode of binge eating in the 6 months prior to assessment on a self-report questionnaire. Compared with children who did not endorse binge eating, children who reported binge eating became hungrier earlier following a preload, reported a greater desire to eat, and consumed significantly more energy during laboratory test meals (Mirch et al. 2006). These findings were adjusted for covariates, including body fat-free and fat mass, sex, age, and race, suggesting that these findings cannot be attributed to differences in child body size. In other words, overweight children who self-report binge eating eat more at laboratory test meals and remain sated for less time than overweight youth who do not report binge eating.

In summary, a clear and consistent literature suggests that binge eating begins as early as middle childhood with considerable prevalence. Pediatric binge eating appears to be negatively associated with children's physical and emotional well-being. A positive relationship exists between binge eating in community children and adolescents and increased body weight. Children who report binge eating appear to differ in their eating behavior in laboratory meal studies. Finally, regardless of treatment-seeking status, youth with binge eating appear to struggle with increased disturbed eating attitudes and psychological distress compared with their peers without binge eating.

Question 2: Does Binge Eating Predict the Development of Adverse Physiological and Psychological Outcomes?

Binge eating behaviors have been shown to predict weight gain in a number of longitudinal, pediatric studies. Among adolescent girls from a community sample, binge eating according to interview assessment was associated with elevated weight gain (Stice et al. 1999) and obesity onset (Stice et al. 2002) over a 4-year period. In a large community cohort of youth 9–14 years of age, boys, but not girls, who self-reported binge eating in a survey gained significantly more weight compared with those who reported no binge eating (Field et al. 2003). Among 6- to 12-year-old children at heightened risk for adult obesity by virtue of their own overweight status or parental overweight, self-reported binge eating episodes predicted greater gains in body fat mass approximately 4 years later (Tanofsky-Kraff et al. 2006).

Despite the ample data demonstrating that binge eating predicts fat gain and obesity, it is not well understood how binge eating might impact physiological correlates of adiposity. There are data in adults demonstrating a relationship between BED and physical illnesses (Javaras et al. 2008; Johnson et al. 2001). Although there are preliminary data showing a trend association between binge eating and fasting insulin in youth (Lourenco et al. 2008), the relationship between binge eating and medical conditions independent of adiposity is largely unexplored. Future research on the potential impact binge eating has on the development or worsening of insulin resistance, high triglycerides, and other components of the metabolic syndrome is warranted.

The literature on the psychological outcomes of children and adolescents who report binge eating is surprisingly sparse. Prospective data from a community sample of adolescents suggest that binge eating is predictive of increases in depressive symptoms (Presnell et al. 2009). However, the authors of that study also found that depressive symptoms were predictive of eating pathology, suggesting that depressive and binge eating symptoms may contribute reciprocally over time.

Clearly, more prospective data on the psychological outcome of binge eating during childhood are required. Specifically, studies are needed to determine the natural history of childhood binge episodes. In particular, it is often assumed, but has not been empirically tested, that reports of binge eating during youth are a precursor to a full-syndrome DSM-IV eating disorder, especially BED. Additionally, research is needed to investigate whether such behaviors during childhood predict the development of psychological disturbance such as major depressive disorder and other mood- and anxiety-related syndromes often comorbid with BED in adulthood.

Question 3: Does Size of the Episode Matter?

A great deal of attention has been paid to the relevance of the DSM-IV binge size criterion among children and adolescents. In concordance with the DSM-IV criteria, traditional interview assessments of binge eating behavior require that a binge episode be diagnosed *only* if the amount of food consumed is deemed *unambiguously* large (Bryant-Waugh et al. 1996; Fairburn and Cooper 1993). However, a substantial proportion of youth who describe experiencing LOC over eating do not report having consumed an *unambiguously* large amount of food. In part, it is often difficult for an interviewer to make a size criterion determination for children of different ages, because physically developing boys and girls have vastly varying energy needs. For example, the consumption of an entire large pizza by a child or adolescent of any age would likely be considered *unambiguously* large. By contrast, five slices of pizza eaten by a 16-year-old boy might be less clear and thus deemed an *ambiguously* large amount of food that, even if accompanied by a sense of LOC over eating, might not be classified as an objective binge eating episode. Furthermore, in younger children the size of eating episodes may be limited by parental controls, masking how much a child might have eaten given the opportunity.

Few studies have directly examined the relevance of episode size in pediatric samples, but recent data point to the possibility that the experience of LOC over eating itself, regardless of the reported eating episode size, may be most relevant for determining disordered eating pathology among youth (Shomaker et al. 2009a). Shomaker et al. (2009a) examined 367 non-treatment-seeking youth (ages 6–17 years) who were categorized as reporting objective binge eating, subjective binge eating (LOC over eating while consuming *ambiguously* large amounts of food or less), objective overeating without LOC, or no episodes, according to responses to a structured interview. Children with objective and subjective binge eating generally did not differ in their reports of disordered eating attitudes, emotional eating, eating in the absence of hunger, depressive and anxiety symptoms, or adiposity (Shomaker et al. 2009a). However, both groups that experienced feelings of LOC (i.e., objective and subjective episodes) had significantly greater disordered eating attitudes, emotional eating, eating in the absence of hunger, depressive and anxiety symptoms, and adiposity compared with those reporting objective overeating or no aberrant eating.

Findings from a large, multisite study on the phenomenology of pediatric eating episodes bolster the contention that the experience of LOC, regardless of reported episode size, is the most salient aspect of binge eating behaviors among youth (Tanofsky-Kraff et al. 2007a). Four hundred forty-five children and adolescents from four sites in the United States and Belgium were interviewed to assess aspects of aberrant eating. Episodes involving the experience of LOC (regardless of amount of food reportedly consumed), but not those involving overeating or any eating without LOC, were associated with eating forbidden food before the episode, eating when not hungry, eating alone, and experiencing a desire for secrecy, negative emotions, and a sense of *numbing* while eating (Tanofsky-Kraff et al. 2007a). Despite these consistent data, it should be noted that episode size has been suggested to be of relevance in studies that have examined populations of weight loss treatment–seeking adolescents. Three studies involving interview methodology reported that some, but not all, domains of psychological distress were greater among youth who reported classic binge episodes as compared with those reporting LOC episodes that were *ambiguously* large (Glasofer et al. 2007; Goldschmidt et al. 2008; Goossens et al. 2007). It is plausible that the size of the episode has more relevance to heavier children who are actively attempting to reduce their food intake; alternatively, the failure to find that binge eating episodes are associated with greater psychopathology among non-treatment-seeking samples may be a function of the power of the investigations, because individuals who report classic binge eating episodes and/or meet criteria for BED are more prevalent among those who seek specialized weight reduction treatment.

The notion that the experience of LOC is the most relevant component of a binge episode is often adopted in child studies. A number of research groups use the umbrella term *LOC eating* to refer to both classic objective binge episodes as well as those that involve an *ambiguously* large amount of food. The emerging data on LOC eating suggest its prevalence ranges from 4% to 45%, with higher estimates found among overweight youth (vs. non-overweight) and adolescents (vs. preadolescents) and when a questionnaire (vs. a semistructured interview) was used for the assessment (Tanofsky-Kraff 2008). Youth with LOC—both those reporting objective and subjective episodes—are more likely to be heavier and/or have greater fat mass than youth with no LOC episodes (Shomaker et al. 2009a; Tanofsky-Kraff et al. 2007a).

Children and adolescents with LOC eating, whether assessed by questionnaire or interview, also exhibit greater psychological symptoms and disordered eating cognitions and behaviors (Goossens et al. 2007; Morgan et al. 2002; Tanofsky-Kraff et al. 2004, 2007b, 2008b), as well as dysfunctional emotion regulation strategies (Czaja et al. 2009), compared with their counterparts without LOC. Collectively, these data support the premise that in work with children and adolescents with LOC eating, the size of the episode is often a less salient feature of such aberrant eating episodes.

There are also naturalistic and observational data of pediatric LOC eating that lend support to the behavior as a distinct phenotype. Using ecological momentary assessment (EMA) methodology in a sample of children (8–13 years), Hilbert et al. (2009) found that LOC episodes were associated with greater overall energy intake compared with regular meals. Using this same sample with a different paradigm, the authors found that youth who reported LOC during an interview consumed more snacks following a parent-child test meal than those without LOC eating (Hilbert et al. 2010). In another laboratory study of non-treatment-seeking overweight and non-overweight 8- to 17-year-olds, youth with LOC eating according to interview consumed a greater percentage of calories from carbohydrates, consumed a smaller percentage from protein, ate more snack and dessert-type foods, and ate less meat and dairy across two test meals compared with those without LOC eating (Tanofsky-Kraff et al. 2009b). Furthermore, those with LOC eating experienced greater increases in state negative affect following the meals.

LOC eating may be, in part, a genetically determined behavior. Bolstering the premise that LOC eating may be a highly important marker of disordered eating and excess body weight are data linking children and adolescents with *FTO* rs9939609 obesity-risk alleles and LOC eating according to interview report (Tanofsky-Kraff et al. 2009a). This finding is notable because the relationship was significant after accounting for the contribution of BMI. Taken together, the literature is relatively consistent that both reported and observational data support the view that LOC eating, regardless of the amount of food consumed, appears to be a salient marker of aberrant eating among youth and a distinct behavioral phenotype.

Question 4: Does Loss-of-Control Eating With or Without Consumption of a Large Amount of Food Predict Development of an Adverse Physiological and Psychological Outcome?

To our knowledge, there is only one published study that prospectively examined the naturalistic outcome of children with LOC eating regardless of whether the amount of food reportedly consumed was unambiguously large. A sample of 6- to 12-year-old children, all of whom were at high risk for adult obesity, was administered an interview to assess LOC eating and other constructs of disordered eating, including dietary restraint (Tanofsky-Kraff et al. 2009d). The authors obtained 772 measurements of height and weight from 143 children over 4.5 years. LOC eating, but not disordered eating attitudes or dietary restraint, predicted an increased rate of BMI growth over time. Compared with children without LOC eating, those reporting LOC eating gained an additional mean 2.4 kg of weight per year (Tanofsky-Kraff et al. 2009d). These data suggest that LOC eating, regardless of baseline disordered eating attitudes or dietary restraint, is a potent predictor of excessive body weight gain during middle childhood.

Further research is required to determine whether childhood LOC eating, with or without an unambiguously large amount of food consumed, tends to persist without intervention and is a precursor to clinically significant adverse physiologic and psychological outcomes.

Question 5: What Is the Impact of Binge and/or Loss-of-Control Eating on Weight Loss in Youth?

Given the relationship between binge and LOC eating and increased body weight as well as adult studies suggesting that baseline binge eating may adversely affect weight loss treatment (Sherwood et al. 1999; Yanovski et al. 1994), several studies have explored how such eating behaviors may impact weight loss treatment outcome in youth. There are very preliminary, and somewhat inconsistent, results on this relationship in pediatric samples. Two studies in obese children (collectively ranging in age from 8 to 16 years) reported no significant relationship between pretreatment LOC eating based upon interview assessment and weight loss following behavioral-based programs (Goossens et al. 2009a; Levine et al. 2006). However, although the sample size was small ($N=27$) in the study by Levine et al. (2006), the authors observed a pattern of lower retention among youth with LOC: only 50% of the children with LOC eating completed treatment, compared with 70% of those without such behaviors. By contrast, Goossens et al. (2009a) found that LOC eating was positively, significantly related to program completion among 132 obese youngsters. Yet a third study of 66 adolescents found that the presence of any psychological disorder at baseline predicted less weight loss; however, binge eating episodes examined separately had no impact on treatment outcome and were, in fact, reduced following an inpatient obesity program (Vlierberghe et al. 2009). In another very recent study, questionnaire-assessed binge eating appeared to have an adverse impact on weight change in the short term (Wildes et al. 2010); among a sample of 192 severely obese children (ages 8–12 years), improvements in percent overweight after a family-based weight loss program were observed only for youth without self-reported binge eating.

Taken together, the current findings on the impact of binge or LOC eating and weight loss treatment are inconsistent. Based upon the findings of one study (Wildes et al. 2010), binge eating may be associated with poorer obesity treatment compliance and less weight loss in the short term. Alternatively, weight loss interventions that address and improve maladaptive eating behaviors may reduce such episodes and result in more effective weight outcomes for certain youth, especially if improvement in binge eating is maintained over the long term. Given the dearth of data and inconsistencies in the existing literature, further research is essential to test these hypotheses. In particular, future study in this area requires an examination of the impact of binge and LOC eating on weight loss treatment that involve larger samples and makes use of more precise and/or multiple assessment methods. For instance, rather than the sole reliance on self-report measures of changes in binge or LOC eating, the evaluation of eating behavior via structured clinical interviews, EMA methods, and observation of eating behavior in the laboratory may provide more complete operationalizations of the effects that such eating patterns may have on weight management. Furthermore, adult studies suggest that the persistence or resolution of binge eating during the course of treatment impacts weight loss outcome (Gorin et al. 2008). Similar investigations are required among children. Another area of exploration that is greatly needed is the examination of interventions specifically targeting LOC eating behaviors in youth. There is a significant literature demonstrating that the treatment of BED can be quite effective in reducing binge eating episodes in adults (Brownley et al. 2007; Tanofsky-Kraff et al. 2007c). Building on this body of research, there are preliminary data indicating that reducing binge and LOC eating may be effective for both weight loss (Jones et al. 2008) and obesity prevention (Tanofsky-Kraff et al. 2009b) in youth. Additional exploration of these and other interventions targeting LOC eating is needed to determine if such approaches are also effective for the treatment and prevention of BED in youth.

Question 6: Should There Be a Child-Specific Conceptualization of Loss-of-Control Eating?

Over the past decade, eating disorder experts have considered whether a different conceptualization of binge and/or LOC eating among children is warranted. In 2003, Marcus and Kalarchian pioneered this dialogue by raising the concern that the DSM-IV criteria for BED may not adequately capture binge eating behaviors among children. They proposed provisional BED research criteria for children 14 years of age and younger (Table 15–1, left column). To date, only one study has tested this provisional criteria set (Shapiro et al. 2007). A brief interview measure designed specifically to assess the proposed criteria was administered to 55 overweight children (5–13 years of age) seeking weight loss treatment. The authors diagnosed 30% of the sample with pediatric BED according to Marcus and Kalarchian's (2003) provisional criteria (Shapiro et al. 2007). Given that this prevalence rate somewhat parallels that of adult weight loss treatment–seeking samples (Wilfley et al. 2001;

Yanovski et al. 1993), the authors concluded that these data preliminarily supported Marcus and Kalarchian's contention that child-specific criteria for BED may be warranted.

Building on Marcus and Kalarchian's proposal, we previously recommended that binge and LOC eating among youth be more clearly elucidated (Tanofsky-Kraff 2008; Tanofsky-Kraff and Yanovski 2004). Since pediatric researchers typically make use of adaptations of measures that assess disturbed eating patterns among adults, there is the likelihood that the child-specific features of LOC eating have been potentially overlooked. To address this concern, a multisite investigative team analyzed a number of behavioral, physical, and emotional variables surrounding aberrant eating episodes among 445 children and adolescents ranging in age from 8 to 18 years. The sample included overweight participants initiating weight loss treatment as well as non-treatment-seeking overweight and non-overweight youth (Tanofsky-Kraff et al. 2007a). Hierarchical cluster analysis revealed a small but cohesive subgroup of participants (3% of the sample; $n=15$), 87% of whom had reported engaging in LOC eating behaviors. Behaviors that were reported by this group included having an event (e.g., an argument) trigger the LOC episode, eating alone, and eating while watching television. Additionally, these individuals described the episode as a snack, reported eating despite a lack of hunger, sought secrecy and felt a sense of "numbing out" while eating, were unsure of how much they were eating, and experienced negative emotions before and after eating, including feelings of shame and guilt. Seventy-five percent of these youth were participating in a weight loss treatment study, 80% were overweight, and 80% were adolescent females. Furthermore, almost half of these participants met full or subthreshold frequency criteria (on average, at least four classic binge episodes or eight ambiguously large LOC episodes per month) for DSM-IV BED, compared with 6% for the rest of the sample. Thus, among adolescent females, DSM-IV BED may present in a similar fashion as in adulthood (Tanofsky-Kraff et al. 2007a).

However, a follow-up hierarchical cluster analysis of only the participants age 12 years and younger revealed a somewhat different set of characteristics from results generated by the entire sample. These 15 children, 12 of whom endorsed LOC eating episodes, tended to report that the episode took place at a home other than their own and in the afternoon, and that they were eating more than others (Tanofsky-Kraff et al. 2007a). Similar to the cluster for the entire group, younger children also reported experiencing a negative emotion and a trigger occurring prior to the episode, eating in secret, and feeling numb while eating. Quite notably, however, only 13% of this subgroup met full or subthreshold frequency criteria for DSM-IV BED, suggesting that the current criteria for adults may not adequately identify youth with aberrant LOC eating patterns. Using responses to several interview and self-report assessments, Hilbert and Czaja (2009) conducted a hierarchical cluster analysis in a sample of 120 non-treatment-seeking children ages 8–13 years with and without reported LOC eating behaviors. In addition to endorsing several be-

TABLE 15–1. Criteria for binge eating disorder (BED) in children and loss-of-control eating disorder (LOC-ED) in children 12 years of age and older

Provisional research criteria for diagnosing BED in children (Marcus and Kalarchian 2003)	Provisional criteria for LOC-ED in children 12 years and younger (Tanofsky-Kraff et al. 2008a)
A. Recurrent episodes of binge eating. An episode of binge eating is characterized by both of the following: 1. Food seeking in absence of hunger (e.g., after a full meal) 2. A sense of lack of control over eating (e.g., endorse "When I start to eat, I just can't stop")	A. Recurrent episodes of loss-of-control (LOC) eating. An episode of LOC eating is characterized by both of the following: 1. A sense of lack of control over eating 2. Food seeking in the absence of hunger or after satiation
B. Binge episodes are associated with one or more of the following: 1. Food seeking in response to negative affect (e.g., sadness, boredom, restlessness) 2. Food seeking as a reward 3. Sneaking or hiding food	B. The LOC eating episodes are associated with three or more of the following: 1. Eating in response to negative affect 2. Secrecy regarding the episode 3. Feelings of numbness (lack of awareness) while eating 4. Eating more, or the perception of eating more, than others 5. Negative affect following eating (e.g., shame/guilt)
C. Symptoms persist over a period of 3 months.	C. The LOC eating episodes occur, on average, at least twice a month for 3 months.
D. Eating is not associated with the regular use of inappropriate compensatory behaviors (e.g., purging, fasting, excessive exercise) and does not occur exclusively during the course of anorexia nervosa or bulimia nervosa.	D. Eating is not associated with the regular use of inappropriate compensatory behaviors and does not occur exclusively during the course of anorexia nervosa, bulimia nervosa, or binge eating disorder.

havioral symptoms of adult BED, children with LOC were more likely to report seeking food in the absence of hunger and in response to negative affect and sneaking or hiding food compared with those without LOC. Given these data, the notion of further research examining a child-specific manifestation of LOC eating problems appears reasonable.

Based on the available research on child-specific LOC eating, its characteristics and correlates, we proposed a revised set of criteria (Tanofsky-Kraff et al. 2008a) that extends Marcus and Kalarchian's (2003) provisional criteria. Table 15–1 (right column) lists provisional criteria that require further testing for Loss of Control Eating Disorder (LOC-ED) in children age 12 years and younger. Working from Marcus and Kalarchian's conceptualization, we made a number of modifications. In order to avoid redefining the term *binge, LOC eating* is used to describe consumption of food while experiencing a lack of control over eating *independent* of the amount of food consumed. Criterion A2 has been extended to include "food seeking in the absence of hunger *or after satiation*" because many children report feeling hungry when LOC episodes are initiated (Tanofsky-Kraff et al. 2007a) and do not distinguish between eating in the absence of hunger and eating past satiation during LOC eating episodes (Tanofsky-Kraff et al. 2008b). Criterion B (associated characteristics) has been modified based upon findings from the multisite investigation (Tanofsky-Kraff et al. 2007a). Finally, although current data suggest that episodes of LOC eating occurring once a month or more are associated with distress, we opted for a proposed Criterion C cutoff of two episodes per month to provide a more conservative estimate of the frequency of LOC eating required for a psychiatric diagnosis. Finally, because some children may meet full DSM-IV criteria for BED (Morgan et al. 2002), we have included in Criterion D that LOC-ED should not be diagnosed if BED is present. Validation testing of these proposed criteria is under way.

The existence of a childhood conceptualization of LOC eating patterns and its utility are as yet unclear and require extensive exploration. Nevertheless, the current literature provides evidence that the prevalence of LOC eating during middle childhood is substantial and appears to be associated with psychological distress, overweight, and potentially adverse health outcomes. Therefore, future research into the utility and clinical significance of LOC-ED and other proposed conceptualizations should be undertaken to determine if a syndrome distinguishes children uniquely in need of intervention for further eating disturbances and risk of inappropriate weight gain and psychopathology.

Conclusion

LOC eating appears to be a distinct construct that is prevalent among children and adolescents and is associated with, and predictive of, increased body weight. Furthermore, such episodes in youth are associated with increased disordered eating attitudes and behaviors, and psychological distress. Among youth, LOC eating episode size appears to be less relevant in community samples but may have greater import among overweight adolescents seeking weight loss treatment. Further research is required to elucidate the impact of LOC eating patterns on physical and psychological outcomes as well as in response to weight loss therapy. Consideration of a child-specific conceptualization of LOC eating behaviors may be warranted.

References

Abbott DW, de Zwaan M, Mussell MP, et al: Onset of binge eating and dieting in overweight women: implications for etiology, associated features and treatment. J Psychosom Res 44:367–374, 1998

Ackard DM, Neumark-Sztainer D, Story M, et al: Overeating among adolescents: prevalence and associations with weight-related characteristics and psychological health. Pediatrics 111:67–74, 2003

American Psychiatric Association: Diagnostic and Statistical Manual of Mental Disorders, 4th Edition. Washington, DC, American Psychiatric Association, 1994

American Psychiatric Association: Diagnostic and Statistical Manual of Mental Disorders, 4th Edition, Text Revision. Washington, DC, American Psychiatric Association, 2000

Binford RB, Pederson Mussell M, Peterson CB, et al: Relation of binge eating age of onset to functional aspects of binge eating in binge eating disorder. Int J Eat Disord 35:286–292, 2004

Brownley KA, Berkman ND, Sedway JA, et al: Binge eating disorder treatment: a systematic review of randomized controlled trials. Int J Eat Disord 40:337–348, 2007

Bryant-Waugh RJ, Cooper PJ, Taylor CL, et al: The use of the Eating Disorder Examination with children: a pilot study. Int J Eat Disord 19:391–397, 1996

Czaja J, Rief W, Hilbert A: Emotion regulation and binge eating in children. Int J Eat Disord 42:356–362, 2009

Fairburn CG, Cooper Z: The Eating Disorder Examination, 12th edition, in Binge Eating: Nature, Assessment and Treatment. Edited by Fairburn CG, Wilson GT. New York, Guilford, 1993, pp 317–360

Field AE, Colditz GA, Peterson KE: Racial differences in bulimic behaviors among high school females. Ann N Y Acad Sci 817:359–360, 1997

Field AE, Camargo CA Jr, Taylor CB, et al: Overweight, weight concerns, and bulimic behaviors among girls and boys. J Am Acad Child Adolesc Psychiatry 38:754–760, 1999

Field AE, Austin SB, Taylor CB, et al: Relation between dieting and weight change among preadolescents and adolescents. Pediatrics 112:900–906, 2003

Flegal KM, Carroll MD, Ogden CL, et al: Prevalence and trends in obesity among US adults, 1999–2008. JAMA 303:235–241, 2010

Glasofer DR, Tanofsky-Kraff M, Eddy KT, et al: Binge eating in overweight treatment-seeking adolescents. J Pediatr Psychol 32:95–105, 2007

Goldschmidt AB, Jones M, Manwaring JL, et al: The clinical significance of loss of control over eating in overweight adolescents. Int J Eat Disord 41:153–158, 2008

Goossens L, Braet C, Decaluwé V: Loss of control over eating in obese youngsters. Behav Res Ther 45:1–9, 2007

Goossens L, Braet C, Van Vlierberghe L, et al: Weight parameters and pathological eating as predictors of obesity treatment outcome in children and adolescents. Eat Behav 10:71–73, 2009a

Goossens L, Soenens B, Braet C: Prevalence and characteristics of binge eating in an adolescent community sample. J Clin Child Adolesc Psychol 38:342–353, 2009b

Gorin AA, Niemeier HM, Hogan P, et al: Binge eating and weight loss outcomes in overweight and obese individuals with type 2 diabetes: results from the Look AHEAD trial. Arch Gen Psychiatry 65:1447–1455, 2008

Grilo CM, Masheb RM: Onset of dieting vs binge eating in outpatients with binge eating disorder. Int J Obes Relat Metab Disord 24:404–409, 2000

Hilbert A, Czaja J: Binge eating in primary school children: towards a definition of clinical significance. Int J Eat Disord 42:235–243, 2009

Hilbert A, Rief W, Tuschen-Caffier B, et al: Loss of control eating and psychological maintenance in children: an ecological momentary assessment study. Behav Res Ther 47:26–33, 2009

Hilbert A, Tuschen-Caffier B, Czaja J: Eating behavior and familial interactions of children with loss of control eating: a laboratory test meal study. Am J Clin Nutr 91:510–518, 2010

Javaras KN, Pope HG, Lalonde JK, et al: Co-occurrence of binge eating disorder with psychiatric and medical disorders. J Clin Psychiatry 69:266–273, 2008

Johnson JG, Spitzer RL, Williams JB: Health problems, impairment and illnesses associated with bulimia nervosa and binge eating disorder among primary care and obstetric gynaecology patients. Psychol Med 31:1455–1466, 2001

Jones M, Luce KH, Osborne MI, et al: Randomized, controlled trial of an internet-facilitated intervention for reducing binge eating and overweight in adolescents. Pediatrics 121:453–462, 2008

Lamerz A, Kuepper-Nybelen J, Bruning N, et al: Prevalence of obesity, binge eating, and night eating in a cross-sectional field survey of 6-year-old children and their parents in a German urban population. J Child Psychol Psychiatry 46:385–393, 2005

Levine MD, Ringham RM, Kalarchian MA, et al: Overeating among seriously overweight children seeking treatment: results of the children's eating disorder examination. Int J Eat Disord 39:135–140, 2006

Lourenco BH, Arthur T, Rodrigues MD, et al: Binge eating symptoms, diet composition and metabolic characteristics of obese children and adolescents. Appetite 50:223–230, 2008

Marcus MD, Kalarchian MA: Binge eating in children and adolescents. Int J Eat Disord 34(suppl):S47–S57, 2003

Marcus MD, Moulton MM, Greeno CG: Binge eating onset in obese patients with binge eating disorder. Addict Behav 20:747–755, 1995

Mirch MC, McDuffie JR, Yanovski SZ, et al: Effects of binge eating on satiation, satiety, and energy intake of overweight children. Am J Clin Nutr 84:732–738, 2006

Morgan C, Yanovski S, Nguyen T, et al: Loss of control over eating, adiposity, and psychopathology in overweight children. Int J Eat Disord 31:430–441, 2002

Mussell MP, Mitchell JE, Weller CL, et al: Onset of binge eating, dieting, obesity, and mood disorders among subjects seeking treatment for binge eating disorder. Int J Eat Disord 17:395–401, 1995

Neumark-Sztainer D, Story M, French SA, et al: Psychosocial concerns and health-compromising behaviors among overweight and nonoverweight adolescents. Obes Res 5:237–249, 1997

Ogden CL, Carroll MD, Curtin LR, et al: Prevalence of high body mass index in US children and adolescents, 2007–2008. JAMA 303:242–249, 2010

Presnell K, Stice E, Seidel A, et al: Depression and eating pathology: prospective reciprocal relations in adolescents. Clin Psychol Psychother 16:357–365, 2009

Shapiro JR, Woolson SL, Hamer RM, et al: Evaluating binge eating disorder in children: development of the children's binge eating disorder scale (C-BEDS). Int J Eat Disord 40:82–89, 2007

Sherwood NE, Jeffery RW, Wing RR: Binge status as a predictor of weight loss treatment outcome. Int J Obes Relat Metab Disord 23:485–493, 1999

Shomaker LB, Tanofsky-Kraff M, Elliott C, et al: Salience of loss of control for pediatric binge episodes: does size really matter? Int J Eat Disord October 13, 2009a [Epub ahead of print]

Shomaker LB, Tanofsky-Kraff M, Young-Hyman D, et al: Psychological symptoms and insulin sensitivity in adolescents. Pediatr Diabetes November 11, 2009b [Epub ahead of print]

Spurrell EB, Wilfley DE, Tanofsky MB, et al: Age of onset for binge eating: are there different pathways to binge eating? Int J Eat Disord 21:55–65, 1997

Stice E, Cameron RP, Killen JD, et al: Naturalistic weight-reduction efforts prospectively predict growth in relative weight and onset of obesity among female adolescents. J Consult Clin Psychol 67:967–974, 1999

Stice E, Presnell K, Spangler D: Risk factors for binge eating onset in adolescent girls: a 2-year prospective investigation. Health Psychol 21:131–138, 2002

Stice E, Marti CN, Shaw H, et al: An 8-year longitudinal study of the natural history of threshold, subthreshold, and partial eating disorders from a community sample of adolescents. J Abnorm Psychol 118:587–597, 2009

Tanofsky-Kraff M: Binge eating among children and adolescents, in Handbook of Child and Adolescent Obesity. Edited by Jelalian E, Steele R. New York, Springer, 2008, pp 41–57

Tanofsky-Kraff M, Yanovski SZ: Eating disorder or disordered eating? Non-normative eating patterns in obese individuals. Obes Res 12:1361–1366, 2004

Tanofsky-Kraff M, Yanovski SZ, Wilfley DE, et al: Eating disordered behaviors, body fat, and psychopathology in overweight and normal weight children. J Consult Clin Psychol 72:53–61, 2004

Tanofsky-Kraff M, Cohen ML, Yanovski SZ, et al: A prospective study of psychological predictors of body fat gain among children at high risk for adult obesity. Pediatrics 117:1203–1209, 2006

Tanofsky-Kraff M, Goossens L, Eddy KT, et al: A multisite investigation of binge eating behaviors in children and adolescents. J Consult Clin Psychol 75:901–913, 2007a

Tanofsky-Kraff M, Theim KR, Yanovski SZ, et al: Validation of the emotional eating scale adapted for use in children and adolescents (EES-C). Int J Eat Disord 40:232–240, 2007b

Tanofsky-Kraff M, Wilfley DE, Young JF, et al: Preventing excessive weight gain in adolescents: interpersonal psychotherapy for binge eating. Obesity (Silver Spring) 15:1345–1355, 2007c

Tanofsky-Kraff M, Marcus MD, Yanovski SZ, et al: Loss of control eating disorder in children age 12 years and younger: proposed research criteria. Eat Behav 9:360–365, 2008a

Tanofsky-Kraff M, Ranzenhofer LM, Yanovski SZ, et al: Psychometric properties of a new questionnaire to assess eating in the absence of hunger in children and adolescents. Appetite 51:148–155, 2008b

Tanofsky-Kraff M, Han JC, Anandalingam K, et al: The FTO gene rs9939609 obesity-risk allele and loss of control over eating. Am J Clin Nutr 90:1483–1488, 2009a

Tanofsky-Kraff M, McDuffie JR, Yanovski SZ, et al: Laboratory assessment of the food intake of children and adolescents with loss of control eating. Am J Clin Nutr 89:738–745, 2009b

Tanofsky-Kraff M, Wilfley DE, Young JF, et al: A pilot study of interpersonal psychotherapy for preventing excess weight gain in adolescent girls at-risk for obesity. Int J Eat Disord October 30, 2009c [Epub ahead of print]

Tanofsky-Kraff M, Yanovski SZ, Schvey NA, et al: A prospective study of loss of control eating for body weight gain in children at high risk for adult obesity. Int J Eat Disord 42:26–30, 2009d

Vlierberghe LV, Braet C, Goossens L, et al: Psychological disorder, symptom severity and weight loss in inpatient adolescent obesity treatment. Int J Pediatr Obes 4:36–44, 2009

Wildes JE, Marcus MD, Kalarchian MA, et al: Self-reported binge eating in severe pediatric obesity: impact on weight change in a randomized controlled trial of family-based treatment. Int J Obes (Lond) 34:1143–1148, 2010

Wilfley DE, Pike KM, Dohm FA, et al: Bias in binge eating disorder: how representative are recruited clinic samples? J Consult Clin Psychol 69:383–388, 2001

Yanovski SZ, Nelson JE, Dubbert BK, et al: Association of binge eating disorder and psychiatric comorbidity in obese subjects. Am J Psychiatry 150:1472–1479, 1993

Yanovski SZ, Gormally JF, Leser MS, et al: Binge eating disorder affects outcome of comprehensive very-low-calorie diet treatment. Obes Res 2:205–212, 1994

16

DIAGNOSTIC CLASSIFICATION OF EATING DISORDERS IN CHILDREN AND ADOLESCENTS

How Does DSM-IV-TR Compare to Empirically Derived Categories?

Kamryn T. Eddy, Ph.D.
Daniel Le Grange, Ph.D.
Ross D. Crosby, Ph.D.

The authors wish to acknowledge Leanna Delhey for her assistance with data compilation and entry.

This chapter was first published in Eddy KT, Le Grange D, Crosby RD, et al.: "Diagnostic Classification of Eating Disorders in Children and Adolescents: How Does DSM-IV-TR Compare to Empirically Derived Categories?" *Journal of the American Academy of Child and Adolescent Psychiatry* 49(3):277–287. Copyright Elsevier, 2010.

Support for this research was provided by grants to the first author (K.T.E.) through the National Institute of Mental Health (F32MH084396), Harvard Medical School (Livingston Fellowship Award), and the Harris Center at Massachusetts General Hospital.

This work was presented at the Conference on the Classification and Diagnosis of Eating Disorders, Washington, D.C., March 2009 (NIMH R13MH081447 [Wonderlich]) and at the Eating Disorders Research Society Meeting, Brooklyn, NY, September 2009.

Renee Rienecke Hoste, Ph.D.
Angela Celio Doyle, Ph.D.
Angela Smyth, M.D.
David B. Herzog, M.D.

The phenomenology of eating disorders in children and adolescents is understudied and poorly understood. The current classification system of eating disorders (DSM-IV; American Psychiatric Association 1994, 2000) recognizes three diagnoses: anorexia nervosa (AN), bulimia nervosa (BN), and eating disorder not otherwise specified (EDNOS). AN and BN are defined by specific physical, cognitive, and behavioral criteria; EDNOS is defined instead by eating disorder symptoms that do not meet full criteria for either AN or BN. DSM-IV does not make specific provisions for the diagnosis of eating disorders in children and adolescents. To inform DSM-5, research is needed to determine whether the same symptom clusters and diagnostic presentations observed in adults can be found in children and adolescents.

Indeed, limited empirical work has examined the appropriateness and applicability of the DSM-IV categories to youth, but it has been suggested that different diagnostic thresholds or categories may be needed for younger populations. The Work Group for Classification of Eating Disorders in Children and Adolescents reviewed the literature relevant to nosology in children and adolescents, identifying potential problems with the diagnostic criteria as they are applied to youth (Bravender et al. 2007, 2010). For example, growth and weight gain are expected in children and adolescents, which can challenge application of a strict weight criterion required for the AN diagnosis. Similarly, children and adolescents may be premenarcheal or have not yet established regular menstrual cycles, which makes the AN amenorrhea criterion irrelevant. Importantly, the cognitive eating disorder criteria—extreme fear of weight gain, body image disturbance, and overvaluation of weight and shape—are also difficult to assess and apply in younger patients, who may have limited insight into their motives for eating disorder behaviors, due in part to an underdeveloped capacity for abstract reasoning (Rosso et al. 2004; Yurgelun-Todd 2007). Furthermore, in both adults and youth alike, the twice-weekly frequency criterion for binge eating and purging required for the diagnosis of BN is not empirically based and may be too strict a threshold (Thomas et al. 2009).

Descriptive clinical studies indicate that EDNOS is the most common eating disorder in clinical settings (Eddy et al. 2008; Nicholls et al. 2000; Peebles et al. 2006; Turner and Bryant-Waugh 2004), perhaps as a result of the challenges involved in applying the current eating disorder diagnoses to younger patients. The EDNOS diagnosis is problematic due to its heterogeneity, rendering the amount of specific information conveyed by the EDNOS label minimal. This problem is not unique to youth—EDNOS similarly predominates in adult clinical samples (Fairburn et al. 2007)—but the reasons younger patients are assigned this diagnosis may be distinct, as suggested by the Work Group (Bravender et al. 2007).

Preliminary studies have suggested a lack of clinically meaningful differences between youth with AN and BN and those with EDNOS who narrowly miss criteria for either of the other two disorders (Eddy et al. 2008; Peebles et al. 2006). These study findings support the Work Group's position that the current thresholds for AN and BN may be overly narrow and that relaxing the criteria would allow a subset of youth with EDNOS to be meaningfully reclassified within broadened forms of AN or BN. However, research from our group also demonstrated that a subset of youth with EDNOS did not resemble either AN or BN (Eddy et al. 2008). Indeed, youth with eating problems may present with a distinct set of symptoms including selective or picky eating, for example, which are not currently included within DSM-IV examples of EDNOS (Bravender et al. 2007). Taken together, the literature suggests that the current classification system of eating disorders may be inadequate for categorizing eating pathology in youth.

Empirical approaches can be used to investigate nosology. One such approach utilizes the statistical technique of latent class analysis (LCA) or latent profile analysis (LPA). LCA and LPA identify underlying (or latent) groups of individuals on the basis of their patterned responses across a set of eating disorder features (Wonderlich et al. 2007). LPA has the advantage of allowing for the inclusion of continuous indicators, whereas LCA is limited to categorical indicators. To date, this empirical classification research has been limited to adult samples (Bulik et al. 2000; Duncan et al. 2007; Eddy et al. 2009; Keel et al. 2004; Mitchell et al. 2007; Striegel-Moore et al. 2005; Sullivan et al. 1998; Wade et al. 2006), with the exception of one recent report combining adolescents and young adults (Pinheiro et al. 2008). In adult samples, this research has demonstrated that LCA and LPA reliably identify clinically meaningful subgroups of individuals with eating disorders, including those that resemble AN and BN and one particular type of EDNOS characterized by binge eating without purging (binge eating disorder [BED]) (Bulik et al. 2000; Eddy et al. 2009; Keel et al. 2004; Striegel-Moore et al. 2005). However, the resemblance is imperfect, and subthreshold presentations cluster with similar full-syndrome disorders (Bulik et al. 2000; Keel et al. 2004; Striegel-Moore et al. 2005).

Because developmental differences between children, adolescents, and adults may result in unique sets of challenges related to the fit of the DSM-IV eating disorder criteria (Bravender et al. 2007, 2010; Eddy et al. 2008), empirical studies are needed to characterize the full range of individuals who seek treatment for eating disorders. Although it is possible that similar eating disorder phenotypes will be identified in younger samples as have been identified in adults, unique child or adolescent phenotypes may emerge. Because the onset of eating disorders most often occurs in adolescence, failure to characterize younger patients with eating disorders (and to examine them separately from adults) is problematic.

Given that the diagnostic classification system plays a critical role in guiding clinical practice and research, ensuring that this system accurately organizes and includes the full range of psychopathology in individuals of all ages is imperative. This study was designed to examine diagnostic classification in children and adolescents using an empirical approach that has been useful in nosological studies of adult samples. Specifically, we sought 1) to determine whether an empirical classification system of eating disorders in adolescents could be derived using LPA, 2) to examine the concordance of latent profile group membership with DSM-IV eating disorder diagnoses, and 3) to compare the validity of the two classification systems across cross-sectional and outcome indices. On the basis of the descriptive child and adolescent literature and the adult LCA/LPA studies, we hypothesized that LPA would successfully identify eating disorder phenotypes in youth and that these would resemble the DSM-IV diagnoses imperfectly.

Method

PARTICIPANTS

Data were collected from 401 consecutive children and adolescents evaluated through the Eating Disorders Program at the University of Chicago Medical Center between October 2001 and April 2009. The Eating Disorders Program is a specialist outpatient treatment setting at a tertiary medical institution. Three hundred sixty-three girls (90.5%) and 38 boys (9.5%) participated. The mean age of participants was 15.14 ± 2.35 years. The majority (73.9%) were Caucasian, 12.4% were Hispanic, 8.9% were African American, and 2.0% were Asian; 2.8% identified as another race/ethnicity.

Follow-up data were available for a subset of these participants who had completed more than 3 months of treatment (n=229; 57.1%). The mean duration between pretreatment and follow-up was 11.19 ± 5.59 months.

PROCEDURE

This study was approved by the Institutional Review Board at The University of Chicago Medical Center. Data were collected at baseline, prior to the initiation of treatment, as well as at the end of treatment or the last available follow-up point for a subset. Each child/adolescent gave written assent, and a parent/guardian gave written consent for protocol participation. Fewer than 10% of youth presenting for treatment during this time period did not consent to have their data included in this research database; nonparticipants did not differ from participants with regard to demographics.

MEASURES

Intake (Pretreatment)

Eating Disorder Examination Version 12.0D/C.2 or Version Adapted for Children.
Both the adult and child versions of the Eating Disorder Examination (EDE; Bryant-Waugh et al. 1996; Fairburn and Cooper 1993) assess eating-related behaviors and cognitions to diagnose specific DSM-IV eating disorders and yield four dimensional scales: Dietary Restraint, Eating Concern, Shape Concern, and Weight Concern; a global scale is calculated as the average of the four scales. For each of the scales, scores range from 0 to 6, with higher scores indicating increased eating disorder pathology. The presence and frequency of specific eating and compensatory behaviors during the 3 months before the assessment are collected, including objective binge eating, subjective binge eating (collected only 1 month before the assessment), self-induced vomiting, misuse of laxatives or diuretics, excessive exercising, and fasting. The EDE has shown excellent reliability and validity (Cooper et al. 1989; Fairburn and Cooper 1993), and studies indicate that the child interview also demonstrates good reliability and validity (Bryant-Waugh et al. 1996; Tanofsky-Kraff et al. 2004; Watkins et al. 2005). Interviewers were trained in the administration of both the adult and child versions of the interview, which capture the same sets of symptoms, and were able to use the more simple language in the child version to ensure comprehension by children and younger adolescents.

DSM-IV diagnoses of AN and BN were assigned based on EDE-generated behavioral and cognitive symptoms. Eating disorder presentations that did not meet DSM-IV criteria for AN or BN were categorized as EDNOS. Due to its heterogeneity, we divided EDNOS into clinically meaningful categories of subthreshold AN, subthreshold BN, BED, and purge disorder, along with an EDNOS "other" category that included individuals who could not be classified elsewhere (Eddy et al. 2008).

Beck Depression Inventory.　The Beck Depression Inventory (BDI; Beck 1987) is a self-report measure of depressive symptoms; scores range from 0 to 63; a score of 10–18 suggests mild/moderate depressive symptoms and a score higher than 18 indicates moderate/severe depressive symptoms. This measure is widely used and has demonstrated good psychometric properties and strong associations with clinical depression; it has recently been used in two randomized, controlled clinical trials of adolescent AN (Lock et al. 2005) and BN (le Grange et al. 2007).

Rosenberg Self-Esteem Scale.　The Rosenberg Self-Esteem Scale (Rosenberg 1965) is a self-report measure of overall self-esteem; scores range from 0 to 30; scores less than 15 suggest low self-esteem. This measure has demonstrated adequate reliability and validity in adolescents (Hagborg 1996).

Follow-Up

Self-reported frequency of objective binge eating and purging (by self-induced vomiting, misuse of laxatives or diuretics) during the past 4 weeks was ascertained.

Physical assessment.   At both pretreatment and follow-up, participants were weighed on a calibrated digital or balance-beam scale in light indoor clothing; height was obtained using a calibrated stadiometer.

STATISTICAL ANALYSIS

Latent Profile Analysis

Four hundred one cases were included in the LPA (Lazarsfeld and Henry 1968). The analyses were also run with male participants excluded, and the results were unchanged. LPA posits that a heterogeneous group can be broken down to a finite number of homogeneous subgroups through minimizing associations among responses across multiple indicators. In doing so, LPA identifies the number and composition of unobserved latent groups, which themselves are mutually exclusive. The number of latent profiles was determined by three information criterion indices: the Bayesian information criterion (BIC) parsimony index (Sclove 1987), the sample-size adjusted BIC (ABIC; Croudace et al. 2003), and the consistent Akaike information criterion (CAIC), which was suggested by Bozdogan (1987). The BIC expresses model fit as a function of log-likelihood, sample size, and number of model parameters. The CAIC is derived from the Akaike information criterion (Akaike 1987), which determines model fit on the basis of log-likelihood of the model and number of estimated parameters; the advantage of using the CAIC is that it includes a penalty for models having larger numbers of parameters. The BIC, the ABIC, and the CAIC were used for comparing plausible models, where the lowest value of a given index indicates the best fitting model.

Analysis was performed using Latent Gold Version 4.5 software (Vermunt and Magidson 2000). Eight indicators of eating disorder pathology were selected from the EDE to represent the DSM-IV eating disorder criteria sets for AN and BN. Indicators included percent ideal body weight (IBW), defined as current body mass index (BMI)/50th centile BMI for age and gender using Centers for Disease Control and Prevention (2002) growth charts (<86% IBW; ≥86% IBW and <95% IBW; ≥95% IBW and <105% IBW; ≥105% IBW); objective binge eating episodes, subjective binge eating episodes, self-induced vomiting, laxative or diuretic abuse (combined as a summary variable due to their non-independence), excessive exercising (all rated in clinically relevant ordered categories: never or <1×/month; 1–7×/month; ≥8×/month); and fear of weight gain and weight and shape overvaluation (both rated: not at all or slightly; moderately; very much or extremely). Missing values were estimated with full information maximum-likelihood estimation.

Validation Analyses

Cross-sectional validators included the EDE scales, depressive symptoms measured by the BDI, and self-esteem measured by the Rosenberg Self-Esteem Scale. Outcome variables relevant to eating disorders were measured as percent IBW, binge frequency, and purge frequency at follow-up. Validation analyses were run using general linear models for cross-sectional and outcome indices; age and gender were controlled in all analyses. Note that for the outcome variables, only participants for whom the variable was relevant were included (i.e., for percent IBW, only those who were below 95% IBW at intake were included; for binge eating, only those who reported objective binge eating more than once a month at intake were included; and for purging, only those who reported purging more than once a month at intake were included). For outcome analyses, both relevant pretreatment variables (e.g., percent IBW, binge frequency, purge frequency) and duration of treatment were additionally included as covariates. Post hoc comparisons were made using Bonferroni-corrected significance levels (i.e., for each of the 10 validators, we made three between-group comparisons, and significance levels were adjusted to reflect multiple comparisons). Direct comparisons of the latent profiles to the DSM-IV diagnoses were made based on the size of partial η^2, representing the unique portion of variance in the dependent variable accounted for by group membership (i.e., DSM-IV or latent profile). All validation analyses were conducted using SPSS Version 17.0.

Results

LATENT PROFILE ANALYSIS

LPA models varying the number of latent profiles from one to seven were evaluated. Fit indices were lowest for a three-profile solution ($\chi^2_{362} = 11,171.17$; $P > 0.99$) with 39 parameters, indicating that a three-profile (i.e., LP1, LP2, LP3) solution was the best-fitting model (see Table 16–1). Of the total sample, 144 (35.9%) were members of LP1, 126 (31.4%) were members of LP2, and 131 (32.7%) were members of LP3. Table 16–2 presents the frequency and severity of the indicators by latent profile.

LP1 resembled BN, wherein patients were mostly in the healthy weight range and endorsed objective binge eating, purging by self-induced vomiting, and high levels of eating disorder cognitions; we labeled LP1 "binge-purge." In contrast, LP2 and LP3 were both characterized by low frequencies of objective binge eating and purge behaviors. LP2 was low to normal weight and endorsed excessive exercise and extreme eating disorder cognitions, whereas LP3 included individuals of all weights who generally endorsed minimal eating disorder behaviors and cognitions. Accordingly, we labeled LP2 "exercise-extreme cognitions," and LP3 "minimal behaviors/cognitions."

TABLE 16–1. Fit indices for latent profile analysis

Class	Parameters	BIC	ABIC	CAIC	LL
1	17	5618.65	5564.70	5635.65	−2758.37
2	28	5300.49	5211.64	5328.49	−2566.33
3	39	5246.79	5123.03	5285.79	−2506.51
4	50	5282.46	5123.80	5332.46	−2491.38
5	61	5325.62	5216.70	5386.62	−2480.00
6	72	5366.59	5138.12	5438.59	−2467.51
7	83	5411.34	5147.97	5484.34	−2456.92

Note. Lower BIC, ABIC, and CAIC indicate better model fit.
ABIC=sample-size adjusted BIC; BIC=Bayesian information criterion; CAIC=consistent Akaike information criterion; LL=log-likelihood.

TABLE 16–2.   Frequency of eating disorder pathology in latent profiles

	LP1 (*n*=144), %	LP2 (*n*=126), %	LP3 (*n*=131), %
Percent ideal body weight			
<86%	1.6	36.5	47.7
≥86% and <95%	20.7	27.3	20.1
≥95% and <105%	22.3	21.4	8.7
≥105%	55.32	14.7	23.5
Objective binge episodes			
0 (<1×/month)	22.6	91.4	93.9
1 (1–7×/month)	35.0	8.1	5.8
2 (≥8×/month)	42.4	0	0
Subjective binge episodes			
0 (<1×/month)	41.4	61.2	80.3
1 (1–7×/month)	23.6	20.6	13.6
2 (≥8×/month)	35.0	18.2	6.1
Vomiting			
0 (<1×/month)	13.9	78.7	85.6
1 (1–7×/month)	16.3	12.7	9.7
2 (≥8×/month)	70.8	8.6	4.7
Laxatives/Diuretics			
0 (<1×/month)	80.2	89.7	100
1 (1–7×/month)	12.4	7.7	0
2 (≥8×/month)	7.5	2.6	0
Exercise			
0 (<1×/month)	46.7	24.3	87.2
1 (1–7×/month)	19.1	17.9	8.9
2 (≥8×/month)	34.2	57.8	3.9
Fear			
0 (none/slight)	12.6	15.0	86.0
1 (moderate)	15.9	16.9	9.9
2 (severe)	71.5	68.2	4.1
Shape/Weight concerns			
0 (none/slight)	2.6	3.3	57.3
1 (moderate)	11.9	13.1	25.2
2 (severe)	85.5	83.6	17.5

Figure 16–1 demonstrates the distribution of the DSM-IV diagnoses by latent profile. χ^2 Analyses indicated an association between eating disorder diagnosis and latent
profile ($\chi^2_{12} = 246.36$; $P < 0.001$). Notably, 100% of those with BN and BED along
with the majority of those with EDNOS characterized by binge eating and/or purging
(subthreshold BN, purge disorder) were included in LP1. The diagnostic breakdowns
for LP2 and LP3 were similar to one another, with each including nearly half of those
with AN or subthreshold AN and nearly half of those with EDNOS "other."

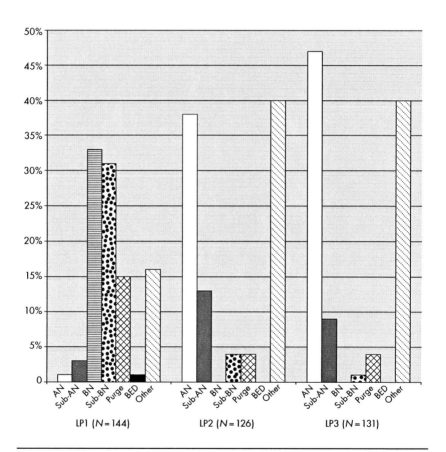

FIGURE 16–1.   Distribution of DSM-IV diagnoses across latent profile (LP) groups
(LP1 = "binge-purge," LP2 = "exercise-extreme cognitions," and LP3 = "minimal behav-
iors/cognitions").

Percentage of individuals with a given diagnosis within each LP group.
AN = anorexia nervosa ($n = 111$); BED = binge eating disorder ($n = 2$); BN = bulimia nervosa
($n = 47$); Other = eating disorder not otherwise specified, other type ($n = 126$); Purge = purge
disorder ($n = 32$); sub-AN = subthreshold anorexia nervosa ($n = 33$); Sub-BN = subthreshold
bulimia nervosa ($n = 50$).

VALIDATION ANALYSES

Latent profiles differed in age ($F_{2,398} = 20.0$; $P < 0.001$), gender ($\chi^2_2 = 6.46$; $P = 0.04$), and current percent IBW ($F_{2,394} = 15.82$; $P < 0.001$). Post hoc contrasts indicated that compared with LP2 and LP3, LP1 was older (16.10 ± 1.80 years vs. 14.82 ± 2.17 years in LP2 and 14.44 ± 2.72 in LP3). All three groups differed in percent IBW ($111.31\% \pm 21.17\%$ in LP1; $91.35\% \pm 15.19\%$ in LP2; $102.44\% \pm 42.98\%$ in LP3). Although all groups were within a healthy weight range on average, individuals who were below the fifth centile for age and gender (representing 20.2% of the entire sample) were more likely to be included in LP2 and LP3 (representing 28.0% and 33.1% of LP2 and LP3, respectively) than LP1 (1.4% of LP1). Those who were overweight ($\geq$95th centile for age and gender; 5.5% of the entire sample) or at risk for overweight ($\geq$85th centile and <95th centile for age and gender; 7.1% of the entire sample) were represented across all groups but least likely in LP2 (1.6% overweight, 1.6% at risk for overweight) compared with LP1 (4.9% overweight, 12.6% at risk for overweight) and LP3 (10.0% overweight, 6.2% at risk for overweight). Although females predominated across groups, males were most likely to be classified in LP3, comprising 13.7% of LP3 compared with 10.3% in LP2 and only 4.9% in LP1.

Pretreatment

General linear models demonstrated that both the identified latent profile groups and the DSM-IV groups were differentiated on all pretreatment validators, including eating disorder psychopathology measured by the EDE scores, depressive symptoms, and self-esteem (Figure 16–2). Across the EDE scales, BDI, and Rosenberg Self-Esteem Scale, the latent profile groups were more differentiated than the DSM-IV groups. Among the groups, LP3 reported less severe or fewer symptoms compared with LP1 and LP2 (all $P < 0.01$). LP1 reported significantly greater pathology than LP2 on EDE Eating Concern, Weight Concern, and Global scales.

Follow-Up

General linear models indicated that the groups were differentiated on percent IBW at follow-up (controlling for pretreatment percent IBW, duration of treatment, age, and gender) ($\eta^2 = 0.068$; $F = 4.29$; $df = 123$; $P = 0.016$). Compared with LP2, LP3 gained less weight between pretreatment and follow-up and was less likely to be in a healthy weight range at follow-up ($P < 0.01$); LP1 did not differ significantly from either group. DSM-IV diagnoses were not differentiated on percent IBW at follow-up. Neither the latent profile groups nor the DSM-IV categories were differentiated on binge eating or purging at follow-up.

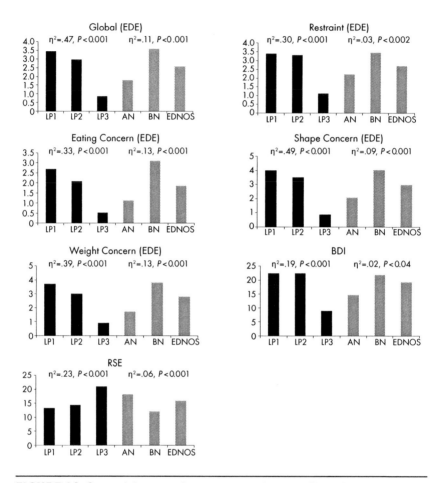

FIGURE 16–2.   Validation analyses comparing latent profile (LP) groups (denoted by darker shading) with DSM-IV diagnoses (denoted by lighter shading) on pretreatment assessments.

AN = anorexia nervosa; BDI = Beck Depression Inventory; BN = bulimia nervosa; EDE = Eating Disorder Examination; EDNOS = eating disorder not otherwise specified; LP1, LP2, LP3 = latent profile groups; RSE = Rosenberg Self-Esteem Scale.

Discussion

LPA identified three groups of children and adolescents presenting for treatment through a specialty eating disorders clinic. We labeled these groups "binge-purge," "exercise-extreme cognitions," and "minimal behaviors/cognitions." These empirically derived groups bore resemblance to the DSM-IV categories as well as to latent groups identified in the adult eating disorders literature, yet important differences emerged.

The largest group identified ("binge-purge") resembled BN: all youth with BN were included in this group, along with the majority of those with EDNOS characterized by bingeing and/or purging. This empirical work suggests that these EDNOS types, including subthreshold BN, purge disorder, and BED, can be grouped together with BN. Both of the remaining latent profile groups resembled AN in terms of their inclusion of low-weight individuals; however, neither group included predominantly low-weight individuals. Furthermore, only the "exercise-extreme cognitions" group was characterized by the hallmark fear of weight gain that defines DSM-IV AN, whereas the "minimal behaviors/cognitions" group instead was marked by a relative absence of the cognitive eating disorder symptoms. These latter two latent groups were further differentiated from one another by the presence of excessive exercise, endorsed by three-quarters of those in the group with the characteristic eating disorder cognitions compared with a small minority in the minimal cognitions group. Similar to the way in which full-syndrome BN clustered with similar EDNOS presentations, individuals with AN and subthreshold AN clustered together and were likely to be included in one of these two latent groups. These findings are consistent with the descriptive child and adolescent literature that suggests few differences between full-syndrome AN or BN and similar EDNOS presentations (Eddy et al. 2008; Peebles et al. 2006), which may support the notion of relaxing the current thresholds for AN and BN in youth (Bravender et al. 2007).

It is noteworthy, however, that in contrast to those with BN and similar EDNOS variants who were organized into a single latent group, youth with AN and EDNOS resembling AN were organized into two groups. DSM-IV distinguishes two types of individuals with AN on the basis of binge-purge symptoms. In this sample, two groups that included low-weight individuals emerged but were instead distinguished by severity of eating disorder–related cognitions and excessive exercise. Furthermore, in addition to including AN and subthreshold AN, these two latent groups included individuals with a truly residual EDNOS "other" diagnosis, which could not be described as any of the other EDNOS types.

The three latent profile groups were differentiated in clinically meaningful ways at treatment presentation. Consistent with the descriptive literature, youth in the "binge-purge" group tended to be older and were less likely to be in the low weight range compared with the other two groups. Interestingly, although there were a minority of boys in this sample, they were relatively more common in the group with the fewest typical eating disorder symptoms ("minimal behaviors/cognitions"). This finding raises the possibility that boys with eating disorders may be more likely to exhibit atypical presentations than girls. Significant eating disorder pathology, depressive symptoms, and problems with self-esteem were evident in the "binge-purge" and the "exercise-extreme cognitions" latent groups. In contrast, the "minimal behaviors/cognitions" group endorsed little eating disorder or general psychopathology. A striking finding was that across these clinical indices at treatment presentation, the empirically derived groups were more differentiated than the DSM-IV groups, suggesting that these empirical groupings may have more clinical utility. In individuals with eating disorders, it is clinically useful to note the presence of symptoms such as binge eating, purging, and low weight; these findings suggest that in youth, it may also be particularly meaningful to note the presence of cognitive symptoms and excessive exercise.

In this sample, we examined a subset of youth for whom pretreatment and follow-up data were available. Providing further support for the validity of the identified groups, outcome analyses demonstrated that low-weight youth in the "minimal behaviors/cognitions" group gained less weight at follow-up compared with low-weight youth in either of the other two groups. Latent profile group membership—but not DSM-IV diagnosis—was associated with change in percent IBW at follow-up. Although individuals with low-weight eating disorders are, by definition, resistant to weight gain, these low-weight youth with minimal eating disorder cognitions and nondepressed mood may be particularly reluctant to gain weight because they deny or minimize their experience of psychopathology/distress.

Our identified latent profile groups were somewhat similar to those reliably found in the adult literature. However, rather than identifying several different bulimic spectrum latent groups (e.g., BN-like, purge disorder, BED-like), we found that youth with a predominance of any of these symptoms (binge eating and/or purging) clustered in a single latent group. The separation of our groups containing low-weight patients into two non–binge eating or purging latent groups is consistent with some of the adult findings (Eddy et al. 2009; Keel et al. 2004). Two of the adult studies identified latent groups resembling AN that were distinguished by level of psychopathology (Eddy et al. 2009; Keel et al. 2004), with one of these being a group that endorsed low levels of both eating disorder cognitions and depression and anxiety but at the same time reported treatment seeking and medical concerns at levels that were comparable with the other latent groups (Eddy et al. 2009).

Yet even if the groups identified in this youth sample resemble those empirically derived in adults, they may not be the same. In youth, in particular, it can be difficult to parse out denial from inability to comprehend. It is possible that the "minimal behaviors/cognitions" group is heterogeneous, including youth who have minimal psychopathology or who lack the developmental capacity to endorse psychopathology along with youth who deny or minimize their symptoms for other reasons (Becker et al. 2009). More sensitive assessment tools are needed to parse out denial/minimization, limited insight due to cognitive development, and absence of symptoms. One such recommendation is the collection of collateral reports, particularly by parents. Preliminary reports suggest that the addition of a parent-report component to the EDE can be clinically useful in addressing minimization of eating disorder psychopathology in youth (Couturier et al. 2006). Furthermore, given the preliminary findings herein that these youth may gain less weight during treatment, increased attention to understanding and describing this group is needed.

Study strengths include the application of LPA to investigate nosology in a child and adolescent clinical sample of girls and boys with the full range of eating disorders. To our knowledge, no published studies have utilized this statistical method in a child and adolescent eating disorders sample. Furthermore, this is the first LPA study to include longitudinal data, allowing for the consideration of the predictive validity of identified phenotypes. However, important limitations warrant acknowledgment. First, the identified eating disorder phenotypes were defined by the indicators of eating disorder pathology included in the analyses. The measurement of eating disorder symptoms (e.g., delineation of weight status, cognitive criteria) is challenging in youth. Although a study strength was the assessment of eating disorder pathology through a gold standard clinical interview, it is possible that this measure did not assess the full range of clinical signs and symptoms of eating disorder pathology specific to youth. It is possible that different subtypes of youth with eating disorders would have been identified if other types of indicators (e.g., picky/selective eating, taste/tactile sensitivities) had been included. Second, this study included a limited range of pretreatment and follow-up clinical validators, and outcome data were not available for all youth. Third, this sample included treatment-seeking youth collected through a single clinical site, which may limit external validity of findings. Finally, although LPA identified the optimal number and composition of classes, it did not address whether the relationship between classes was taxonic versus dimensional (Wonderlich et al. 2007). It is possible that some of the identified groups (e.g., LP2 and LP3) differ along a continuum rather than existing as distinct categories. Taxometric analyses would address this question and may be an approach utilized in future research (Beauchaine 2003; Meehl 1995).

This study suggests that LPA can be used to identify meaningful eating disorder phenotypes in a clinical sample of children and adolescents. Youth who regularly engage in binge eating and/or purging are distinguished from those who do not; those who do not are more likely to be low weight and are organized into two groups distinguished by the presence of typical eating disorder cognitions and excessive exercise. These empirically derived groups demonstrate both concurrent and predictive validity, supporting their candidacy as clinically meaningful groups. Our findings are consistent with the recommendations of the Work Group for Classification of Eating Disorders in Children and Adolescents, in which there is a focus on the need for diagnostic criteria to recognize that symptom expression—both cognitive and behavioral—may differ on the basis of development and that comprehensive eating disorder assessment and diagnosis should include collateral (e.g., parent) report (Bravender et al. 2007, 2010). Furthermore, the empirical groupings of full-syndrome AN or BN with similar EDNOS presentations are consistent with the Work Group's recommendations that strict thresholds be relaxed (Bravender et al. 2007, 2010). Ongoing research focused on the nosology of eating disorders in children and adolescents utilizing developmentally sensitive assessment tools and a broad range of clinical indicators and both cross-sectional and treatment outcome validators is needed to replicate and extend these findings in preparation for DSM-5.

References

Akaike H: Factor analysis and AIC. Psychometrika 52:317–332, 1987

American Psychiatric Association: Diagnostic and Statistical Manual of Mental Disorders, 4th Edition. Washington, DC, American Psychiatric Association, 1994

American Psychiatric Association: Diagnostic and Statistical Manual of Mental Disorders, 4th Edition, Text Revision. Washington, DC, American Psychiatric Association, 2000

Beauchaine TP: Taxometrics and developmental psychopathology. Dev Psychopathol 15:501–527, 2003

Beck AT: Beck Depression Inventory. San Antonio, TX, Psychological Corporation, 1987

Becker AE, Eddy KT, Perloe A: Clarifying criteria for cognitive signs and symptoms for eating disorders in DSM-V. Int J Eat Disord 42:611–619, 2009

Bozdogan H: Model selection and Akaike's information criterion: the general theory and its analytical extensions. Psychometrika 52:345–370, 1987

Bravender T, Bryant-Waugh R, Herzog D, et al: Classification of child and adolescent eating disturbances. Workgroup for Classification of Eating Disorders in Children and Adolescents (WCEDCA). Int J Eat Disord 40:S117–S122, 2007

Bravender T, Bryant-Waugh R, Herzog D, et al: Classification of eating disturbance in children and adolescents: proposed changes for the DSM-V. Workgroup for Classification of Eating Disorders in Children and Adolescents (WCEDCA). Eur Eat Disord Rev 18:79–89, 2010

Bryant-Waugh RJ, Cooper PJ, Taylor CL, et al: The use of the Eating Disorder Examination with children: a pilot investigation. Int J Eat Disord 19:391–397, 1996

Bulik CM, Sullivan PF, Kendler KS: An empirical study of the classification of eating disorders. Am J Psychiatry 157:886–895, 2000

Centers for Disease Control and Prevention: CDC Growth Charts for the United States: Development and Methods. Atlanta, GA, Centers for Disease Control and Prevention, 2002. Available at: http://www.cdc.gov/growthcharts/percentile_data_files.htm. Accessed April 1, 2009.

Cooper Z, Cooper PJ, Fairburn CG: The validity of the Eating Disorder Examination and its subscales. Br J Psychiatry 154:807–812, 1989

Couturier J, Lock J, Forsberg S, et al: The addition of a parent and clinician component to the EDE for children and adolescents. Int J Eat Disord 40:472–475, 2006

Croudace TJ, Jarvelin M-R, Wadsworth MEJ, et al: Developmental typology of trajectories to nighttime bladder control: epidemiologic application of longitudinal latent class analysis. Am J Epidemiol 157:834–842, 2003

Duncan AE, Bucholz KK, Neuman RJ, et al: Clustering of eating disorder symptoms in a general population female twin sample: a latent class analysis. Psychol Med 37:1097–1107, 2007

Eddy KT, Celio Doyle A, Hoste RR, et al: Eating disorder not otherwise specified (EDNOS): an examination of EDNOS presentations in adolescents. J Am Acad Child Adolesc Psychiatry 47:156–164, 2008

Eddy KT, Crosby RD, Keel PK, et al: Empirical identification and validation of eating disorder phenotypes in a multisite clinical sample. J Nerv Ment Dis 197:41–49, 2009

Fairburn CG, Cooper Z: The Eating Disorder Examination (12th edition), in Binge Eating: Nature, Assessment and Treatment. Edited by Fairburn CG, Wilson GT. New York, Guilford, 1993, pp 333–360

Fairburn CG, Cooper Z, Bohn K, et al: The severity and status of eating disorder NOS: implications for DSM-V. Behav Res Ther 45:1705–1715, 2007

Hagborg WJ: Scores of middle-school-age students on the Rosenberg Self-Esteem Scale. Psychol Rep 78:1071–1074, 1996

Keel PK, Fichter M, Quadflieg N, et al: Application of a latent class analysis to empirically define eating disorder phenotypes. Arch Gen Psychiatry 61:192–200, 2004

Lazarsfeld PF, Henry NW: Latent Structure Analysis. Boston, MA, Houghton Mifflin, 1968

le Grange D, Crosby RD, Rathouz PJ, et al: A randomized controlled comparison of family based treatment and supportive psychotherapy for adolescent bulimia nervosa. Arch Gen Psychiatry 64:1049–1056, 2007

Lock J, Agras WS, Bryson S, et al: A comparison of short- and long-term family therapy for adolescent anorexia nervosa. J Am Acad Child Adolesc Psychiatry 44:632–639, 2005

Meehl P: Bootstraps taxometrics: solving the classification problem in psychopathology. Am Psychol 50:266–275, 1995

Mitchell JE, Crosby RD, Wonderlich SA, et al: Latent profile analysis of a cohort of patients with eating disorder not otherwise specified. Int J Eat Disord 40:S95–S98, 2007

Nicholls D, Chater R, Lask B: Children into DSM don't go: a comparison of classification systems for eating disorders in childhood and early adolescence. Int J Eat Disord 28:317–324, 2000

Peebles R, Wilson JL, Lock JD: How do children with eating disorders differ from adolescents with eating disorders at initial evaluation? J Adolesc Health 39:800–805, 2006

Pinheiro AP, Bulik CM, Sullivan PF, et al: An empirical study of the typology of bulimic symptoms in young Portuguese women. Int J Eat Disord 41:251–258, 2008

Rosenberg M: Society and the Adolescent Self-Image. Princeton, NJ, Princeton University Press, 1965

Rosso IM, Young AD, Femia LA, et al: Cognitive and emotional components of frontal lobe functioning in childhood and adolescence. Ann N Y Acad Sci 1021:355–362, 2004

Sclove S: Application of model-selection criteria to some problems in multivariate analysis. Psychometrika 52:333–343, 1987

Striegel-Moore RH, Franko DL, Thompson D, et al: An empirical study of the typology of bulimia nervosa and its spectrum variants. Psychol Med 35:1563–1572, 2005

Sullivan PF, Bulik CM, Kendler KS: The epidemiology and classification of bulimia nervosa. Psychol Med 28:599–610, 1998

Tanofsky-Kraff M, Yanovski SZ, Wilfley DE, et al: Eating disordered behaviors, body fat, and psychopathology in overweight and normal weight children. J Consult Clin Psychol 72:53–61, 2004

Thomas JJ, Vartanian LR, Brownell KD: The relationship between eating disorder not otherwise specified (EDNOS) and officially recognized eating disorders: meta-analysis and implications for DSM-V. Psychol Bull 135:407–433, 2009

Turner H, Bryant-Waugh R: Eating disorder not otherwise specified (EDNOS): profiles of clients presenting at a community eating disorders service. Eur Eat Disord Rev 12:18–26, 2004

Vermunt JK, Magidson J: Latent GOLD User's Guide. Belmont, MA, Statistical Innovations Inc, 2000

Wade TD, Crosby RD, Martin NG: Use of latent profile analysis to identify eating disorder phenotypes in an adult Australian twin cohort. Arch Gen Psychiatry 63:1377–1384, 2006

Watkins B, Frampton I, Lask B, et al: Reliability and validity of the child version of the Eating Disorder Examination: a preliminary investigation. Int J Eat Disord 38:183–197, 2005

Wonderlich SA, Joiner TE, Keel PK, et al: Eating disorder diagnoses: empirical approaches to classification. Am Psychol 62:167–180, 2007

Yurgelun-Todd D: Emotional and cognitive changes during adolescence. Curr Opin Neurobiol 17:251–257, 2007

PART 4

CULTURAL CONSIDERATIONS IN THE CLASSIFICATION OF EATING DISORDERS

17

CULTURE AND EATING DISORDERS CLASSIFICATION

Anne E. Becker, M.D., Ph.D., Sc.M.

The classification and measurement of eating disorders across culturally diverse populations present major challenges to policymakers, researchers, and clinicians. These challenges are inherent to cross-cultural measurement of mental illnesses and their associated symptoms, but assessing eating disorders is especially difficult given the wide variation in cultural values, practices, and norms concerning food and body experience and, by extension, symptoms related to eating disorders. The phenomenological heterogeneity of eating disorders identified in culturally diverse populations also raises questions about core symptoms of the illnesses. Greater flexibility and dimensionality in classification encompassing cultural diversity in symptom presentations should enhance opportunities for equitable access to treatment.

Cross-Cultural Variation in Illness Experience and Presentation

Variation in cultural norms for both recognition and articulation of psychological distress and treatment seeking is well recognized in the literature of cross-cultural

Reprinted from Becker AE: "Culture and Eating Disorders Classification." *International Journal of Eating Disorders* 40(Nov suppl):S111–S116, 2007. Used with permission from John Wiley & Sons.

The author thanks Lauren Richards for her contributions to the literature search on ethnicity and epidemiology of eating disorders.

psychiatry (Kleinman 1980) and may result in a highly culturally particular idiom of distress (Nichter 1981) in illness presentation. Conversely, signs or symptoms may remain unmarked as illness when they are not culturally salient, despite their clinical significance in other contexts. These sources of variation can undermine case detection in both clinical and research settings, resulting in ethnic disparities in access to health care and biased prevalence estimates, respectively (Alarcón et al. 2002). Furthermore, when symptoms are not recognized locally as a culturally salient pattern of illness, an indigenous category corresponding to a Western biomedical nosologic correlate may not exist. Without such an indigenous illness category, treatment seeking may be comparatively low, notwithstanding serious symptoms. Prevalence estimates based upon clinic samples would underestimate pathology under this scenario.

Dissonance between universal and local nosologies for and manifestations of illness is generally a key consideration driving cross-cultural research in mental illness. This problem of both measurement and meaning very often involves a dialectic between "etic" (encompassing the universal or outsider perspective) and "emic" (encompassing the local, insider, or indigenous perspective) approaches. An etic perspective on mental illness conventionally focuses on the problem of how to accurately measure an illness category that is presumed to be universal across diverse cultural settings. Notwithstanding language barriers as well as cultural differences in recognizing and reporting physical states, emotions, attitudes, and so forth (Kirmayer and Young 1998), presumed universal diagnostic criteria are applied to distinguish cases from noncases. Measurement concerns inherent to this approach center on finding a locally valid method for eliciting symptoms. Strategies for optimizing accuracy of measurement include careful idiomatic translation of assessments, back translation to establish congruity with the initial language version (Canino et al. 1997), and establishing both reliability and validity of the instrument (Regier and Burke 2000).

In contrast, an emic approach conventionally begins "from the ground up" by identifying indigenous illness categories and relating these to universal categories. Illness meaning relates to how individual signs and symptoms are attended to, amplified, disregarded, and organized into a locally salient illness category (Kleinman 1988). Indigenous illness nosologies may include illness categories that have little overlap with Western psychiatric categories for mental illness, and/or may not recognize biomedical illnesses as locally relevant (Good 1977). Illnesses distinct from known Western biomedical categories may be glossed as "culture-bound syndromes" to designate them as culturally unique. On the other hand, some illnesses may have considerable overlap in core symptoms yet maintain a distinctive presentation—including manifestation of symptoms and course. Such incomplete overlap presents a special challenge for classification and, by extension, measurement of prevalence and identification of risk factors. For example, if an illness presents with incomplete phenomenological overlap in another cultural setting, the prevalence estimate may be biased because of systematic misclassification of cases as noncases. Screening for cases would be unlikely to have meaningful clinical impact in the absence of negotiation of local clinical reality that would promote help seeking, because individuals may be reluctant to seek or accept treatment for an illness they do not recognize (Kleinman 1980).

In the absence of a universal norm for body image, body experience, diet, and use of purgatives, meaningful designation of particular attitudes and behaviors as pathological must evaluate them relative to local cultural practices. Implicit in diagnostic criteria for bulimia nervosa (BN) and anorexia nervosa (AN) in DSM-IV (American Psychiatric Association 1994, 2000) are behaviors and attitudes that carry meaning as symptoms in relation to their social context. For example, to the extent that core cultural values are represented in body shape ideals and dietary norms, rationale for food refusal, concern with body shape, and distress associated with overeating will be culturally particular (Becker 1995; Lee et al. 1993). The physical and social environments also impose constraints on dietary choices and opportunities to engage in inappropriate compensatory behaviors (Lee 1996). Surveillance of food intake and limiting opportunities to overeat or purge following meals constitute a cornerstone of behavioral treatment for eating disorders. The abundance of food resources, access to modern plumbing, and space configurations that allow for privacy that characterize many affluent, modern lifestyles globally are absent across many other social environments.

Cultural variation in phenotypes of eating disorders has been described at length in the literature. The most notable example is the absence of fat phobia among Hong Kong Chinese individuals who otherwise appear to meet diagnostic criteria for AN (Lee et al. 1993). Similar presentations of AN without fat phobia have been described in populations in Japan, Singapore, Malaysia, and India (Lee 1994). The Hong Kong patients with AN, but without fat phobia, were misclassified as noncases on the Eating Attitudes Test (EAT; Lee et al. 1998, 2002). Likewise, cases of AN described in India differed with respect to the body image disturbance that characterizes the disorder in DSM-IV (American Psychiatric Association 1994; Khandelwal et al. 1995).

There is also potential for misclassification of noncases as cases. For example, le Grange et al. (2004) in follow-up interviews of five impoverished, black South African adolescents who had screened positive on the EAT clarified that their preoccupation with food was related to poverty, food shortage, and hunger rather than to an eating disorder. Similarly, investigators screening North Indian girls with the EAT found a very large percentage scored above their study cut score but also that respondents had misinterpreted many of the questions (King and Bhugra 1989).

Phenomenological variation is also evident in an ethnic Fijian population, where motivation for the recently emerging purging and dieting behaviors among adolescent girls relates to a pragmatic concern with obtaining a wage-earning job, given their perception that being slim will enhance social and economic opportunities

(Becker 2004). A similar finding has been reported among cases of Belizean girls with disordered eating (Anderson-Fye 2004). Moreover, use of indigenous herbal preparations as purgatives to compensate for culturally sanctioned feasting in Fiji is routine. Despite the prevalence of some disordered eating behaviors comparable with those of adolescents in Western societies, there is no indigenous nosologic correlate of an eating disorder in this society, and these behaviors are not organized and experienced as illness, notwithstanding their potential impact on physical health (Becker 1995; Becker et al. 2002). Culturally sanctioned overeating—sometimes associated with distress—as well as purging in this society in the absence of indigenous recognition of illness suggests that variation in universal behaviors may sometimes be recognized as symptoms only in relation to the social context (Becker et al. 2003a). In addition, there is an indigenous category—commonplace in Pacific societies, but without a clear analogue in Western biomedical nosology—for an appetite disorder (*macake,* Fijian) that is characterized by poor appetite and food refusal and arouses intense social concern and intervention (Becker 1995) but otherwise bears little resemblance to any DSM-established eating disorder. Individuals with *macake* are characteristically distressed by the poor appetite and generally willingly take prophylactic or therapeutic doses of traditional herbal medicines to restore appetite. Usually, the illness episode is brief. Likewise, body size and shape ideals worldwide are diverse. Moreover, both gender roles and social conventions that moderate personal care in relation to these ideals vary considerably (Becker 1995; Furnham and Baguma 1994; Mackenzie 1985). Without appropriate social context, application of diagnostic criteria for eating disorders risks misclassification.

Phenomenological diversity may well characterize eating disorders within Western populations as well. That is, the most common presentation of an eating disorder is eating disorder not otherwise specified—a diagnostic category comprising patients with quite heterogeneous symptom presentations (Fairburn and Bohn 2005). This means that the majority of individuals with an eating disorder present with "atypical" symptom patterns—which may emerge with some frequency. For example, Keel et al. (2005) identified a pattern of recurrent purging behavior in the absence of binge eating behavior. This variant suggests that DSM-IV classification for eating disorders may be too coarse-grained to reflect the full range of phenomenological diversity even within a relatively homogeneous population.

Consistent with reports from other studies that eating disorders often remain unrecognized in clinical settings or untreated (Cachelin et al. 2000; Whitehouse et al. 1992), Hudson et al. (2007) reported that more than half of the individuals identified in their study who met criteria for BN or binge eating disorder (BED) never received care for their illness. If there is a systematic bias in missing cases that are phenomenological outliers—which seems very plausible—then there is a risk for reification of a subtype that is more likely to access treatment in the current classification system. Because only a small percentage (6%) of articles published in high-impact psychiatric journals report on studies based in regions that compose more than 90% of the global population, the majority of clinical observational and trial data reflect a minority of the world's population (Patel and Sumathipala 2001). Thus, Western biomedical psychiatry provides the presumed nosologic standard for prevalence studies and there is selective attention to and reification of "universal" patterns of mental illness, resulting in a kind of cultural hegemony of DSM-IV. Clinical features of illness in understudied populations are both underrepresented and potentially unrecognized, a potential observational bias that may impact perceived prevalence and phenomenology of the eating disorders. This underrepresentation extends to ethnic minority populations within European and North American societies as well (Cummins et al. 2005).

Challenges to the Interpretation of Epidemiological and Phenomenological Data Across Ethnically Diverse Populations

Several key factors curtail our understanding of the prevalence and phenomenological diversity of eating disorders across ethnically diverse populations: 1) general difficulties in characterizing diverse populations for study; 2) a dearth of research on ethnicity, epidemiology, and eating disorders; 3) limited attention to and data on validity and reliability of assessments for disordered eating across ethnically diverse populations; and 4) treatment access patterns that may reinforce clinical stereotypes.

Characterization of ethnic diversity in populations is problematic across epidemiological studies. Census categories may be used for bureaucratic reasons (e.g., a description of the study population using these categories is required for federally funded research in the United States), yet provide only a poor proxy for ethnicity. First, the categories do not convey consistent meanings outside of the United States. Second, these terms do not allow for respondents' plural ethnic identities. Third, census categories do not reflect the considerable ethnic heterogeneity within them. A study reporting on a "Latino" study population excludes important detail about South American versus Central American versus Caribbean ethnicity—populations that are culturally quite distinct despite sharing a common language. Data from the National Survey of American Life indicating higher rates of BN and BED in Caribbean blacks than in African American respondents (Taylor et al. 2006) illustrate the heterogeneity of risk within a single census category.

Next, the impact of ethnic and cultural factors is rarely studied in relation to mental illness. A recent study that screened seven major U.S. psychiatric journals for their use of ethnicity-related terms reported that only 8% of papers identified contained a term related to race, ethnicity, or culture in the title or abstract (Lewis-Fernandez et al. 2005). Likewise, there are few epidemiological studies on eating disorders in which ethnicity is a central consideration. To confirm the infrequency of epidemiological studies on eating disorders featuring a discussion of diverse populations, we searched the MEDLINE database from 1950 through 2006 for papers addressing the epidemiology of eating disorders. We identified all papers published in English and relating to human subjects that contain *both* a term relating to epidemiology (for the purpose of this survey, we used the terms: *epidemiolog[y]*,[1] *prevalence, incidence*) and a term relating to eating disorders (*eating disorder*,[1] *bulimia nervosa, anorexia nervosa, binge-eating, binge eating*, or *disordered eating*) in the title. We identified 179 papers meeting these criteria. Among these, we identified the subset of papers containing terms in either the title or abstract relating to major racial and ethnic census categories (*African [American], Black, Latin[o]*,[1] *Hispan[ic]*,[1] *Asian, Native [American], Indian, Pacific [Islander]*) as well as some additional ethnicity terms (*Caribbean, Dominican, Mexican*, and *Puerto Ric[an]*[1]). For the former group, we identified just seven papers (<4% of the total) containing a major census category term related to ethnic minority populations. For the latter group of additional terms relating to ethnicity, we identified no papers. Despite limitations in the scope and specificity of our search terms, this survey of the literature on the epidemiology of eating disorders provides strong evidence of the infrequency of studies with ethnicity as a central focus.

Inconsistency among studies of assessments to measure disordered eating limits comparability of prevalence, phenomenology, and severity of eating disorder symptoms across study populations. The problem of limited comparability is compounded for ethnic minority populations by the sparseness of psychometric data evaluating performance of standardized assessments in ethnically diverse populations (Becker and Fay 2006). A notable exception is the study by Franko et al. (2004), who reported differences in Eating Disorder Inventory factor structure between black and white girls. Additionally, inadequate sample sizes for some ethnic populations limit statistical power in detecting differences between groups (Cummins et al. 2005; Wildes et al. 2001). The assessment of variation in microcultural norms across ethnically diverse populations requires increased methodological sophistication and breadth (Canino et al. 1997; Striegel-Moore and Bulik 2007). For example, the integration of systematic qualitative assessment of illness experience with semistructured interview techniques, such as use of the Explanatory Model Interview Catalogue, with population-based quantitative data can assist in integrating culturally particular and universal perspectives on eating disorders (Weiss 1997).

Finally, data suggesting that the majority of individuals with an eating disorder do not seek specialty care for their illness are of deep concern (Cachelin et al. 2000;

---

[1]For the purpose of this survey we combined this term with like stem words with different suffixes. The material in brackets augments the stem terms here to indicate the ethnic or other category sought by this method.

Hudson et al. 2007). Treatment access patterns for eating disorders in the United States also suggest ethnic disparities (Becker et al. 2003b; Cachelin et al. 2001; Pike et al. 2001). Whereas these are consistent with patterns observed in health care access in the United States (American College of Physicians 2004), they underscore the importance of identifying diverse patterns of presentation of illness and representing them in the DSM classification schema. Differences in access to treatment relate not only to clinician and patient factors (e.g., misrecognition of illness and treatment-seeking patterns) but also to a poor fit between conventional nosology and diverse presentations of illness (Good 1993). Patterns of symptom presentation (e.g., the relative frequency of specific purging behaviors) that may be more common among certain populations than others require further investigation with both population and qualitative data (Cachelin et al. 2000; Cummins et al. 2005; Striegel-Moore and Bulik 2007). Similarly, the relation between body dissatisfaction, which does appear to vary significantly across ethnic groups (Wildes et al. 2001), and disordered eating may vary (Anderson-Fye and Becker 2003) and reflects culturally particular etiological pathways for an eating disorder (Striegel-Moore and Bulik 2007). The lack of information on diversity of presentation among ethnic minority populations likely contributes to poorer access to care.

Research Priorities and Future Directions

The salience of behaviors and cognitions related to eating disorders can best be interpreted in relation to their cultural context, especially in the case of body image, because of considerable cultural diversity in body ideals and body experience across geographically and ethnically diverse populations. It is also true for dietary patterns and weight control behaviors, which are best understood as pathological when they deviate from cultural norms. Standardized self-report assessments risk both false-positive and false-negative misclassification when not validated locally. In addition to validation against Western population-based diagnostic criteria, evaluation of these assessments should identify whether culturally unique phenotypes are captured.

The higher than expected prevalence of BED in the National Survey of American Life study (5.02% lifetime prevalence for African Americans and 5.78% for Caribbean blacks; Taylor et al. 2006) suggests that more nationally representative studies of prevalence of, risk of, and service use for eating disorders in ethnic minority populations are desirable. More research establishing psychometric properties of conventional assessments for diverse populations is also urgently needed in order to provide data on comparative risk and risk factors within and between these populations. As a corollary, better international population and ethnographic data are needed to establish patterns of phenomenological diversity and prevalence.

In particular, qualitative data are essential to relating symptoms to indigenous categories and local salience. There must be a dialectical relation between clinically observed phenotypes and Western biomedical nosologic standards to avoid misclassification and to enhance cultural sensitivity of care delivery. This will promote identification of clinician practice patterns that fail to recognize need for care and to deliver it. Optimal access to care for diverse populations will include 1) ethnographically informed identification of idioms of distress and illness experience; 2) dialectical consideration of both universal and culturally particular presentations of illness; 3) improved assessment through valid and reliable measures relevant to the local population that incorporate questions to capture locally salient illness presentations; and 4) increased attention to ethnically and culturally diverse populations in epidemiological studies.

The inherently dimensional nature of body shape preoccupation and dietary behaviors poses special classificatory challenges when interpreted against a culturally particular social context. Eating disorders are both biological and social realities. Moreover, both social expectations and the physical environment will shape and constrain symptom presentations, attribution of meaning, and treatment seeking for these disorders. As a result, there is a critical need to understand and recognize cultural diversity in presentation in order to render all individuals in need of treatment—and especially those from underserved populations—visible in clinical settings. A more flexible and dimensional classificatory system for the eating disorders may be desirable in order to encompass their culturally based phenomenological diversity. This, in turn, will stimulate research that can facilitate culturally sensitive and strategic prevention strategies and reduce ethnic disparities in access to care.

References

Alarcón RD, Bell DD, Kirmayer LJ, et al: Beyond the funhouse mirrors, in A Research Agenda for DSM-V. Edited by Kupfer DJ, First MB, Regier DA. Washington, DC, American Psychiatric Association, 2002, pp 219–289

American College of Physicians: Racial and ethnic disparities in health care: a position paper of the American College of Physicians. Ann Intern Med 141:226–232, 2004

American Psychiatric Association: Diagnostic and Statistical Manual of Mental Disorders, 4th Edition. Washington, DC, American Psychiatric Association, 1994

American Psychiatric Association: Diagnostic and Statistical Manual of Mental Disorders, 4th Edition, Text Revision. Washington, DC, American Psychiatric Association, 2000

Anderson-Fye EP: A "coca-cola" shape: cultural change, body image, and eating disorders in San Andrés, Belize. Cult Med Psychiatry 28:561–595, 2004

Anderson-Fye EP, Becker AE: Eating disorders across cultures, in Handbook of Eating Disorders and Obesity. Edited by Thompson JK. New York, Wiley, 2003, pp 565–589

Becker AE: Body, Self, and Society: The View from Fiji. Philadelphia, University of Pennsylvania Press, 1995

Becker AE: Television, disordered eating, and young women in Fiji: negotiating body image and identity during rapid social change. Cult Med Psychiatry 28:533–559, 2004

Becker AE, Fay K: Socio-cultural issues and eating disorders, in Annual Review of Eating Disorders. Edited by Wonderlich S, de Zwaan M, Steiger H, et al. Chicago, IL, Academy for Eating Disorders, 2006, pp 35–63

Becker AE, Burwell RA, Gilman SE, et al: Eating behaviours and attitudes following prolonged television exposure among ethnic Fijian adolescent girls. Br J Psychiatry 180:509–514, 2002

Becker AE, Burwell RA, Navara K, et al: Binge-eating and binge-eating disorder in a small-scale indigenous society: the view from Fiji. Int J Eat Disord 34:423–431, 2003a

Becker AE, Franko D, Speck A, et al: Ethnicity and differential access to care for eating disorder symptoms. Int J Eat Disord 33:205–212, 2003b

Cachelin FM, Veisel C, Barzegarnazari E, et al: Disordered eating, acculturation, and treatment-seeking in a community sample of Hispanic, Asian, black, and white women. Psychol Women Q 24:244–253, 2000

Cachelin FM, Rebeck R, Veisel C, et al: Barriers to treatment for eating disorders among ethnically diverse women. Int J Eat Disord 30:269–278, 2001

Canino G, Lewis-Fernandez R, Bravo M: Methodological challenges in cross-cultural mental health research. Transcult Psychiatry 34:163–184, 1997

Cummins LH, Simmons AM, Zane WS: Eating disorders in Asian populations: a critique of current approaches to the study of culture, ethnicity, and eating disorders. Am J Orthopsychiatry 75:533–574, 2005

Fairburn CG, Bohn K: Eating disorder NOS (EDNOS): an example of the troublesome "not otherwise specified" (NOS) category in DSM-IV. Behav Res Ther 43:691–701, 2005

Franko DL, Striegel-Moore RH, Barton BA, et al: Measuring eating concerns in black and white adolescent girls. Int J Eat Disord 35:179–189, 2004

Furnham A, Baguma P: Cross-cultural differences in the evaluation of male and female body shapes. Int J Eat Disord 15:81–89, 1994

Good BJ: The heart of what's the matter: the semantics of illness in Iran. Cult Med Psychiatry 1:25–58, 1977

Good BJ: Culture, diagnosis and comorbidity. Cult Med Psychiatry 16:427–446, 1993

Hudson JI, Hiripi E, Pope HG Jr, et al: The prevalence and correlates of DSM-IV eating disorders in the National Comorbidity Survey Replication. Biol Psychiatry 61:348–358, 2007

Keel PK, Haedt A, Edler C: Purging disorder: an ominous variant of bulimia nervosa? Int J Eat Disord 38:191–199, 2005

Khandelwal SK, Sharan P, Saxena S: Eating disorders: an Indian perspective. Int J Soc Psychiatry 41:132–146, 1995

King M, Bhugra D: Eating disorders: lessons from a cross-cultural study. Psychol Med 19:955–958, 1989

Kirmayer LJ, Young A: Culture and somatization: clinical, epidemiological, and ethnographic perspectives. Psychosom Med 60:420–430, 1998

Kleinman A: Patients and Healers in the Context of Culture. Berkeley, University of California Press, 1980, pp 104–118

Kleinman A: The Illness Narratives: Suffering, Healing, and the Human Condition. New York, Basic Books, 1988

le Grange D, Louw J, Breen A, et al: The meaning of 'self-starvation' in impoverished black adolescents in South Africa. Cult Med Psychiatry 28:439–461, 2004

Lee S: The Diagnostic Interview Schedule and anorexia nervosa in Hong Kong. Arch Gen Psychiatry 51:251–252, 1994

Lee S: Reconsidering the status of anorexia nervosa as a Western culture–bound syndrome. Soc Sci Med 42:21–34, 1996

Lee S, Ho TP, Hsu LKG: Fat phobic and non–fat phobic anorexia nervosa: a comparative study of 70 Chinese patients in Hong Kong. Psychol Med 23:999–1017, 1993

Lee S, Lee AM, Leung T: Cross-cultural validity of the Eating Disorder Inventory: a study of Chinese patients with eating disorder in Hong Kong. Int J Eat Disord 23:177–188, 1998

Lee S, Kwok K, Liau C, et al: Screening Chinese patients with eating disorders using the Eating Attitudes Test in Hong Kong. Int J Eat Disord 32:91–97, 2002

Lewis-Fernandez R, Oquendo M, Schmidt A, et al: The inclusion of race, culture, and psychiatry in current psychiatric literature. Presented at the annual meeting of the American Psychiatric Association, Atlanta, GA, May 2005

Mackenzie M: The pursuit of slenderness and addiction to self control, in Nutrition Update, Vol 2. Edited by Weininger J, Briggs GM. New York, John Wiley, 1985

Nichter M: Idioms of distress—alternatives in the expression of psychosocial distress: a case study from South India. Cult Med Psychiatry 5:379–408, 1981

Patel V, Sumathipala A: International representation in psychiatric literature: survey of six leading journals. Br J Psychiatry 178:406–409, 2001

Pike KM, Dohm FA, Striegel-Moore RH, et al: A comparison of black and white women with binge eating disorder. Am J Psychiatry 158:1455–1460, 2001

Regier DA, Burke JD: Epidemiology, in Kaplan & Sadock's Comprehensive Textbook of Psychiatry, 7th Edition, Vol 1. Edited by Sadock BJ, Sadock VA. Philadelphia, PA, Lippincott, Williams & Wilkins, 2000, pp 500–522

Striegel-Moore RH, Bulik C: Risk factors for eating disorders. Am Psychol 62:181–198, 2007

Taylor JY, Caldwell CH, Jackson JS, et al: Eating disorders in African Americans and Caribbean blacks: findings from the National Survey of American Life. Paper presented at the NIMH Workshop on the Classification of Eating Disorders, National Institute of Mental Health, Bethesda, MD, June 2006

Weiss M: Explanatory Model Interview Catalogue (EMIC): framework for comparative study of illness. Transcult Psychiatry 34:235–263, 1997

Whitehouse AM, Cooper PJ, Vize CV, et al: Prevalence of eating disorders in three Cambridge general practices: hidden and conspicuous morbidity. Br J Gen Pract 42:57–60, 1992

Wildes JE, Emery RE, Simons AD: The roles of ethnicity and culture in the development of eating disturbance and body dissatisfaction: a meta-analytic review. Clin Psychol Rev 21:521–551, 2001

18

EATING DISORDERS IN NATIVE AMERICAN POPULATIONS

A Review of Prevalence Studies

Ruth H. Striegel-Moore, Ph.D.
Wesley C. Lynch, Ph.D.
Olga Levin
Anne E. Becker, M.D., Ph.D., Sc.M.

Epidemiological research on eating disorders has lagged behind research on other mental disorders. Even the most basic questions typically addressed in epidemiological studies such as prevalence in major demographic subgroups of a population have been left unanswered for eating disorders. Notably, in the United States, nationally representative data on prevalence of eating disorders were unavailable as late as 2006 because the diagnostic interviews used in the major psychiatric epidemiological surveys excluded questions about disordered eating. Until the publication of findings from the National Comorbidity Survey II (NCS II; Hudson et al. 2007), there were no data based on nationally representative samples regarding the prevalence of eating disorders in the United States. This gap in knowledge stood in stark contrast to the extensive scientific data that had accumulated in the United States in other areas of eating disorder research.

As part of the NCS II, which was conducted between 2001 and 2003, a subsample was administered a survey related to diagnostic criteria for anorexia nervosa (AN), bulimia nervosa (BN), and binge eating disorder (BED). Findings confirmed what had long been clear from nonrepresentative samples and from epidemiological studies conducted in Europe: lifetime prevalence estimates for AN and BN were much higher in women (0.9% and 1.5%, respectively) than in men (0.3% and 0.5%, respectively). The gender difference in prevalence of BED was considerably less marked (3.5% in women vs. 2.0% in men); this finding provided an important signal that eating disorders without inappropriate compensatory behaviors as a core feature might have a different demographic profile from eating disorder syndromes for which purging or extreme dietary restriction is the defining feature. The NCS II sample size recruited for the eating disorder assessment was too small to report differential prevalence estimates across racial or ethnic minorities (Hudson et al. 2007).

Likewise, community-based prevalence data on eating disorders have been limited in Europe. A 2005 review of 27 major epidemiological studies of mental disorders conducted in Europe showed that only nine studies assessed eating disorders, and of these four were done in Germany, two in Italy, two in the Netherlands, and one in Iceland (Wittchen and Jacobi 2005). The importance of community-based data for an unbiased description of prevalence, correlates, and course and outcome of disorders has been amply documented (Fairburn and Beglin 1990). In light of the limited community-based data, it should come as no surprise that information about eating disorders experienced by racial or ethnic minority populations in the United States has been particularly sparse.

A growing number of studies conducted among nonwhite and Latino samples have established that eating disorders occur across racial and ethnic populations represented in the United States. Experts have called for a more detailed examination of ethnic or racial variations in symptom expression, correlates, or treatment response (Franko et al. 2007; Pike et al. 2001; Striegel-Moore and Bulik 2007). Epidemiological studies conducted in parallel to the NCS II for the purpose of describing mental health problems in U.S. minority populations reported prevalence estimates for eating disorders in African Americans and Caribbean blacks (Taylor et al. 2007), Hispanic Americans (Alegria et al. 2007), and Asian Americans (Nicdao et al. 2007). Notwithstanding these important studies, there was no comparable effort to conduct an "NCS II–like" study among Indigenous peoples, often referred to as "American Indian" or "Native American," "Alaska Native," and "Native Hawaiian" (for brevity, we use the abbreviation AI/NA in this review). An earlier large-scale epidemiological study, the American Indian Service Utilization, Psychiatric Epidemiology, Risk and Protective Factors Project, which surveyed a probability sample of enrolled members of Southwest and Northern Plains tribes between 1997 and 2000 (Beals et al. 2005), used a similar diagnostic interview to what later was used in the NCS II, but did not include the diagnostic items needed for measuring eating disorders. We are unaware of any study to date that that has examined eating disorder pathology based on a representative sample of AI/NA in the United States.

Documentation of epidemiological data relating to eating disorders in AI/NA populations is warranted for several reasons. First of all, such information would complement epidemiological data concerning other major mental disorders experienced by AI/NA individuals and guide policy and strategies for optimizing resource allocation for interventions to enhance mental health and reduce the burden of suffering arising from mental disorders. Second, given that eating disorders are highly comorbid with psychiatric disorders, including mood, anxiety, and substance disorders, in white populations (Hudson et al. 2007; Javaras et al. 2008; Lewinsohn et al. 2000), there is reason for concern that eating disorders may be especially prevalent among AI/NA adolescents and adult populations, in which anxiety and substance use disorders are prevalent (Beals et al. 2005; Whitbeck et al. 2008). Moreover, studies of white samples have found significantly elevated rates of obesity among individuals with BED, and vice versa (Javaras et al. 2008; Wonderlich et al. 2009). Given that obesity is a major health problem among AI/NA individuals (Denny et al. 2003; Rutman et al. 2008; Steele et al. 2008), its comorbidity with BED in AI/NA populations is critical to determine. Furthermore, an epidemiological survey of Native American and Alaska Native adolescents representing 50 different tribes found that "body pride" was a significant correlate both of self-reported emotional health and physical health in girls and boys (Cummins et al. 1999).

In this review, we endeavor to identify and offer a succinct review of research on eating disorder symptoms and syndromes in AI/NA populations. We emphasize the important caveat that any effort to paint a summary picture of eating disorders among Indigenous peoples in the United States is inherently limited in light of the substantial cultural heterogeneity among AI/NA populations. More than 500 AI/NA tribes are recognized within the United States and studies of health disparities have documented large variations across regions (and therefore, presumably, tribes) in health or mental health indicators such as obesity, excessive alcohol intake, or suicide (Steele et al. 2008; Storck et al. 2009). Our description of published studies on eating disorders in AI/NA populations therefore needs to be considered preliminary.

Because an earlier review summarized the literature through 1991 (Crago et al. 1996), in the present chapter we focus on publications dated 1992 or later. Additionally, we excluded from review studies based on data collected prior to 1990 because the nomenclature for eating disorders and associated signs and symptoms has undergone considerable revision since then, rendering earlier study data more challenging to interpret with respect to current diagnostic criteria.

Methods

We identified scientific papers for this review by searching PubMed for English language articles published after 1991, using the following search terms: "Native

American," "American Indian," "Alaska," "eating disorder," "binge eating," "vomiting," "anorexia nervosa," and "bulimia nervosa." Additionally, we reviewed the reference lists of all articles identified by this search approach to identify additional relevant studies. After deleting papers that did not report on eating disorders, we found only 10 papers reporting original research. We examined each paper with respect to year(s) when the data were collected, sample characteristics (sex, age), questions and time frame (e.g., "ever"; past 12 months) used to measure presence of eating disorder signs and symptoms, and prevalence estimates for core eating disorder symptoms. Two papers were eliminated because they did not report specific data on prevalence of eating disorder syndromes or symptoms (Lynch et al. 2007, 2008); however, we were able to obtain unpublished prevalence data from the study author (W. Lynch, personal communication, April 17, 2010). We also were able to obtain unpublished data (S. Rutman, personal communication, March 26, 2010) from the author of a publication reporting epidemiological data on mental health concerns among AI/NA youth (Rutman et al. 2008). Of the remaining eight publications, one paper reported findings from a study specifically assessing Native American populations, the Indian Adolescent Health Survey (Story et al. 1994), and one paper reported prevalence of eating disorders in a consecutive case series of Indigenous people presenting for treatment at a community mental health center in Alaska (Aoun and Gregory 1998); neither of these papers included a white comparison sample. Two of the eight publications reported findings from the same database, the 1996 National Eating Disorders Screening Program (Becker et al. 2003; Franko et al. 2007). Although some of the studies reported data on other ethnic or racial minorities, our focus was limited to AI/AN and white samples. The literature on health disparities uses white samples as the reference group given the widely established finding of better health in the United States among white individuals (e.g., Rutman et al. 2008). Unpublished data were added from one study of AI/AN schoolchildren in southwest Montana (Lynch et al. 2007, 2008) provided to us by the study author (W. Lynch, personal communication, April 24, 2010).

Results

Table 18–1 summarizes key data regarding sampling, assessment, and major findings relevant to eating pathology of the studies included in our review. None of these studies reported prevalence data on full-syndrome eating disorders using DSM criteria based on a community sample, leaving unanswered the question of how common DSM-IV (American Psychiatric Association 1994, 2000) eating disorder diagnoses are among AI/NA populations. The authors of the one study reporting on the prevalence of eating disorders among Eskimo patients in a case series of community mental health center patients noted that eating disorders, in their opinion, were underrepresented in this population (Aoun and Gregory 1998). However, subsequent research (conducted among members of other ethnic minority populations) has documented numerous barriers for ethnic minority patients seeking treatment for eating disorders or, even when they do seek treatment, being diagnosed with an eating disorder (Becker et al. 2003; Cachelin and Striegel-Moore 2006; Cachelin et al. 2006). Therefore, the prevalence estimate reported by Aoun and Gregory (1998) should not be taken as representative of Indigenous peoples of Alaska.

Another major limitation is that these study findings are notably dated, with no data having been collected in the past 5 years. Only three of the published studies and one of the unpublished studies reported findings from data collected since 2000, with the remaining five studies reporting on data collected from the late 1980s and 1990s. The lack of more current data on eating pathology in AI/AN is an important gap in this literature because of indications of secular trends in changing prevalence of eating disorders. Some studies report an overall decrease in recent years (Keel et al. 2007), some report an increase in eating disorders in male populations (Wiseman et al. 2001), and yet others report an increase in binge eating behaviors but not other eating disorder symptoms (Hay et al. 2008).

Although previous reviews concluded that AI/NA samples were more likely than white samples to report eating disorder symptoms (Crago et al. 1996), the present review cannot support this generalization because of the small number of statistically significant differences in direct comparisons for symptom prevalence between AI/NA and white populations of comparable age. That said, in no reported comparisons were the symptoms significantly *lower* in the AI/NA populations than in a white population, and several comparisons demonstrated significantly higher prevalence of symptoms in AI/NA males when compared with white males. For example, AI/NA males were significantly more likely to report symptoms consistent with any disordered eating (Croll et al. 2002) and "any extreme weight control" (Neumark-Sztainer et al. 2002) than were white male respondents in adjusted analyses reported in the respective studies. Studies that tested for between-group differences in AI/NA females compared with white females reported only two significant differences—greater prevalence of exercising more than once daily among high school students participating in a national eating disorder screening program (Austin et al. 2008) and embarrassment due to eating too much among adult women participants in the Add Health Wave III study (Bennett and Dodge 2007)—although Lynch, in an unpublished study, found significant differences between NA females and white females for dieting, fasting, and vomiting (Table 18–1).

Setting aside the limited statistical comparison data, with few exceptions (as reported in Table 18–1), the prevalence of self-reported eating disorder *symptoms* was either higher for AI/NA samples than for white samples or very similar, supporting a conclusion that eating disorder symptoms are at least as common among AI/NA populations as among white populations in the United States. Prevalence of key symptoms was also quite high among AI/NA female youth, warranting clinical con-

TABLE 18–1. Prevalence studies of eating disorder symptoms in Indigenous populations of the United States: 1992–2010

Study	Population[a]	Sample size	Key eating disorder assessments	Major findings of comparisons of NA vs. non-Hispanic WH female or male participants
Story et al. 1994	Indian Adolescent Health Survey (1988–1990) representing eight Indian Health Service areas, grades 7–12 (1), and survey of Minnesota rural youth (2) Mean age not reported No WH comparison data	(1) N=13,454 (2) N=17,322 NAF, n=6,695 Minnesota rural sample: no further information	Weight dissatisfaction ("at present"), weight control behaviors and eating disorder symptoms ("ever")	Weight dissatisfaction: NAF 49.9%; NAM: 31.7% Dieting: NAF: 47.9%; NAM: 30% Diet pills: NAF: 5.1%; NAM: 1.8% Diuretics: NAF: 1.2%; NAM: 0.8% Laxatives: NAF: 0.6%; NAM: 1.2% Vomiting: NAF: 27.1%; NAM: 11.8% Ever been on a food binge: NAF: 41.8%; NAM: 31.5%
Aoun and Gregory 1998	Consecutive series of adult Eskimo patients (Inuit, Inupiat, Yupik, and Siberian Yupik) presenting at a community mental health center in Nome, Alaska, between 1990 and 1993 Mean age, 37 years No WH comparison data	NAF, n=115 NAM, n=140	Chart review to identify DSM-III-R diagnoses based on psychiatrists' evaluation	Eating disorder: NAF: 2.9%; NAM: 0%

TABLE 18–1. Prevalence studies of eating disorder symptoms in Indigenous populations of the United States: 1992–2010 *(continued)*

Study	Population[a]	Sample size	Key eating disorder assessments	Major findings of comparisons of NA vs. non-Hispanic WH female or male participants
Croll et al. 2002	Minnesota Student Survey (1998) subsample of 9th and 12th graders Mean age not reported	NA, *n*=641 WH, *n*=69,544 NAF, *n*=294 WHF, *n*=35,255 NAM, *n*=347 WHM, *n*=34,289	Unhealthy weight control behaviors[b] and binge eating[c] in the past 12 months; "any disordered eating" (yes to any of[b-c]) was used to examine group differences	Fasting: NAF: 47.6%, WHF: 43.0%; NAM: 18.2%, WHM: 13.9% Cigarettes: NAF: 29.4%, WHF: 18.2%; NAM: 20.5%, WHM: 9.8% Diet pills: NAF: **13.2%**, WHF: 9.4%; NAM: **5.4%**, WHM: 2.0% Laxatives: NAF: 2.4%, WHF: 1.8%; NAM: 3.1%, WHM: 1.3% Vomiting: NAF: **14.2%**, WHF: 8.7%; NAM: **2.6%**, WHM: 1.3% Binge eating: NAF: **27.1%**, WHF: 25.2%; NAM: 21.4%, WHM: 11.6% "Any disordered eating": NAF: **62.9%**, WHF: 55.9%, n.s.; NAM: **46.4%**, WHM: 27.9%, *P*<0.05, adjusted for socioeconomic differences

TABLE 18–1. Prevalence studies of eating disorder symptoms in Indigenous populations of the United States: 1992–2010 *(continued)*

Study	Population[a]	Sample size	Key eating disorder assessments	Major findings of comparisons of NA vs. non-Hispanic WH female or male participants
Neumark-Sztainer et al. 2002	Project EAT (1998) middle and high school students Mean age not reported	$N = 4,746$ NAF, $n=91$ WHF, $n=1,057$ NAM, $n=74$ WHF, $n=1,206$	Unhealthy weight control behaviors[b] and binge eating[c] in the past year; "any disordered eating" (yes to any of[b–c]) was used to examine group differences	Fasting: NAF: 22.7%, WHF: 19.3%; NAM: **14.5%**, WHM: 7.4% Diet pills: NAF: **6.6%**, WHF: 7.1%; NAM: **2.8%**, WHM: 1.3% Diuretics: NAF: **1.1%**, WHF: 1.1%; NAM: **5.6%**, WHM: 1.2% Laxatives: NAF: **3.3%**, WHF: 1.3%; NAM: **0%**, WHM: 0.4% Vomiting: NAF: **13.3%**, WHF: 7.2%; NAM: **5.6%**, WHM: 1.2% Binge eating: NAF: **20.9%**, WHF: 25.2%; NAM: **6.0%**, WHM: 4.8% "Any extreme weight control"[r]d. NAF OR=1.13 (CI=0.57, 2.25), n.s.; NAM OR=4.02 (CI=1.53, 10.57), $P<0.05$ Binge eating[d]: NAF OR = 1.11 (CI=0.59, 2.09), n.s.; NAM OR = 0.99 (CI=0.30, 3.28), n.s.

TABLE 18–1. Prevalence studies of eating disorder symptoms in Indigenous populations of the United States: 1992–2010 *(continued)*

Study	Population[a]	Sample size	Key eating disorder assessments	Major findings of comparisons of NA vs. non-Hispanic WH female or male participants
Becker et al. 2003	National Eating Disorder Screening Program (1996) A subsample of subjects who completed both stages of screening interview was used in this study Mean age=23.57 years (SD=10.1, range=17–58)	*N*=5,787 84% female (no gender stratification) NA, *n*=82 (0.9%) WH, *n*=7,254 (81.6%)	DSM-IV eating disorder criteria	Received a diagnosis and/or treatment for an eating disorder: NA: 12.8%, WH: 9.7%, n.s. NA were significantly *less likely to be referred for further evaluation* relative to WH (χ^2=4.16, *P*=0.04; OR=0.514, CI=0.271, 0.974)

TABLE 18–1. Prevalence studies of eating disorder symptoms in Indigenous populations of the United States: 1992–2010 (continued)

Study	Population[a]	Sample size	Key eating disorder assessments	Major findings of comparisons of NA vs. non-Hispanic WH female or male participants
Franko et al. 2007[e]	National Eating Disorders Screening Program (1996) A subsample of participants who opted to meet with a counselor; recruited on college campuses Mean age = NA = 29.4 years, WH = 23.9 years ($P < 0.001$)	NA, $n=55$ WH, $n=4,652$ NAF, $n=42$ (76.4%) WHF, $n=4,082$ (87.8%)	DSM-IV behavioral eating disorder symptoms present at least once in the past 6 months Distress due to eating and weight concerns (0 = never, 4 = all the time)	Restricting: NA: 25.5%, WH: 30.1%, n.s. Diuretics: NA: 5.5%, WH: 4.9%, n.s. Laxatives: NA: 16.4%, WH: 6.1%, n.s. Exercise > 2 hours/day: NA: 18.9%, WH: 18.9%, n.s. Vomiting: NA: 13%, WH: 8.7%, n.s. Binge eating: NA: 41.8%, WH: 36.2%, n.s. Distress: NA: mean = 2.54 (SD = 2.63), WH: mean = 1.91 (SD = 2.13), n.s.

TABLE 18–1. Prevalence studies of eating disorder symptoms in Indigenous populations of the United States: 1992–2010 *(continued)*

Study	Population[a]	Sample size	Key eating disorder assessments	Major findings of comparisons of NA vs. non-Hispanic WH female or male participants
Austin et al. 2008	National Eating Disorders Screening Program (2000), high school students Mean age not reported	NAF, *n*=49 WHF, *n*=2,751 NAM, *n*=44 WHM, *n*=1,878	Eating disorder symptoms present at least once in the past 3 months	Vomiting: NAF: **17.8%**, WHF: 12.4%, OR=1.5, CI=0.7, 3.3, n.s.; NAM: **11.8%**, WHM: 2.9%, OR=4.5 (CI=1.6, 13.1), $P<0.05$ Exercise > 1 time/day: NAF: **15.2%**, WHF: 2.8%, OR=6.2 (CI=2.8, 14.1), $P<0.05$; NAM: **2.7%**, WHM: 2.1%, OR=1.3 (CI=0.1, 12.0), n.s. Binge eating: NAF: **10.2%**, WHF: 7.5%, OR= 1.4 (CI=0.7, 2.7), n.s.; NAM: **19.3%**, WHM: 6.4%, OR=3.5 (CI=1.5, 8.4), $P<0.05$ "Any eating disorder symptom": NAF: **34.5%**, WHF: 25%, OR=1.6 (CI=1.0, 2.6), n.s.; NAM: **22%**, WHM: 9.8%, OR=2.6 (CI=1.1, 5.9), $P<0.05$ "Ever treated for an eating disorder": NAF: **15.6%**, WHF: 4.0%, OR=4.4 (CI=1.3, 14.7), n.s.; NAM: **5.3%**, WHM: 1.1%, OR=5.0 (CI=1.6, 15.6), $P<0.05$

TABLE 18–1. Prevalence studies of eating disorder symptoms in Indigenous populations of the United States: 1992–2010 *(continued)*

Study	Population[a]	Sample size	Key eating disorder assessments	Major findings of comparisons of NA vs. non-Hispanic WH female or male participants
Bennett and Dodge 2007	Add Health Wave III (2001/2002) Mean age, 22 years	A subsample of 5,726 women NAF, *n*=34 WHF, *n*=3,956	Fear of losing control over eating Eating so much that you would feel embarrassed	"Fear of losing control": NAF: **3.0%**, WHF: 2.6%, n.s. "Embarrassed": NAF: **13.5%**, WHF: 7.1%, *P*<0.05 (adjusted for family income and maternal education)
Rutman et al. 2008[f]	Youth Risk Behavior Survey (1997–2003); a subsample of urban youth Mean age not given	WH, *n*=19,189 NA, *n*=513 NAF, *n*=224 WHF, *n*=9,338 Analyses not stratified by gender	Dieting,[g] compensatory behaviors (past 30 days)	Dieting: NA: 36.4%, WH: 43.7%, n.s Fasting: NA: **13.8%**, WH: 12.4%, n.s Diet pills: NA: **10%**, WH: 7.6% ,n.s. Diuretics: NA: 1.1%, WH: 1.1%, n.s. Laxatives: NA: 3.3%, WH: 1.3%, n.s Vomiting: NA: 7.7%, WH: 4.8% , n.s.
W. Lynch, unpublished, April 17, 2010[h]	NA adolescents (2003–2004) collected in southwest Montana schools; grades 5–10	WHM, *n*=675 NAM, *n*=179 WHF, *n*=580 NAF, *n*=197	McKnight Risk Factor Survey, version 4 (All items: "In the past year, how often…" percent reported reflect "sometimes, usually, or always")	Felt Fat: NAF: **48.3%**, WHF: 49.4%, n.s.; NAM: **23.2%**, WHM: 17.5%, n.s. Dieting: NAF: **36.9%**, WHF: 27.3%, *P*<0.009; NAM: **32.5%**, WHM: 12.1%, *P*<0.001 Fasting: NAF: **15.9%**, WHF: 10.8%, *P*<0.05; NAM: **11.0%**, WHM: 6.8%, *P*<0.05

(continued)

TABLE 18–1. Prevalence studies of eating disorder symptoms in Indigenous populations of the United States: 1992–2010 *(continued)*

Study	Population[a]	Sample size	Key eating disorder assessments	Major findings of comparisons of NA vs. non-Hispanic WH female or male participants
W. Lynch, unpublished, April 17, 2010[h] *(continued)*	Mean age: NAF, 13.7 years; NAM, 13.6 years; WHF, 13.9 years; WHM, 14.0 years			Diet pills: NAF: 4.3%, WHF: 4.9%, n.s.; NAM: 4.7%, WHM: 2.0%, $P < 0.04$ Laxatives or water pills: NAF: **2.9%**, WHF: **2.2%**, n.s.; NAM: **3.2%**, WHM: **1.1%**, $P < 0.05$ Vomiting: NAF: **7.2%**, WHF: **3.9%**, $P < 0.05$; NAM: **3.7%**, WHM: **1.7%**, n.s. Exercise to lose weight: NAF: **51.2%**, WHF: **57.8%**, n.s.; NAM: **50.0%**, WHM: **37.7%**, $P < 0.002$ Binge eating: NAF: **25.1%**, WHF: **25.1%**, n.s.; NAM: **18.8%**, WHM: **24.5%**, n.s.

Note. BMI=body mass index; NA=Native American; NAF=Native American female; NAM=Native American male; WH=white; WHF=white female; WHM=white male.

[a]Information is shown only for non-Hispanic white and NA participants, even when a study may have included other ethnic or racial groups. [b]"During the last 12 months, have you done any of the following to lose or control your weight (mark all that apply): fasting or skipping meals; smoking cigarettes; using diet pills or speed; vomiting (throwing up) on purpose after eating; and using laxatives?" [c]"During the last 12 months, have you ever eaten so much in a short period of time that you felt out of control (binge eating)?" (Shisslak et al. 1999). [d]WH is reference group; adjusted for differences in school level, socioeconomic status, and BMI. [e]Analysis sample drawn from the same 1996 NEDSP participants as the study by Becker et al. 2003. [f]Prevalence data were not included in the published report (Rutman et al. 2008) but were provided by personal communication (March 26, 2010). [g]Dieting: "Ate less food, fewer calories, or foods low in fat to lose weight or keep from gaining weight during the past 30 days." [h]Data based on mean symptom scale scores that were previously reported in Lynch et al. 2007.

cern. For example, the lifetime prevalence of vomiting for weight control purposes was 27% in a large sample (Story et al. 1994); 12-month prevalence was between 7% and 14% in three smaller samples (Croll et al. 2002; W. Lynch, unpublished, April 17, 2010; Neumark-Sztainer et al. 2002), and the 1-month point prevalence was 7.7% (Rutman et al. 2008) for AI/NA female youth in these studies, respectively. Likewise, the lifetime prevalence of binge eating was high at 27.1% (Story et al. 1994), as were reported 12-month prevalence estimates (27.1% and 20.9%) among AI/NA female youth (Croll et al. 2002; Neumark-Sztainer et al. 2002).

These summary statements based on reported findings need to be qualified by a detailed consideration of methodological differences—including both sampling and analytic approaches—that limit their comparability with data reported for other demographic sectors of the U.S. population. First, studies targeted different age groups and used different sampling approaches. Most of the studies recruited in school or college settings, and we could not find any study that encompassed non–college attending adults. Hence, the prevalence of core eating disorder signs and symptoms in adults representing Indigenous peoples in the United States is unknown. Three of the studies that we identified recruited participants in the context of a screening initiative for eating disorders among college (Becker et al. 2003; Franko et al. 2007) or high school (Austin et al. 2008) students, whereas the remaining studies collected information on a broad range of health or mental health issues (Story et al. 1994) or used convenience samples (e.g., survey distribution as part of a classroom activity) without making case finding an explicit study goal for participation. The National Eating Disorder Screening Day studies' prevalence estimates should not be directly compared with estimates reported by studies without an explicit focus on eating disorders, because of the unknown selection bias inherent to the study design.

Second, in most of these studies, AI/NA participants represented a small proportion of all respondents. With the exception of one paper presenting findings from the Indian Adolescent Health Survey that reported data from an exclusively AI/NA sample ($n=13,454$) and a comparison white sample ($n=17,322$) (Story et al. 1994), the studies included relatively small numbers of AI/NA respondents (sample sizes ranging from 34 to 641). As a result, their sample sizes likely were inadequate either to be representative of the AI/NA communities from which they were drawn or to be powered for statistical significance testing for between-group differences. Indeed, the one study that recruited a nationally representative sample of youth and included 224 female and 289 male AI/NA participants did not stratify analyses by gender because of sample size considerations (S. Rutman, personal communication, March 26, 2010). When studies calculated between-group differences, few adjusted for demographic variables and none adjusted for urban versus rural residence. This latter limitation is salient because urban location has been identified as an important risk correlate in samples of European women, with higher eating disorder prevalence estimates obtained in urban compared with rural dwelling samples (van Son et al. 2006).

Third, key variables were defined and measured differently across the various studies. The time frames used for identifying presence of various symptoms ranged from "ever" (Story et al. 1994) to the "past year" (Croll et al. 2002; W. Lynch, unpublished, April 17, 2010; Neumark-Sztainer et al. 2002), "past 6 months" (Franko et al. 2007), "past 3 months" (Austin et al. 2008), "past 30 days" (Rutman et al. 2008), and "past 7 days" (Bennett and Dodge 2007). Not surprisingly, prevalence estimates for symptoms tended to be higher in studies using a longer time frame than in studies basing the estimates on a shorter time period. Comparisons across studies were also rendered difficult by differences in phrasing of the items addressing symptomatic behaviors, ranging from precise (Franko et al. 2007; Rutman et al. 2008) to vague (W. Lynch, unpublished, April 17, 2010; Story et al. 1994) in the case of dieting or involving distinctive content for the items assessing binge eating. Moreover, all but one study (Bennett and Dodge 2007) did not measure symptoms using interview methods but rather relied on self-report, an approach deemed less reliable especially for assessing binge eating (Fairburn and Beglin 1990).

Fourth, none of the studies explicitly addressed the validity of the assessments for eating pathology in AI/NA populations. For example, it is unknown whether between-group differences for an item probing whether respondents had "eaten so much in a short period that you would have been embarrassed if others had seen you do it" (Bennett and Dodge 2007) might reflect cultural differences in perceived social acceptability for eating quickly or a large amount or culturally diverse attribution of food consumption to social mores.

Although the published data are insufficient to interpret the relative prevalence of eating pathology and associated symptoms in AI/NA samples compared with other demographic groups in the United States, the data we reviewed document that signs and symptoms of eating disorders are present—and apparently prevalent—among AI/NA samples in this country.

Discussion

Representative prevalence estimates of full-syndrome eating disorders among AI/NA populations in the United States are unavailable. The few studies reporting descriptive or comparative data with respect to eating disorder signs and symptoms for AI/NA populations are insufficient to draw conclusions about the relative prevalence in these populations compared with other sociodemographic groups in the United States. Moreover, prevalence data are largely available for AI/NA adolescent populations. However, in aggregate, the small number of studies identified and examined for this review support that eating disorder symptoms are *at least* as prevalent among AI/NA female youth and, in some cases, may be even more prevalent among male youth than in white male youth. These studies also confirm that specific behaviors characteristic of eating disorders—for example, vomiting and binge eating—are prevalent in the AI/NA samples studied to date.

Our review identifies scientific and health equity gaps warranting special concern. First, there are inadequate descriptive data on eating pathology within AI/NA populations. Given the high mortality and associated medical comorbidity of eating disorders, comprehensive mental health services delivery must encompass identification and therapeutic interventions for eating disorders in all sectors of the population at risk. Behavioral symptoms consistent with eating disorders appear to be prevalent, especially among AI/NA female youth. Moreover, relative to white male youth, these symptoms may be more prevalent among AI/NA male youth. Given the potential clinical implications of these findings, additional research is urgently needed that will address sampling concerns with respect to representativeness and cultural heterogeneity among AI/NA populations. In particular, future research should specifically address cultural diversity across these populations with respect to prevalence and presentation of symptoms. This review is limited because our search included only generic, but not specific, terms for AI/NA populations in the United States. Validation of self-report assessment of eating disorder symptoms and the correspondence of presentation of eating pathology with the present DSM-IV classification scheme will also be essential to estimating the burden associated with eating pathology in AI/NA populations. This may be especially critical to ensuring optimal recognition and referrals for care for these populations (Becker et al. 2003). Finally, additional epidemiological studies identifying risk factors—especially with respect to sociocultural mediators and moderators of treatment course and outcome—will advance understanding of social contributions to pathogenesis and will also inform future preventive and therapeutic interventions for AI/NA populations at risk for eating disorders.

References

Alegria M, Woo M, Cao Z, et al: Prevalence and correlates of eating disorders in Latinos in the United States. Int J Eat Disord 40:S15–S21, 2007

American Psychiatric Association: Diagnostic and Statistical Manual of Mental Disorders, 4th Edition. Washington, DC, American Psychiatric Association, 1994

American Psychiatric Association: Diagnostic and Statistical Manual of Mental Disorders, 4th Edition, Text Revision. Washington, DC, American Psychiatric Association, 2000

Aoun SL, Gregory RJ: Mental disorders of Eskimos seen at a community mental health center in western Alaska. Psychiatr Serv 49:1485–1487, 1998

Austin SB, Ziyadeh NJ, Forman S, et al: Screening high school students for eating disorders: results of a national initiative. Prev Chronic Dis 5:A114, 2008

Beals J, Manson SM, Whitesell NR, et al: Prevalence of DSM-IV disorders and attendant help-seeking in 2 American Indian reservation populations. Arch Gen Psychiatry 62:99–108, 2005

Becker AE, Franko DL, Speck A, et al: Ethnicity and differential access to care for eating disorder symptoms. Int J Eat Disord 33:205–212, 2003

Bennett S, Dodge T: Ethnic-racial differences in feelings of embarrassment associated with binge eating and fear of losing control. Int J Eat Disord 40:454–459, 2007

Cachelin FM, Striegel-Moore RH: Help seeking and barriers to treatment in a community sample of Mexican American and European American women with eating disorders. Int J Eat Disord 39:154–161, 2006

Cachelin FM, Striegel-Moore RH, Reagan PC: Factors associated with treatment seeking in a community sample of European American and Mexican American women with eating disorders. Eur Eat Disord Rev 14:422–429, 2006

Crago M, Shisslak CM, Estes LS: Eating disturbances among American minority groups. Int J Eat Disord 19:239–248, 1996

Croll J, Neumark-Sztainer D, Story M, et al: Prevalence and risk and protective factors related to disordered eating behaviors among adolescents: relationship to gender and ethnicity. J Adolesc Health 31:166–175, 2002

Cummins J, Ireland M, Resnick M, et al: Correlates of physical and emotional health among Native American adolescents. J Adolesc Health 24:38–44, 1999

Denny CH, Holtzman D, Cobb N: Surveillance for health behaviors of American Indians and Alaska Natives: findings from the Behavioral Risk Factor Surveillance System, 1997–2000. MMWR Surveill Summ 352:1–13, 2003

Fairburn CG, Beglin SJ: Studies of the epidemiology of bulimia nervosa. Am J Psychiatry 147:401–408, 1990

Franko D, Becker A, Thomas J, et al: Cross-ethnic differences in eating disorder symptoms and related distress. Int J Eat Disord 40:156–164, 2007

Hay PJ, Mond J, Buttner P, et al: Eating disorder behaviors are increasing: findings from two sequential community surveys in South Australia. PLoS One 3:e1541, 2008

Hudson J, Hiripi E, Pope HG Jr, et al: The prevalence and correlates of eating disorders in the National Comorbidity Survey Replication. Biol Psychiatry 61:348–358, 2007

Javaras KN, Pope HG, Lalonde JK, et al: Co-occurrence of binge eating disorder with psychiatric and medical disorders. J Clin Psychiatry 69:266–273, 2008

Keel PK, Baxter MG, Heatherton TF, et al: A 20-year longitudinal study of body weight, dieting, and eating disorder symptoms. J Abnorm Psychol 116:422–432, 2007

Lewinsohn PM, Striegel-Moore RH, Seeley JP: The epidemiology and natural course of eating disorders in young women from adolescence to young adulthood. J Am Acad Child Adolesc Psychiatry 39:1284–1292, 2000

Lynch WC, Heil DP, Wagner E, et al: Ethnic differences in BMI, weight concerns, and eating behaviors: comparisons of Native American, white, and Hispanic adolescents. Body Image 4:179–190, 2007

Lynch WC, Heil DP, Wagner E, et al: Body dissatisfaction mediates the association between body mass index and risky weight control behaviors among white and Native American adolescent girls. Appetite 51:210–213, 2008

Neumark-Sztainer D, Croll J, Story M, et al: Ethnic/racial differences in weight-related concerns and behaviors among adolescent girls and boys: findings from Project EAT. J Psychosom Res 53:963–974, 2002

Nicdao EG, Hong S, Takeuchi DT: Prevalence and correlates of eating disorders among Asian Americans: results from the National Latino and Asian American Study. Int J Eat Disord 40(suppl):S22–S26, 2007

Pike KM, Dohm FA, Striegel-Moore RH, et al: A comparison of black and white women with binge eating disorder. Am J Psychiatry 158:1455–1460, 2001

Rutman S, Park A, Castor M, et al: Urban American Indian and Alaska Native youth: Youth Risk Behavior Survey 1997–2003. Matern Child Health J 12:S76–S81, 2008

Shisslak CM, Renger R, Sharpe T, et al: Development and validation of the McKnight Risk Factor Survey for assessing potential risk and protective factors for disordered eating in preadolescent and adolescent girls. Int J Eat Disord 25:195–214, 1999

Steele CB, Cardinez CJ, Richardson LC, et al: Surveillance for health behaviors of American Indians and Alaska Natives: findings from the Behavioral Risk Factor Surveillance System, 2000–2006. Cancer 113:1131–1141, 2008

Storck M, Beal T, Bacon JG, et al: Behavioral and mental health challenges for indigenous youth: research and clinical perspectives for primary care. Pediatr Clin North Am 56:1461–1479, 2009

Story M, Hauck FR, Broussard BA, et al: Weight perceptions and weight control practices in American Indian and Alaska Native adolescents: a national survey. Arch Pediatr Adolesc Med 148:567–571, 1994

Striegel-Moore R, Bulik C: Risk factors for eating disorders. Am Psychol 62:181–198, 2007

Taylor JY, Caldwell CH, Baser RE, et al: Prevalence of eating disorders among blacks in the National Survey of American Life. Int J Eat Disord 40(suppl):S10–S14, 2007

van Son GE, van Hoeken D, Bartelds AI, et al: Urbanisation and the incidence of eating disorders. Br J Psychiatry 189:562–563, 2006

Whitbeck LB, Yu M, Johnson KD, et al: Diagnostic prevalence rates from early to mid-adolescence among indigenous adolescents: first results from a longitudinal study. J Am Acad Child Adolesc Psychiatry 47:890–900, 2008

Wiseman CV, Sunday SR, Klapper F, et al: Changing patterns of hospitalization in eating disorder patients. Int J Eat Disord 30:69–74, 2001

Wittchen HU, Jacobi F: Size and burden of mental disorders in Europe: a critical review and appraisal of 27 studies. Eur Neuropsychopharmacol 15:357–376, 2005

Wonderlich SA, Gordon KH, Mitchell JE, et al: The validity and clinical utility of binge eating disorder. Int J Eat Disord 42:687–705, 2009

19

EATING DISORDER SYMPTOMS OF NATIVE AMERICAN AND WHITE ADOLESCENTS

Wesley C. Lynch, Ph.D.
Ross D. Crosby, Ph.D.
Stephen A. Wonderlich, Ph.D.
Ruth H. Striegel-Moore, Ph.D.

In the past two decades numerous surveys of eating attitudes, weight perceptions, or weight control behaviors have concluded that Native American (NA) adolescents are less satisfied with their body weight and shape, show more disturbed eating behaviors, and may be at greater risk for eating disorders than most other ethnic groups (Auker 1993; Davis and Yager 1992; Neumark-Sztainer et al. 1997a, 1997b; Rosen et al. 1988; Snow and Harris 1989; Story et al. 1986, 2001). Comparisons with whites (Crago et al. 1996; Story et al. 1997), Hispanics (Smith and Krejci 1991), and certain other ethnic groups (Story et al. 1995) have led to conclusions similar to those of Crago et al. (1996), who noted that "compared to Caucasian females, eating disturbances are equally common among Hispanic females, more frequent among Native Americans, and less frequent among Black and Asian American females" (p. 239). In a recent school-based survey of 81,247 Minnesota high school students (Croll et al. 2002), the authors concluded that "consistent with other studies…, both Hispanic and Native American females reported a higher prevalence of disordered eating than white females, and black and Asian females reported the lowest prevalence" (p. 172).

Despite this general consensus, data on the nature of these eating problems remain limited. In particular, the prevalence of specific symptoms among NA adolescents and the degree to which they may experience full-syndrome eating disorders are unknown. Several of the largest previous surveys have not included direct comparison of NA and non-NA groups (Neumark-Sztainer et al. 1997b; Story et al. 1994, 1997), and studies including NA participants as part of larger health surveys have typically included only a limited range of items related to weight concerns or eating behaviors (French et al. 1995; Neumark-Sztainer et al. 1997a; Story et al. 1991, 1994, 1995). In one of the few studies using validated eating disorder instruments, Smith and Krejci (1991) administered the Eating Disorder Inventory (Garner et al. 1983) and the Bulimia Test (Smith and Thelen 1984) to samples of Hispanic ($n=327$), NA ($n=129$), and Caucasian ($n=89$) high school students. They reported that "Native Americans consistently scored the highest on each of seven items representing disturbed eating behaviors and attitudes" (p. 179). However, statistically significant differences were found for only four of these seven items: "Any episodes of binge eating"; "Induced vomiting at least once per month"; "Always terrified of weight gain"; and "Never satisfied with body weight." Because of the small sample sizes, gender differences were not explored in this study. The few studies directly comparing NA females with their peers from other ethnic groups have tended to confirm the Smith and Krejci findings. Thus, compared with white females (and most other ethnic groups), NA females are generally less satisfied with their bodies, more likely to perceive themselves as overweight (French et al. 1997; Neumark-Sztainer et al. 1997a), and equally or more likely to engage in dieting or fasting to lose weight (Croll et al. 2002; Neumark-Sztainer et al. 1997a; Story et al. 1995), although at least one study found NA girls to be significantly less likely to engage in dieting (Story et al. 1994). In terms of more serious eating problems, NA girls were also more likely to engage in binge eating (Croll et al. 2002) and to vomit, smoke cigarettes, or use diuretics (Croll et al. 2002; Story et al. 1995) as methods of weight control. In addition, the extent of these "symptoms" appears to increase in NA girls with increases in body mass index (BMI; Davis and Lambert 2000; Neumark-Sztainer et al. 1997a, 1997b; Rosen et al. 1988; Story et al. 1986). This may be particularly important in light of the greater levels of overweight and obesity among NA children and adolescents (Broussard et al. 1995; Crawford et al. 2001; Story et al. 1999). Few previous studies of differences comparing NA and white girls have controlled for BMI, and those that have generally report fewer symptoms in BMI-controlled or matched groups (Lynch et al. 2004; Neumark-Sztainer et al. 2002). In a previous study, we noted that BMI and NA ethnicity may each contribute, somewhat independently, to increased eating disorder symptoms (Lynch et al. 2004).

Based on the evidence, it appears that NA adolescents may be experiencing potentially serious eating and weight-management problems—at least as serious as those affecting their white peers. In a recent review, limited to studies reporting eating disorder symptoms that were based on data collected since 1990 (i.e., omitting early studies), Striegel-Moore and colleagues (Chapter 18) concluded that evidence points to the *absence* of ethnic group differences among girls. They also noted, however, that many studies included small sample sizes of NA participants and measured a limited range of attitudes and behaviors. Thus, the goal of the present study was to survey a relatively large sample of NA boys and girls. We further were interested in examining the degree to which ethnic group differences in BMI contributed to differences in eating disorder symptoms.

Method

PARTICIPANTS

Students from 13 public schools in south-central Montana participated in the study. Schools were selected on the basis of their historically high enrollment of NA students. Eight schools were located in Billings; four in Hardin; and one in Ashland. All students in grades 5–10 were eligible to participate. Parental consent was obtained using a passive consent method approved by the Institutional Review Board at Montana State University in Bozeman, Montana, and by the school board (Billings) or individual school administrators (Hardin and Ashland). Among the NA (two NA parents) and NA-mixed (one NA parent) groups, the tribes represented were mainly those of the U.S. Central Plains, primarily the Crow (approximately 64%) and Northern Cheyenne (approximately 7%) but also including numerous other Plains tribes (e.g., Apache, Arapaho, Assiniboine, Blackfeet, Chippewa, Flathead, Gros Ventre, Mandan, Plains Ojibwe, Shoshone, Sioux). Individuals affiliated with virtually all of these tribes are descendants of the nomadic peoples of the Great Plains. The degree to which these tribal groups are representative of other indigenous peoples in North America is unclear. However, it is true that obesity and a variety of eating-related problems have been reported among widely dispersed NA tribes in the United States, ranging from the Pueblo people of the Southwest (Snow and Harris 1989), to the Cherokee tribes of the Southeast (Story et al. 1986), to the Chippewa of the Northeast (Rosen et al. 1988). In 1997, Story and colleagues reported eating and weight-related symptoms based on data collected from more than 12,000 NA youth living on or near reservations in 12 states. Unfortunately, no studies have examined differences among tribal groups in eating disorder symptoms.

Ethnic group and gender distributions of participants in the current study were as follows: 59.4% were white, 19.1% had two biological parents who were NA, 7.7% reported only one NA biological parent (NA-mixed), 7.3% were Hispanic, and 6.5% were of other or mixed ethnic backgrounds. Selected data from this study have been reported previously (Lynch et al. 2007, 2008). The present report used only data from white and NA participants.

Ethnic identity was determined by answers to several questions about self and parent. First, all participants were asked to identify their own ethnicity using a list of eight major groups, including white/Caucasian and American Indian/Alaska Native. Those of mixed ethnicity were given the opportunity to choose two ethnic groups to describe themselves. Those who self-identified as American Indian/Alaska Native were next asked which tribal group they most identified with. For participants who indicated that either parent was at least 50% American Indian/Alaska Native, a second set of questions assessed whether one or both parents were American Indian/Alaska Native and, if so, to which tribe each parent belonged. For the purposes of this data analysis, participants were assigned to the NA group only if they identified themselves and both parents as American Indian/Alaska Native.

ANALYSES AND INSTRUMENTS

Demographic Information

Age (based on date of birth), gender, and ethnicity were self-reported.

McKnight Risk Factor Survey

The McKnight Risk Factor Survey, Version IV (MRFS-IV) is a self-report questionnaire originally designed to assess risk factors for the development of eating disorders among pre- and postadolescents girls (Shisslak et al. 1999). An earlier version (MRFS-III) has been psychometrically validated with individuals ranging in age from 8 to 18 (grades 4–12). Although three forms of the MRFS-IV were available at the time of this study (C.M. Shisslak, personal communication, July 18, 2002), only the form designed for grades 6–12 was used (http://bml.stanford.edu/mcknight/). No attempt was made to modify the language of this instrument for NA participants because all were fluent in English, which is the language used in all the public schools surveyed. Furthermore, 81% of the NA participants reported speaking English at home and only 19% reported speaking their native language at home "some or all of the time." For the purpose of the present report, fourteen items representing potential eating disorder symptoms were selected for analysis. Specifically, five items measured body image disturbance, two items measured dieting for weight control practices, two items assessed binge eating, and five items assessed inappropriate compensatory behaviors (see Table 19–1). Students were asked how often "in the past year" they had experienced each of the symptoms, using a 5-point Likert scale ranging from never (1) to always (5).

Body Mass Index

Height (m) and weight (kg) were derived from digital photographs taken while participants stood barefoot on a Tanita BWB-800S digital balance with their faces covered. Each photo included a meter stick placed beside the participant that was later used to calculate his/her height using ImageJ software (http://rsb.info.nih.gov /ij/). Weight was read directly from the balance. BMI was calculated as kg/m². This photographic method was employed in order to facilitate rapid collection of large amounts of data within the limited time schedule of the participating schools. BMI scores were transformed to z-scores (BMIZ scores) using the 2000 Centers for Disease Control and Prevention growth charts (Centers for Disease Control and Prevention 2009).

Data Analyses

A univariate analysis of variance (ANOVA) was used to assess gender (male, female) and ethnicity (NA, white) differences in BMIZ scores. Furthermore, to examine ethnic group differences in eating disorder symptoms, multivariate analyses were carried out using each of the 14 MRFS-IV items as dependent variables (DVs; Table 19–1). ANOVAs and analyses of covariance (ANCOVAs; BMIZ score as a covariate) were calculated separately for each gender. Because all four multivariate tests indicated significant ethnic group differences ($P<0.01$), only unadjusted between-group differences for individual DVs are reported below. For differences reaching statistical significance ($P<0.05$), partial eta squared (η^2) was used to estimate effect size.

Results

The mean age in years ($\pm$ SD) and number of participants in each group were as follows: white boys, 14.01 ± 1.64 ($n=675$); white girls, 13.87 ± 1.55 ($n=580$); NA boys, 13.62 ± 1.67 ($n=179$); NA girls, 13.66 ± 1.83 ($n=197$). BMIZ score comparisons (ethnic group × gender) yielded significant main effects for ethnic group ($F_{1,1626}=56.57$; $P<0.001$) and gender ($F_{1,1626}=9.39$; $P=0.002$). As can be seen in Table 19–2, mean BMIZ scores were significantly greater for NA participants of both genders, but this difference was greater for boys than for girls, resulting in a significant ethnicity × gender ($F_{1,1626}=5.15$; $P<0.05$) interaction.

Tables 19–1 (girls) and 19–3 (boys) summarize results of ethnic group comparisons on each of the 14 MRFS-IV items, reporting both unadjusted and BMIZ-adjusted results. Among girls, in unadjusted models, ethnic group differences were statistically significant only for four items. Specifically, compared with white girls, NA girls reported ("in the past year") significantly more frequently being on a diet, starving for a day or more, and vomiting intentionally as methods of weight control. On the other hand, white girls were significantly more likely than NA girls to report that weight and shape made a difference in how they felt about themselves (i.e., "importance of weight or shape in how I feel about myself"). In models adjusted for BMIZ scores, only the differences in the importance of weight or shape remained statistically significant.

TABLE 19–1. Item score means and standard deviations for female participants on each of 14 symptom-related items taken from the McKnight Risk Factor Survey (MRFS)

MRFS item number	White		NA		No CoV			BMIZ CoV		
	Mean	SD	Mean	SD	F	P	η^2	F	P	η^2
Dieting										
2: Been on a diet to lose weight?	1.93	1.07	2.09	1.14	4.43	0.036	0.006	1.05	n.s.	
17: Skipped meals to lose weight?	1.69	1.05	1.75	1.06	0.76	n.s.		0.08	n.s.	
Compensatory behaviors										
4: Starved for a day or more?	1.41	0.86	1.55	0.94	4.72	0.030	0.006	2.42	n.s.	
15: Used laxatives or water pills?	1.07	0.39	1.10	0.413	0.96	n.s.		0.52	n.s.	
22: Exercised to lose weight?	2.70	1.21	2.62	1.23	0.46	n.s.		3.00	n.s.	
25: Thrown up intentionally?	1.15	0.55	1.26	0.73	5.96	0.015	0.008	3.52	n.s.	
32: Taken diet pills or speed?	1.16	0.59	1.15	0.57	0.016	n.s.		0.18	n.s.	
Binge/Lack of control										
19: Kept eating and eating and couldn't stop?	1.93	1.06	2.00	1.13	1.04	n.s.		0.47	n.s.	
36: Lot of food, short time, not meal?	1.97	1.00	1.96	1.06	0.06	n.s.		0.01	n.s.	

TABLE 19–1. Item score means and standard deviations for female participants on each of 14 symptom-related items taken from the McKnight Risk Factor Survey (MRFS) *(continued)*

MRFS item number	White		NA		No CoV			BMIZ CoV		
	Mean	SD	Mean	SD	F	P	η^2	F	P	η^2
Weight/shape concerns										
3: Worried about fat on your body?	2.79	1.33	2.79	1.39	0.008	n.s.		1.23	n.s.	
6: Felt fat?	2.68	1.35	2.69	1.36	0.001	n.s.		1.56	n.s.	
8: Thought about not wanting to be fat?	2.86	1.45	3.05	1.44	2.43	n.s.		0.42	n.s.	
39: Worried about gaining 2 lb?	1.91	1.15	1.86	1.13	0.476	n.s.		0.90	n.s.	
41: Weight/shape made a difference in your feelings about yourself?	2.41	1.24	2.14	1.08	5.89	0.015	0.008	8.62	0.003	0.011

Note. Between-subjects differences for ethnicity based on multivariate analyses of variance with and without BMIZ as a covariate (CoV) are shown. Effect size for each significant effect is indicated by partial eta squared (η^2).

BMIZ = body mass index z-score; NA = Native American.

TABLE 19–2.   Mean body mass index z-scores (±SD) of white and Native American adolescent girls and boys

	White		Native American			
	Mean	SD	Mean	SD	*t*	*P*
Girls	0.75	0.88	1.05	0.93	4.07	<0.001
Boys	0.79	1.10	1.36	0.98	6.77	<0.001

NA boys scored higher than white boys on all but one item ("overeating," eating a large amount of food in a short period of time outside of a meal) and with the exception of the frequency of vomiting ("thrown up intentionally"), binge eating ("kept eating and eating and couldn't stop"), and feelings about weight or shape ("weight and shape made a difference in how I feel about myself"), all these group differences were statistically significant. Surprisingly, NA boys reported lower frequency of overeating. In the model adjusted for differences in BMIZ scores, group differences for boys remained statistically significant for frequency of dieting and skipping meals, starving for a day or more, using laxatives or diuretics, and taking diet pills or speed for weight control. Also, after adjustment for BMIZ scores, the group differences in frequency of overeating remained statistically significant, with white boys reporting more frequent overeating than NA boys.

Discussion

The finding that adolescent NA girls appear to be at no greater risk for eating disorders than their white peers (when BMI covariance is removed) is consistent with findings of recent studies that found few or no statistically significant differences between NA and white girls or female college students (for review, see Chapter 18). Previous research (pre-1990) had suggested that NA girls were at greater eating disorder risk than their white peers. There are at least three possible reasons for this apparent discrepancy. One, it may reflect the methodological limitations of earlier studies. As noted earlier, although few previous studies have actually controlled for ethnic differences in BMI, the somewhat independent contributions of ethnicity and BMI to eating disorder symptoms have been noted (Lynch et al. 2004). Failure to take this into account may explain the apparently greater eating disorder risk among NA girls. Two, the increased risk may reflect the fact that the current data were gathered from a somewhat unique group of NA girls (i.e., Northern Plains Tribes) compared with samples in previous studies. Finally, it may be due to actual changes over the past 20 years in the way NA girls are responding to cultural pres-

TABLE 19–3. Item score means and standard deviations for male participants on each of 14 symptom-related items taken from the McKnight Risk Factor Survey (MRFS)

MRFS item number	White Mean	White SD	Native American Mean	Native American SD	No CoV F	No CoV P	No CoV η²	BMIZ CoV F	BMIZ CoV P	BMIZ CoV η²
Dieting										
2: Been on a diet to lose weight?	1.45	0.86	2.05	1.21	63.54	< 0.001	0.069	37.59	< 0.001	0.044
17: Skipped meals to lose weight?	1.28	0.71	1.54	0.98	17.45	< 0.001	0.020	7.61	0.006	0.009
Compensatory behaviors										
4: Starved for a day or more?	1.23	0.68	1.43	0.86	12.65	< 0.001	0.015	6.38	0.012	0.008
15: Used laxatives or water pills?	1.04	0.32	1.14	0.58	7.84	0.005	0.009	6.26	0.013	0.008
22: Exercised to lose weight?	2.21	1.29	2.52	1.35	9.45	0.002	0.011	1.20	n.s	
25: Thrown up intentionally?	1.06	0.40	1.11	0.44	2.78	n.s.		2.04	n.s	
32: Taken diet pills or speed?	1.07	0.44	1.17	0.51	6.92	0.009	0.008	4.25	0.040	0.005
Binge/Lack of control										
19: Kept eating and eating and couldn't stop?	1.75	1.04	1.78	1.04	0.15	n.s.		0.09	n.s	
36: Lot of food, short time, not meal?	1.97	1.12	1.71	1.00	7.00	0.008	0.018	5.31	0.021	0.006

TABLE 19–3. Item score means and standard deviations for male participants on each of 14 symptom-related items taken from the McKnight Risk Factor Survey (MRFS) *(continued)*

MRFS item number	White		Native American		No CoV			BMIZ CoV		
	Mean	SD	Mean	SD	F	P	η^2	F	P	η^2
Weight/shape concerns										
3: Worried about fat on your body?	1.84	1.11	2.20	1.25	16.37	0.000	0.019	3.03	n.s	
6: Felt fat?	1.68	1.05	1.90	1.12	7.09	0.008	0.008	0.23	n.s	
8: Thought about not wanting to be fat?	1.97	1.29	2.26	1.41	9.65	0.002	0.011	2.21	n.s	
39: Worried about gaining 2 lb?	1.28	0.72	1.45	0.90	6.66	0.010	0.008	3.25	n.s	
41: Weight/shape made a difference in your feelings about yourself?	1.72	1.04	1.76	1.08	0.23	n.s.		0.03	n.s	

Note. Between-subjects differences for ethnicity based on multivariate analyses of variance with and without BMIZ as a covariate (CoV) are shown. Effect size for each significant effect is indicated by partial eta squared (η^2).
BMIZ=body mass index z-score.

sures for thinness. Interestingly, in the present study, dieting and engaging in certain compensatory behaviors (starving and vomiting) by NA girls appear to be related to their higher average BMIZ scores, because these differences became nonsignificant when BMIZ score was accounted for statistically. Nevertheless, it is important to recognize that extreme weight control measures, such as vomiting and starving, remain serious public health concerns for NA girls. One group difference that appears not to be related to differences in body weight for height is the greater role that weight and shape perceptions play in how white girls feel about themselves. Despite the fact that white girls have significantly lower average BMIZ scores, they report significantly greater concerns about how weight and shape affect their self-worth than do NA girls. This may suggest that social comparison within local ethnic or community groups plays a greater role in determining how weight and shape are viewed in relation to self-esteem than do the general influences of the larger U.S. culture.

Differences between NA and white boys in eating disorder symptoms were particularly striking and somewhat unexpected. Few previous studies have compared NA and white adolescent boys. In one recent study, substantially higher percentages of NA than white boys reported ("in the past year") engaging in binge eating (21.4% vs. 11.6%), fasting or skipping meals (18.2% vs. 13.9%), using diet pills (5.4% vs. 2.0%) or laxatives (3.1% vs. 1.3%) to control weight, and vomiting after eating (2.6% vs. 1.3%) (Croll et al. 2002). A similar analysis of data from the present study found comparable differences. Analyses such as these, however, do not take account of body weight differences between groups. Nevertheless, when weight differences are accounted for, NA boys report greater frequencies for weight control behaviors, including dieting and skipping meals to lose weight, intentionally starving for a day or more, using laxatives or water pills, and using diet pills to control body weight. Why NA boys are more engaged in these compensatory behaviors than white boys remains unclear, although their very high average BMIZ scores and their concerns about being overweight may be contributing factors.

There was also a significant difference between white and NA boys in overeating; surprisingly, however, it was the white boys in the current study who reported more frequent overeating. This is contrary to the findings of Croll et al. (2002), who reported more frequent binge eating among NA boys. These differences may reflect differences in the wording of questions about binge eating. Unfortunately, because so few studies have included male adolescents, the explanation of these differences remains a matter of speculation. In the future, in-depth interviews of NA boys are needed to better reveal the factors influencing their responses to survey items about eating disorder symptoms.

In summary, there are a few differences in eating disorder symptoms between white and NA girls, but after adjustment for differences in relative weight, only one difference remained significant, indicating that for NA girls, their weight or shape is less important for their sense of self-worth than is true for white girls. On the other hand, compared with white boys, NA boys are engaging much more frequently in dieting, meal skipping, and several inappropriate compensatory behaviors aimed at controlling body weight, and these differences appear to be only partially due to their higher BMIZ scores. More detailed future research focusing on male adolescent eating and weight management behaviors is clearly needed.

References

Auker LM: Binge Eating and Bulimic Behaviors in a Select Native American Adolescent Population. Bozeman, Montana State University, 1993

Broussard BA, Sugarman JR, Bachman-Carter K, et al: Toward comprehensive obesity prevention programs in Native American communities. Obes Res 3(suppl):289s–297s, 1995

Centers for Disease Control and Prevention: A SAS Program for the CDC Growth Charts. Atlanta, GA, Centers for Disease Control and Prevention, updated 2009. Available at: http://www.cdc.gov/nccdphp/dnpao/growthcharts/resources/sas.htm. Accessed October 15, 2003.

Crago M, Shisslak CM, Estes LS: Eating disturbances among American minority groups: a review. Int J Eat Disord 19:239–248, 1996

Crawford PB, Story M, Wang MC, et al: Ethnic issues in the epidemiology of childhood obesity. Pediatr Clin North Am 48:855–878, 2001

Croll J, Neumark-Sztainer D, Story M, et al: Prevalence and risk and protective factors related to disordered eating behaviors among adolescents: relationship to gender and ethnicity. J Adolesc Health 31:166–175, 2002

Davis C, Yager J: Transcultural aspects of eating disorders: a critical literature review. Cult Med Psychiatry 16:377–394, 1992

Davis SM, Lambert LC: Body image and weight concerns among Southwestern American Indian preadolescent schoolchildren. Ethn Dis 10:184–194, 2000

French SA, Story M, Downes B, et al: Frequent dieting among adolescents: psychosocial and health behavior correlates. Am J Public Health 85:695–701, 1995

French SA, Story M, Neumark-Sztainer D, et al: Ethnic differences in psychosocial and health behavior correlates of dieting, purging, and binge eating in a population-based sample of adolescent females. Int J Eat Disord 22:315–322, 1997

Garner DM, Olmsted MP, Polivy J: Development and validation of a multidimensional eating disorders inventory for anorexia nervosa and bulimia. Int J Eat Disord 2:15–34, 1983

Lynch WC, Eppers KD, Sherrodd JR: Eating attitudes of Native American and white female adolescents: a comparison of BMI- and age-matched groups. Ethnic Health 9:253–266, 2004

Lynch WC, Heil DP, Wagner E, et al: Ethnic differences in BMI, weight concerns, and eating behaviors: comparison of Native American, white, and Hispanic adolescents. Body Image 4:179–190, 2007

Lynch WC, Heil DP, Wagner E, et al: Body dissatisfaction mediates the association between body mass index and risky weight control behaviors among white and Native American adolescent girls. Appetite 51:210–213, 2008

Neumark-Sztainer D, Story M, French SA, et al: Psychosocial concerns and health-compromising behaviors among overweight and nonoverweight adolescents. Obes Res 5:237–249, 1997a

Neumark-Sztainer D, Story M, Resnick MD, et al: Psychosocial concerns and weight control behaviors among overweight and nonoverweight Native American adolescents. J Am Diet Assoc 97:598–604, 1997b

Neumark-Sztainer D, Croll J, Story M, et al: Ethnic/racial differences in weight-related concerns and behaviors among adolescent girls and boys. Findings from Project EAT. J Psychosom Res 53:963–974, 2002

Rosen LW, Shafer CL, Dummer GM, et al: Prevalence of pathogenic weight-control behaviors among Native American women and girls. Int J Eat Disord 7:807–811, 1988

Shisslak CM, Renger R, Sharpe T, et al: Development and evaluation of the McKnight Risk Factor Survey for assessing potential risk and protective factors for disordered eating in preadolescent and adolescent girls. Int J Eat Disord 25:195–214, 1999

Smith JE, Krejci J: Minorities join the majority: eating disturbances among Hispanic and Native American youth. Int J Eat Disord 10:179–186, 1991

Smith MC, Thelen MH: Development and validation of a test for bulimia. J Consult Clin Psychol 52:863–872, 1984

Snow JT, Harris MB: Disordered Eating in South-western Pueblo Indians and Hispanics. J Adolesc 12:329–336, 1989

Story M, Tompkins RA, Bass MA, et al: Anthropometric measurements and dietary intakes of Cherokee Indian teenagers in North Carolina. J Am Diet Assoc 86:1555–1560, 1986

Story M, Rosenwinkel K, Himes JH, et al: Demographic and risk factors associated with chronic dieting in adolescents. Am J Dis Child 145:994–998, 1991

Story M, Hauck FR, Broussard BA, et al: Weight perceptions and weight control practices in American Indian and Alaska Native adolescents: a national survey. Arch Pediatr Adolesc Med 148:567–571, 1994

Story M, French SA, Resnick MD, et al: Ethnic/racial and socioeconomic differences in dieting behaviors and body image perceptions in adolescents. Int J Eat Disord 18:173–179, 1995

Story M, French SA, Neumark-Sztainer D, et al: Psychosocial and behavioral correlates of dieting and purging in Native American adolescents. Pediatrics 99:E8, 1997

Story M, Evans M, Fabsitz RR, et al: The epidemic of obesity in American Indian communities and the need for childhood obesity-prevention programs. Am J Clin Nutr 69(suppl):747S–754S, 1999

Story M, Stevens J, Evans M, et al: Weight loss attempts and attitudes toward body size, eating, and physical activity in American Indian children: relationship to weight status and gender. Obes Res 9:356–363, 2001

20

SHOULD NON-FAT-PHOBIC ANOREXIA NERVOSA BE INCLUDED IN DSM-5?

Anne E. Becker, M.D., Ph.D., Sc.M.

Jennifer J. Thomas, Ph.D.

Kathleen M. Pike, Ph.D.

Cultural variation in the presentation of anorexia nervosa (AN) has been reported with respect to the rationale for food refusal. Some of these rationales do not reflect the "intense fear of gaining weight or becoming fat" specified by DSM-IV (American Psychiatric Association 1994, 2000) AN Criterion B. As a result, this atypical presentation—commonly referred to as "non-fat-phobic anorexia nervosa" (NFP-AN)—has raised questions about whether this variant is a *forme fruste* of AN versus a more benign variant of eating disorder not otherwise specified (EDNOS). Likewise, the absence of "fat phobia" in cases that otherwise appear very clinically similar to AN raises questions about whether it is intrinsic to the disorder. Finally, because the diverse rationales for food refusal and low weight—exemplified by patients with NFP-AN—appear associated with particular historical and cultural

This article was co-published by the *International Journal of Eating Disorders* and the American Psychiatric Association. The authors are grateful to Mike Alvarez for his contributions to an earlier version of this article and to the DSM-5 Eating Disorders Work Group for helpful comments on previous drafts.

contexts, this presentation lends support to the possibility that conventional AN is "culture bound."

Given cultural variation in rationales for food refusal, several theorists (Katzman and Lee 1997; Lee 1991; Palmer 1993; Rieger et al. 2001) have advocated for flexibility regarding fear of weight gain as a diagnostic criterion. The countervailing view, however, is that fat phobia is the sine qua non of AN and should be retained as a diagnostic criterion in future nosologic schemata (Habermas 1996). The aim of this review is to synthesize and critique available data on NFP-AN to consider whether and how it might be best represented in eating disorders classification. In doing so, we borrow a framework from a seminal paper examining the diagnostic validity of subtypes of schizophrenia (Robins and Guze 1970). In this article, Robins and Guze proposed five criteria for establishing the diagnostic validity of a putative disorder: 1) clinical description; 2) laboratory studies (including psychological testing); 3) delimitation from other disorders; 4) follow-up studies; and 5) familial aggregation. The current review comprises three aims: 1) to determine whether NFP-AN meets established criteria for diagnostic validity using this standard; 2) to conduct a meta-analytic evaluation of its delimitation from DSM-IV AN; and 3) to consider possible options for inclusion in DSM-5.

Method

SYSTEMATIC SEARCH OF THE LITERATURE

We performed two systematic searches to identify studies in MEDLINE and Psyc-INFO published from 1950 to 2008 with relevance to NFP-AN. First, we identified papers with the search terms "anorexia nervosa" or "EDNOS" as well as one or more of the following stem words (and/or their derivatives): "fat phobia," "weight phobia," "laparophobia," "fear of fatness," "food refusal," "asceticism," and "empty stomach." This search phase identified fewer than 50 relevant papers, many of which discussed data from the same clinic or were reviews. We identified additional articles from the reference sections of articles identified by our search or through personal communication. In a second search, we identified literature describing the clinical and prognostic significance of drive for thinness (DT) in both clinical and nonclinical samples through titles or abstracts containing both the term "anorexia" (and its derivatives) and at least one of the following phrases: "drive for thinness," "thin body ideal," "slim body ideal," "excessive weight loss," "excessive weight reduction," and "desire" (spaced within three words of "thin" or "slim").

META-ANALYSIS

To evaluate whether NFP-AN meets Robins and Guze's third criterion, delimitation from other disorders, we applied meta-analytic techniques to studies presenting quantitative data on the differences in eating pathology between AN versus 1) NFP-AN and 2) AN with low drive for thinness (low-DT-AN). We adapted and expanded upon the methodology from a recent meta-analysis quantifying the differences between EDNOS versus AN, BN, or binge eating disorder (BED) (Thomas et al. 2009).[1]

Study eligibility for inclusion in the current meta-analysis required 1) comparison of a group meeting full DSM-III-R (American Psychiatric Association 1987) or DSM-IV (American Psychiatric Association 1994) criteria for AN with a group meeting all criteria for AN except that fat phobia was absent or they had low DT; 2) publication in English in 1987 or later (i.e., after publication of DSM-III-R); and 3) sufficient information for the calculation of effect sizes (descriptive data or test statistics).

From each study, we extracted data on all possible measures of current eating disorder psychopathology (both attitudinal and behavioral) in the AN, NFP-AN, and low-DT-AN groups. When studies presented multiple measures of eating pathology for the same sample of participants, we averaged those effect sizes to obtain a single effect for that study and then combined effect sizes across studies utilizing a random effects model to obtain the standardized mean difference (Cohen's *d*). Because the majority of measures of eating disorder psychopathology contain at least some items that assess fear of weight gain and overvaluation of shape and weight, and because these measures have therefore been critiqued as potentially lacking cross-cultural validity, we addressed this potential source of confounding in two ways. First, we evaluated the extent to which including these measures altered our results by calculating two separate effect sizes for each study. The "conservative" effect size included only those measures with no potential for conceptual overlap with fat phobia, such as dietary restraint, bingeing, purging, and non-overlapping subscales of multidimensional measures of eating pathology. In contrast, the "broad" effect size combined data on all possible measures of eating pathology, including all subscales of the Eating Disorder Examination (EDE; Fairburn et al. 2008), Eating Disorder Inventory (EDI; Garner et al. 1983), and Eating Attitudes Test (EAT; Garner et al. 1982). Second, to examine the magnitude and direction of effects within each cross-cultural context, we calculated summary effect sizes separately for studies on Western versus non-Western populations. In addition to probing between-group differences in eating pathology, we also meta-

---

[1]We utilize some of the same studies as Thomas et al. (2009) but expand on their methodology in three ways: 1) we applied fewer exclusion criteria on potentially eligible studies (i.e., we did not require diagnoses to be obtained via structured interviews) and increased the search timeline from 1987 to 2008 so as to obtain as large a study set as possible; 2) we present two different measures of effect size (i.e., conservative versus broad) for each study; and 3) we evaluate potential between-group differences in body mass index.

analytically evaluated between-group differences in body mass index (BMI), another marker of AN severity.

Results

CLINICAL DESCRIPTION

Robins and Guze's first criterion for diagnostic validity is a description of the "clinical picture" of the putative disorder, including both distinctive symptoms and associated demographic characteristics. Numerous case studies and case series from a variety of cultural contexts present detailed accounts of volitional self-starvation in the absence of fat phobia; this volume of literature appears to meet this first criterion. Although historical data also suggest the contextual nature of food refusal (Bemporad 1996; Parry-Jones 1985), we focus on contemporary data in this review.

Cultural Variation in Rationales for Food Refusal

Contemporary research provides a modest number of case reports and case series documenting NFP-AN (Table 20–1). Most reports describe NFP-AN in Hong Kong Chinese identified in clinical settings (Chan and Ma 2002; Kam and Lee 1998; Lai 2000; Lee 1991, 1995; Lee et al. 1989, 2001; Ngai et al. 2000). Notably, the majority are authored or co-authored by Professor Sing Lee, a psychiatrist and medical anthropologist credited with characterizing this phenomenological variant. However, NFP-AN has also been reported in other non-Western populations, including in Singapore (Ong et a. 1982; Ung et al. 1997), West Malaysia (Goh et al. 1993), Ghana (Bennett et al. 2004), and India (Khandelwal and Saxena 1990) as well as in Asian patients residing in Australia (Rieger et al. 2001) and in South Asian patients residing in the United Kingdom (Ratan et al. 1998; Tareen et al. 2005). Moreover, two studies reporting the relative frequency of NFP-AN in South Asian versus "white" AN patients in the United Kingdom found that NFP-AN was relatively more common in South Asians (Tareen et al. 2005); however, one of these studies reported that "sensitivity to 'fatness'" was "invariably revealed" during treatment (Soomro et al. 1995).

Although Lee's (1991; Lee et al. 1993) early work in Hong Kong emphasizes that NFP-AN is common, he also recognized that fat phobia and body dissatisfaction were increasing among Chinese adolescent girls in the mid-1990s (Lee and Lee 1996). Moreover, several small studies present data indicating that conventional AN is identified equally, if not more commonly, as NFP-AN, even in non-Western cultures (Goh et al. 1993; Lai 2000; Lee et al. 2001; Ong et al. 1982; Ratan et al. 1998; Ung et al. 1997). In contrast, a community sample of 688 students in Ghana found no fat phobia expressed among 10 cases identified with underweight attributed to self-starvation (Bennett et al. 2004), and two India-based investigators assert that fat phobia is "hardly ever seen" in India (Khandelwal and Saxena 1990). Thus, case series and prevalence studies do not support a categorical absence of conventional AN across non-Western cultures. Moreover, our search parameters may have contributed to bias in the relative frequency of NFP-AN, because the search would not necessarily have identified studies finding no evidence of NFP-AN.

These NFP-AN case reports describe a finite number of alternate rationales for food refusal. Commonly, these are complaints of gastrointestinal symptoms, a somatic idiom of distress more acceptable given local cultural values and expectations (Lee et al. 2001). It has also been asserted that the presentation of AN is socially constructed in clinical encounters (Lee 1995). The motivation for and manifestation of behavioral symptoms reference not only cultural symbols but also deeply personal meanings (Katzman and Lee 1997; Kleinman 1989). Indeed, heterogeneous attribution of weight concerns has been identified in case reports of two American women with AN who drew from personally meaningful symbolism to rationalize dietary restriction with religious—not secular—values (Banks 1992, 1996).

In summary, descriptive data establish the wide geographical distribution of NFP-AN, but the small number of papers recently published does not meet Blashfield et al.'s (1990) suggested standard of at least 50 in the past 10 years. Moreover, descriptive data neither specify clearly whether the absence of fat phobia is regarded as a categorical or dimensional (Hsu and Sobkiewicz 1991) construct nor specify how to classify cases that cross over. Finally, the characterization of NFP-AN is most often based on clinical data from non-Western populations.

PSYCHOLOGICAL TESTING

Robins and Guze's (1970) second criterion for the evaluation of diagnostic validity is the refinement of the clinical picture with laboratory tests (in this case, psychological measures). Several NFP-AN papers have presented scores on well-validated measures of eating pathology, including the EAT, EDI, and EDE. Although NFP-AN has typically been assessed with qualitative clinical interviews in non-Western settings, several studies of Western clinical populations have identified cases of low-weight EDNOS or atypical AN exhibiting low levels of fat phobia on standardized assessment measures (Abbate-Daga et al. 2007; Norvell and Cooley 1986–1987; Ramacciotti et al. 2002; Strober et al. 1999; Willenberg and Krauthauser 2000). Moreover, the majority of a small number of studies reporting on comparative measures of DT and related constructs across culturally distinct populations have supported culturally based differences in DT. With the exception of a study comparing data on schoolgirls in Singapore with previously published American data (Kok and Tian 1994) and an assessment across strata defined by religious identification (Joughin et al. 1992), both of which reported negative findings, these studies have all reported significant between-group differences. Of these, significantly lower DT

TABLE 20–1. Clinical observational data and quantitative comparative data supporting cultural diversity in rationale for food refusal in anorexia nervosa (AN) and drive for thinness

Study	Geographical region(s)	Sample	N	Assessment of AN, fat phobia, drive for thinness	Results	Investigator conclusions
Descriptive clinical data supporting cultural variation in rationales for food refusal in AN						
Ong et al. 1982	Singapore	Clinic-based patients with AN	7	Retrospective clinical data	2/7 patients had no fat phobia	AN cases identified that mostly resembled—but were "less severe"—than AN described in Western populations
Norvell and Cooley 1986–1987	USA	Clinic-based patients referred for "significant" EDs	2	Clinical interview EDI	Both cases had 25% weight loss and psychological basis for poor intake but no discernible fear of weight gain	Cases should be considered "atypical" EDs in absence of weight concerns
Lee et al. 1989	Hong Kong	Clinic-based Chinese patients with AN	3	Clinical data	All three had (varying) relative denial of fat phobia; abdominal discomfort used as rationale for restriction	Contrasting social norms in China may reduce pursuit of thinness in AN
Banks 1992 (overlaps with case report in Banks 1996)	USA	Cases of AN identified through religious groups and a treatment center	2	Patient self-report of AN	Religious idioms provided rationale for food refusal and concerns about weight	Religious rationale can motivate AN behaviors in contemporary USA

TABLE 20–1. Clinical observational data and quantitative comparative data supporting cultural diversity in rationale for food refusal in anorexia nervosa (AN) and drive for thinness *(continued)*

Study	Geographical region(s)	Sample	N	Assessment of AN, fat phobia, drive for thinness	Results	Investigator conclusions
Descriptive clinical data supporting cultural variation in rationales for food refusal in AN (continued)						
Goh et al. 1993	West Malaysia	Clinic-based patients who met 2–3 diagnostic criteria for AN	15	Retrospective chart review	9/15 had chart evidence of body image disturbance	Cases of AN occur in this setting that have body image disturbance resembling AN cases in Western populations
Lee 1991	Hong Kong	Clinic-based patients who only partially fulfilled DSM-III-R criteria for AN due to "inconspicuity" of fat phobia and DBI	16	Semistructured clinical interview BMI DBI assessed by clinical interview, discrepancy in ideal and desired body weights, patients' drawings	15/16 complained of abdominal discomfort (usually epigastric), but "intense fear of obesity" was "inconspicuous" Fear of obesity was obvious only in 3, mild in 8, and absent in 5 13/16 required inpatient treatment; "resistance toward weight gain" was "almost always present" but was rationalized by "'no appetite'" or "bloating," for example Fear of obesity did not emerge in treatment (1–5 years' duration)	Intense fear of fatness and DBI may be culture-bound concepts and inappropriate for identifying AN among Chinese unassimilated to Western pressures to be thin

TABLE 20–1. Clinical observational data and quantitative comparative data supporting cultural diversity in rationale for food refusal in anorexia nervosa (AN) and drive for thinness *(continued)*

Study	Geographical region(s)	Sample	N	Assessment of AN, fat phobia, drive for thinness	Results	Investigator conclusions
Descriptive clinical data supporting cultural variation in rationales for food refusal in AN *(continued)*						
Lee 1995	Hong Kong	Clinic-based, emaciated patients	2	Clinical data EDE	2 cases of emaciation/food refusal with rationales that did not include fat phobia	Raises questions about inflexibility of DSM criteria, reification of symptoms, and lack of attunement to patient experience
Ung et al. 1997	Singapore	Clinic-based patients with AN and BN	50	Retrospective chart review; information from attending psychiatrist "when available"	90% "fear of fatness" 84% "body image disturbance" 96% "compulsive efforts to lose weight"	Weight and body concerns and fat phobia were expressed in the majority of AN and BN patients in this clinical sample
Ratan et al. 1998	UK (South Asians)	Clinic-based patients with EDs	21	Case record data on DSM-III/III-R diagnoses and ICD-10 research criteria	3/21 met AN criteria 3/21 met AN criteria but without fat phobia 2/12 cases of BN lacked "dread of fatness"	Absence of fat phobia observed
Kam and Lee 1998	Hong Kong/Canada	Clinic-based patients with AN	2	Clinical data EDI	One patient never manifested fat phobia and had low DT; the other had fat phobia and high DT	AN can present without fat phobia; this may account for treatment delays in Hong Kong

TABLE 20–1. Clinical observational data and quantitative comparative data supporting cultural diversity in rationale for food refusal in anorexia nervosa (AN) and drive for thinness *(continued)*

Study	Geographical region(s)	Sample	N	Assessment of AN, fat phobia, drive for thinness	Results	Investigator conclusions
Descriptive clinical data supporting cultural variation in rationales for food refusal in AN *(continued)*						
Ngai et al. 2000	Hong Kong	Clinic-based patients with AN	4	Longitudinal clinical data	Description of four distinct courses of fat phobia: present, present and then remitting, absent and then present, and absent	Fat phobia is not a core symptom of AN, nor is it temporally stable
Lai 2000	Hong Kong	Clinic-based patients with AN	16	Chart review, including a semistructured clinical interview	14/16 had fear of fatness 13/16 had weight reduction as rationale for food refusal	Majority of these Hong Kong Chinese AN patients had fat phobia
Rieger et al. 2001	Australia	Clinic-based patients with AN or BN and Asian heritage	14	Chart review	All had "ego-syntonic" emaciation; not all patients had fat phobia [no specific number reported]	Assumptions that weight concerns are central to EDs should be examined
Chan and Ma 2002	Hong Kong	Clinic-based patient with AN	1	Data extraction from eight family therapy session videotapes	Rationale for food refusal assessed as self-discipline and "punishment" for her family	Rationale for food refusal in AN may be specific to cultural context

TABLE 20–1. Clinical observational data and quantitative comparative data supporting cultural diversity in rationale for food refusal in anorexia nervosa (AN) and drive for thinness *(continued)*

Study	Geographical region(s)	Sample	N	Assessment of AN, fat phobia, drive for thinness	Results	Investigator conclusions
Descriptive clinical data supporting cultural variation in rationales for food refusal in AN *(continued)*						
Bennett et al. 2004	Ghana	School-based	688	Clinical interview based on ICD-10 diagnostic criteria following a screen for BMI≤19; EAT-30; BITE	10 cases identified (1.5%) with underweight attributed to self-starvation; Rationale related to religious motives and self-efficacy; no fat phobia/weight management motives identified; EAT and BITE scores did not identify these 10 cases	AN presents without fat phobia in Ghana
Studies presenting quantitative cross-cultural comparative data relating to fat phobia and drive for thinness						
Steinhausen et al. 1992 (overlaps with Neumärker et al. 1992)	East Berlin/West Berlin	Clinic-based School-based	East Berlin AN patients (n=37), West Berlin AN patients (n=44), and East Berlin students (n=362)	EDI	AN respondents in East Berlin scored significantly lower on DT (and 5/8 EDI subscales) compared with AN respondents from West Berlin; DT subscale did not discriminate East Berlin AN and East Berlin non-AN groups	EDI may lack trans-cultural validity

TABLE 20–1. Clinical observational data and quantitative comparative data supporting cultural diversity in rationale for food refusal in anorexia nervosa (AN) and drive for thinness *(continued)*

Study	Geographical region(s)	Sample	N	Assessment of AN, fat phobia, drive for thinness	Results	Investigator conclusions
Studies presenting quantitative cross-cultural comparative data relating to fat phobia and drive for thinness (continued)						
Neumärker et al. 1992 (overlaps with Steinhausen et al. 1992)	East Berlin/ West Berlin	Clinic-based School-based	East Berlin AN patients (*n*=37), West Berlin AN patients (*n*=52), East Berlin students (*n*=364), West Berlin students (*n*=165)	EAT	EAT scores were significantly higher in West vs. East Berlin AN patients	EAT scores are culturally dependent
Kok and Tian 1994	Singapore	School-based	656 (Chinese Singapore schoolgirls)	EDI	No significant DT differences versus American undergraduates Significantly more respondents with high BMI in high than in low DT groups	Chinese Singapore schoolgirls endorse DT despite low prevalence of AN in this population

TABLE 20–1. Clinical observational data and quantitative comparative data supporting cultural diversity in rationale for food refusal in anorexia nervosa (AN) and drive for thinness *(continued)*

Study	Geographical region(s)	Sample	N	Assessment of AN, fat phobia, drive for thinness	Results	Investigator conclusions
Studies presenting quantitative cross-cultural comparative data relating to fat phobia and drive for thinness *(continued)*						
Soomro et al. 1995	UK	Clinic-based patients with AN and partial-syndrome AN	"Non-white" (n=41), "white" (n=944), "non-white" classification included Asians, Afro-Caribbeans, "mixed race," and "others"	Clinical data/ Chart review	12% "non-white" vs. 5% "white" patients denied "sensitivity to fatness" on admission. "Non-white" patients were four times less likely to admit to "sensitivity to fatness" at presentation in age-adjusted regression model. "Sensitivity to fatness" was "invariably revealed" during weight restoration	Symptom profiles of AN/partial-syndrome AN are similar in UK "whites" and "non-whites"
Striegel-Moore et al. 1995	USA	Community-based comparison of black and white preadolescent girls	Black (n=311), white (n=302)	DT	Black girls had significantly higher DT than white girls. DT was significantly associated with adiposity in both groups and with weight criticism in the black group	Social pressure is related to DT in black girls

TABLE 20–1. Clinical observational data and quantitative comparative data supporting cultural diversity in rationale for food refusal in anorexia nervosa (AN) and drive for thinness *(continued)*

Study	Geographical region(s)	Sample	N	Assessment of AN, fat phobia, drive for thinness	Results	Investigator conclusions
Studies presenting quantitative cross-cultural comparative data relating to fat phobia and drive for thinness (continued)						
Lee et al. 1998	Hong Kong	Clinic-based patients with AN-R compared with published Canadian patients with AN-R (*n*=129)	23	Clinical assessment EDI	Chinese patients with AN-R had a significantly lower DT than Canadian patients with AN-R	NFP-AN and AN are phenomenologically distinctive
Sjostedt et al. 1998	Australia/India	University-based	Australian students (*n*=297), Indian students (*n*=249)	EAT-26 Goldfarb Fear of Fat Scale	Indians scored significantly higher than Australians on both measures	ED symptoms may be present among educated, elite Indians

TABLE 20–1. Clinical observational data and quantitative comparative data supporting cultural diversity in rationale for food refusal in anorexia nervosa (AN) and drive for thinness *(continued)*

Study	Geographical region(s)	Sample	N	Assessment of AN, fat phobia, drive for thinness	Results	Investigator conclusions
Studies presenting quantitative cross-cultural comparative data relating to fat phobia and drive for thinness *(continued)*						
Pike and Mizushima 2005	Japan/North American control group	Japanese: Clinic-based AN-R patients (*n*=22), AN-BP (*n*=24); BN (*n*=43); community sample without ED (*n*=54) North American comparison sample: Clinic-based AN-R patients (*n*=129), AN-BP (*n*=103), BN (*n*=657); community sample without ED (*n*=205)	Japanese with AN (*n*=46), North American with AN (*n*=232)	For Japanese participants: semistructured clinical interview based on DSM criteria For all: EDI	Japanese respondents: AN-R, AN-BP, and BN had significantly greater DT than non-ED comparison group Cross-national comparison: Japanese AN-R, BN, and non-ED groups all had significantly lower DT than respective North American comparison groups	DT appears to distinguish ED from non-ED individuals in Japan, but DT is lower in Japanese than in North Americans across most categories

TABLE 20–1. Clinical observational data and quantitative comparative data supporting cultural diversity in rationale for food refusal in anorexia nervosa (AN) and drive for thinness *(continued)*

Study	Geographical region(s)	Sample	N	Assessment of AN, fat phobia, drive for thinness	Results	Investigator conclusions
Studies presenting quantitative cross-cultural comparative data relating to fat phobia and drive for thinness *(continued)*						
Tareen et al. 2005	UK	Clinic-based: BMI <18 and history of "self-induced" weight loss without physical cause	South Asian (n=14), "White English" (n=14)	Clinical data	South Asians were significantly less likely to present with fat phobia or to express weight/food preoccupation; significantly more likely to present with loss of appetite than whites	Symptom profiles for AN may differ for UK South Asians; this may result in their not receiving services
Lee and Lock 2007	USA	Clinic-based: adolescents in family treatment for AN	Asian Americans (n=16), non-Asians (n=76)	EDE	Asian Americans scored significantly lower than non-Asians on EDE restraint and weight concerns subscales notwithstanding similar clinical presentation across groups	Asian Americans may underreport ED symptoms

Note. AN-BP=anorexia nervosa, binge-purge type; AN-R=AN, restricting type; BITE=Bulimic Investigatory Test, Edinburgh; BMI=body mass index; BN=bulimia nervosa; DBI=distorted body image; DT=EDI drive for thinness subscale; EAT=Eating Attitudes Test; ED=eating disorder; EDE=Eating Disorder Examination; EDI=Eating Disorder Inventory; NFP-AN=non-fat-phobic AN.

or weight concern was reported for eating disorder patients in presumably less culturally Western populations compared with reference populations (e.g., AN, restricting Hong Kong patients compared with AN, restricting Canadian patients [Lee et al. 1998], Japanese compared with North Americans [Pike and Mizushima 2005], East Berliners compared with West Berliners [Neumärker et al. 1992; Steinhausen et al. 1992], and Asian Americans compared with non–Asian Americans [Lee and Lock 2007]). Finally, one study demonstrated higher levels of DT in black, compared with white, preadolescents in the United States (Striegel-Moore et al. 1995). Another study found significantly greater fear of fatness in (South Asian) Indian compared with Australian university students (Sjostedt et al. 1998). Despite the consistency of cross-cultural differences, individuals with eating disorders typically exhibit significantly greater DT than non-eating-disordered control subjects within culturally homogeneous groups, such as Hong Kong (Lee et al. 1998) and Japan (Pike and Mizushima 2005). Thus, although sociocultural context may moderate mean DT levels, similar case-control distinctions are found in both Western and non-Western cultural settings.

DELIMITATION FROM OTHER DISORDERS

Robins and Guze's (1970) third criterion for diagnostic validity, delimitation from other disorders, requires that the disorder in question be clearly differentiable from similar disorders. In contrast to the numerous case series and theoretical reviews describing the differential phenomenology of NFP-AN versus typical AN, only a handful of empirical studies have quantified the magnitude and significance of these differences utilizing well-validated measures.

Non-Fat-Phobic Anorexia Nervosa Versus DSM-IV Anorexia Nervosa

The first generation of quantitative studies compared NFP-AN with DSM-IV AN patients in non-Western societies, including China and Japan. Patients were grouped into fat-phobic versus non-fat-phobic presentations via qualitative clinical interviews. Overall, NFP-AN patients scored significantly lower on attitudinal measures of eating pathology than fat-phobic patients in two quantitative studies (Lee et al. 2002; Noma et al. 2006), but not in two others (Lau et al. 2006; Lee et al. 1998). In one study, significantly fewer NFP-AN patients endorsed bingeing and purging than fat-phobic AN patients (Lee et al. 1993); a second study also documented lower rates, but the effect was not significant (Lee et al. 2001). Studies with larger samples were more likely to identify significant differences. Aggregating across studies on all available measures of eating pathology, individuals with typical AN scored two-thirds of a standard deviation higher than individuals with NFP-AN (d [broad] = 0.65, SE = 0.21, P = 0.002). Despite critiques of the cross-cultural validity of self-report questionnaires such as the EDI (Lee et al. 1998), EDE (Lau et al. 2006), and EAT (Lee et al. 2002) in non-Western populations, a significant between-group difference remained even when analyses were restricted to measures without potential overlap with fat phobia (d [conservative] = 0.41, SE = 0.20, P = 0.04. In contrast, although the two groups did not differ on BMI at presentation (d = 0.27, SE = 0.21, P = 0.20), individuals with conventional AN exhibited significantly higher premorbid BMI than those with NFP-AN (d = 0.89, SE = 0.26, P = 0.001) (Table 20–2).

Although early studies comparing AN and NFP-AN in non-Western populations were innovative in providing preliminary data on relative severity, findings were limited by their unclear diagnostic reliability (i.e., no interrater reliability kappas for AN versus NFP-AN diagnoses were presented in the original research reports) and low statistical power to detect between-group differences. In addition, study findings were of uncertain generalizability because the majority came from a single Hong Kong research group, and diagnoses of fat-phobic versus NFP-AN were based on clinical judgment, which may not be replicable outside this setting.

Low Versus High Drive for Thinness Anorexia Nervosa

The second generation of quantitative comparisons featured studies of AN patients in Western populations (Europe and Canada) classified as exhibiting high versus low levels of fat phobia based on a cut point derived from a dimensional measure. Three of these (Abbate-Daga et al. 2007; Ramacciotti et al. 2002; Vervaet et al. 2004) reported comparisons between low-weight, amenorrheic patients who scored ≤7 versus >7 on the EDI Drive for Thinness subscale, whereas another (Dalle Grave et al. 2008) presented comparisons between those scoring <4 and ≥4 on EDE items querying "fear of weight gain," "importance of weight," and "importance of shape." Phenomenologically, Western AN patients endorsing low DT report similar rationales for food refusal to those observed in non-Western samples, such as bloating, nausea, and postprandial discomfort (Dalle Grave et al. 2008; Ramacciotti et al. 2002). Comparative findings indicate that AN patients with low DT exhibit significantly lower levels of attitudinal eating pathology on the EDI (Abbate-Daga et al. 2007; Ramacciotti et al. 2002; Vervaet et al. 2004) and EDE (Dalle Grave et al. 2008) than typical AN patients and provide some evidence for a more benign behavioral profile among AN patients with low DT, featuring lower rates of bingeing (Dalle Grave et al. 2008) and purging (Ramacciotti et al. 2002; Vervaet et al. 2004). On the basis of these data, study investigators concluded that low-DT-AN exhibits lower levels of eating pathology than high-DT AN. To examine the possibility that both NFP and low-DT-AN carry similar diagnostic significance, we compared low-DT-AN with conventional AN across studies. Combining effects across studies, the standardized mean difference in eating pathology between AN versus low-DT-AN in Western samples was similar to

TABLE 20–2. Studies featuring quantitative comparisons of typical anorexia nervosa (AN) versus atypical AN (non-fat-phobic or low drive for thinness presentations)

Study	Country	Sample	N	Diagnostic method	Quantitative measures of eating pathology	Cohen's d (SE)	Investigator conclusions
Cross-sectional studies of fat-phobic vs. non-fat-phobic AN							
Lee et al. 1993	Hong Kong	AN patients	70	Qualitative interview	**Binge eating**	**0.87 (0.34)***	AN-like syndromes can occur in the absence of fat phobia
					Exercising		
					Vomiting	*0.74 (0.32)**	
					Ideal BMI	0.26 (0.27)	
					Current BMI	1.39 (0.31)**	
					Premorbid BMI		
Lee et al. 1998	Hong Kong	AN patients	23	Qualitative interview	EDI bulimia	−0.29 (0.42)	EDI has questionable validity for ED screening in China
					EDI ineffectiveness		
					EDI interoceptive awareness		
					EDI interpersonal distrust		
					EDI maturity fears		
					EDI perfectionism		
					EDI drive for thinness	*0.11 (0.43)*	
					EDI body dissatisfaction		
					Desired BMI		
					Current BMI	0.35 (0.42)	
Lee et al. 2001	Hong Kong	AN patients	48	Qualitative interview	**Bulimia**	**0.64 (0.47)**	Multiple rationales for food refusal are possible in a cross-cultural context
						0.64 (0.47)	
					Current BMI	−0.17 (0.31)	
					Premorbid BMI	0.86 (0.32)*	

TABLE 20–2. Studies featuring quantitative comparisons of typical anorexia nervosa (AN) versus atypical AN (non-fat-phobic or low drive for thinness presentations) *(continued)*

Study	Country	Sample	N	Diagnostic method	Quantitative measures of eating pathology	Cohen's *d* (SE)	Investigator conclusions
Cross-sectional studies of fat-phobic vs. non-fat-phobic AN (continued)							
Lee et al. 2002	Hong Kong	AN patients	109	Qualitative interview	**EAT bulimia**	0.52 (0.20)*	EAT has questionable validity for ED screening in China
					EAT social pressure to eat	0.72 (0.20)**	
					EAT dieting		
					Desired BMI		
					Current BMI	0.79 (0.20)**	
					Premorbid BMI	0.54 (0.20)*	
Lau et al. 2006	Hong Kong	AN patients	18	Structured interview	**EDE restraint**	−0.07 (0.47)	AN and AT scored similarly on the EDE; the fat phobia criterion has questionable validity
					EDE eating concern		
					Objective binge episodes		
					EDE weight concern	0.07 (0.47)	
					EDE shape concern		
					Current BMI	−0.21 (0.47)	
Noma et al. 2006	Japan	AN patients	31	Qualitative interview	*EAT-26 ≥ 15*	**Not included** 2.37 (0.72)**	EAT-26 has questionable validity for identifying EDNOS in Japan

TABLE 20–2. Studies featuring quantitative comparisons of typical anorexia nervosa (AN) versus atypical AN (non-fat-phobic or low drive for thinness presentations) *(continued)*

Study	Country	Sample	N	Diagnostic method	Quantitative measures of eating pathology	Cohen's *d* (SE)	Investigator conclusions
Cross-sectional studies of AN with high *vs.* low drive for thinness							
Ramacciotti et al. 2002	Canada[a]	AN patients	104	EDI-DT≤7 vs. >7	EDI bulimia	0.73 (0.39)	AT group exhibited less severe psychopathology
					EDI ineffectiveness		
					EDI interoceptive awareness		
					EDI interpersonal distrust		
					EDI maturity fears		
					EDI perfectionism		
					Laxative abuse		
					EDI body dissatisfaction	*0.80 (0.38)**	
Vervaet et al. 2004	Belgium	AN patients	226	EDI-DT≤7 vs. >7	DEBQ emotional eating	**0.39 (0.16)***	AT group exhibited less severe psychopathology
					DEBQ external eating		
					DEBQ restrained eating		
					Purging	*0.39 (0.16)**	
					Current BMI	0.07 (0.15)	

TABLE 20–2. Studies featuring quantitative comparisons of typical anorexia nervosa (AN) versus atypical AN (non-fat-phobic or low drive for thinness presentations) *(continued)*

Study	Country	Sample	N	Diagnostic method	Quantitative measures of eating pathology	Cohen's *d* (SE)	Investigator conclusions
Cross-sectional studies of AN with high vs. low drive for thinness *(continued)*							
Abbate-Daga et al. 2007	Italy	AN patients	151	EDI-DT < 7 vs. > 7	**EDI-2 asceticism**	0.75 (0.17)**	AT group exhibited less severe psychopathology
					EDI-2 bulimia		
					EDI-2 impulse regulation		
					EDI-2 ineffectiveness		
					EDI-2 interoceptive awareness		
					EDI-2 interpersonal distrust		
					EDI-2 maturity fears		
					EDI-2 perfectionism		
					EDI-2 body dissatisfaction	*0.78 (0.17)***	
					Current BMI	0.27 (0.17)	
Dalle Grave et al. 2008	Italy	AN patients	88	EDE fear of weight gain and importance of shape/ weight < 4 vs. ≥ 4	**Objective bulimic episodes**	0.48 (0.39)	AT group exhibited less severe psychopathology
					Subjective bulimic episodes		
					Self-induced vomiting		
					Laxative abuse		
					Global EDE-Q	*1.44 (0.41)***	
					Current BMI	0.06 (0.27)	

TABLE 20–2. Studies featuring quantitative comparisons of typical anorexia nervosa (AN) versus atypical AN (non-fat-phobic or low drive for thinness presentations) *(continued)*

Study	Country	Sample	N	Diagnostic method	Quantitative measures of eating pathology	Cohen's *d* (SE)	Investigator conclusions
Longitudinal studies of typical AN vs. non-fat-phobic or low drive for thinness AN							
Strober et al. 1999	USA	AN patients 10–15 years posttreatment	97	Qualitative interview (inter-rater $\kappa = 0.91$)	Achievement of full recovery Prospective onset of bingeing	—	AT group recovered more rapidly and was less likely to develop binge eating
Lee et al. 2003	Hong Kong	AN patients an average of 9 years after ED onset	88	Qualitative interview	Morgan-Russell outcome Prospective onset of BN	—	AT group was more likely to achieve good outcome and less likely to develop BN
Dalle Grave et al. 2008	Italy	AN patients posttreatment	88	EDE fear of weight gain and importance of shape/weight <4 vs. ≥4	Posttreatment BMI, eating pathology, and general psychopathology	—	Response to inpatient CBT was similar for AN and AT groups

TABLE 20–2. Studies featuring quantitative comparisons of typical anorexia nervosa (AN) versus atypical AN (non-fat-phobic or low drive for thinness presentations) *(continued)*

Study	Country	Sample	N	Diagnostic method	Quantitative measures of eating pathology	Cohen's *d* (SE)	Investigator conclusions
Longitudinal studies of typical AN vs. non-fat-phobic or low drive for thinness AN *(continued)*							
Crow et al. 2008	USA	ED patients 13–32 years after initial evaluation	317[b]	Latent class analysis	Mortality (National Death Index)	—	Cluster most resembling AT had mortality rate five times higher than cluster most resembling AN

Note. In the Cohen's *d* column, bold font corresponds to eating pathology (conservative), italic font corresponds to eating pathology (broad), and regular font corresponds to either current or premorbid BMI. The "conservative" effect size includes only those measures with no potential for overlap with fat phobia (i.e., only those measures written in bold), whereas the "broad" effect size includes all possible measures of eating pathology available in the original research report (i.e., all measures in bold and italics).
*P<0.05; **P<0.001.

[a]Only the Canadian subsample was included in the meta-analysis, because some participants in the Italian subsample had BN and EDNOS.
[b]Patients were assigned to categories using latent class analysis. One cluster resembled AN, and the other resembled AT, although not all participants in each latent class met full diagnostic criteria for each.

AT=atypical AN; BMI=body mass index; BN=bulimia nervosa; CBT=cognitive-behavioral therapy; DEBQ=Dutch Eating Behavior Questionnaire; DT=EDI drive for thinness subscale; EAT=Eating Attitudes Test; ED=eating disorder; EDE=Eating Disorder Examination; EDI=Eating Disorder Inventory; EDNOS=eating disorder not otherwise specified.

that observed in non-Western samples. When all measures of eating pathology were considered, patients with low-DT-AN scored three quarters of a standard deviation lower than did patients with AN (d [broad] = 0.74, SE = 0.19, P < 0.001). Restricting analyses to measures with no potential conceptual overlap with fat phobia attenuated the effect only slightly (d [conservative] = 0.56, SE = 0.11, P < 0.001). In contrast, the two groups did not differ on BMI at presentation (d = 0.14, SE = 0.10, P = 0.17), and there were insufficient data in the original studies to meta-analytically evaluate group differences in premorbid BMI.

Key advantages of available Western studies of low-DT-AN include independent replications across multiple research groups, larger samples with sufficient statistical power to detect significant effects, and utilization of quantitative assessment to operationalize "fat phobia." However, classification of "fat-phobic" versus "non-fat-phobic" for these studies utilized somewhat arbitrary cut points in continuous measures of attitudinal pathology that appear unsatisfactory. For example, patients endorsing "a definite fear of weight gain" on up to half the days in the past month could still score <4 on that EDE item (Fairburn et al. 2008) and thus be classified as lacking fat phobia. Similarly, patients reporting "sometimes" feeling "terrified of gaining weight" or being "preoccupied with a desire to be thinner" would earn an average score <7 on the Drive for Thinness subscale (Garner et al. 1983) and thus be classified as "low DT." Thus, patients who demonstrate low scores on measures of weight concern may not necessarily be qualitatively distinct from high-DT patients if they experience fat phobia of moderate intensity and periodicity. It is therefore highly uncertain whether low-DT-AN described in Western populations is comparable with NFP-AN described in non-Western samples. Although NFP-AN is most often represented as a categorical absence of fat phobia, it has also been characterized dimensionally and as temporally unstable (Table 20–1; Lee 1991; Lee et al. 2001).

In summary, limited available quantitative data suggest that both NFP and low-DT-AN are characterized by lesser eating pathology, but similar nutritional compromise (as measured by BMI), compared with AN. Effect sizes for eating pathology remain statistically significant and moderately sized even when analyses are restricted to measures without conceptual overlap with fat phobia. Moreover, analogous differences were manifest in Western samples, suggesting that lesser severity transcends cultural context.

FOLLOW-UP STUDIES

Robins and Guze's (1970) fourth diagnostic validity criterion is the predictive validity of the putative category in follow-up studies. Very few longitudinal studies have examined the course of fat-phobic versus NFP-AN, and available evidence is inconclusive. For example, both groups exhibited significant improvements in body weight and eating pathology in response to a 20-week inpatient/day hospital cognitive-behavioral treatment (Dalle Grave et al. 2008). However, both the lesser pretreatment severity of NFP-AN and the lack of control group in this study raise the question of whether NFP-AN might have responded equally well to a less intensive intervention. Indeed, two long-term AN outcome studies found that lack of fat phobia at initial clinical presentation was predictive of increased likelihood of remission and reduced probability of developing bulimic symptoms 9 years after eating disorder onset (Lee et al. 2003) and 10–15 years after clinical presentation (Strober et al. 1999). However, a recent study utilizing empirically derived latent classes to predict eating disorder outcome found that the latent class most resembling NFP-AN exhibited a standardized mortality rate five times higher than the class most resembling typical AN in a 13- to 32-year follow-up of eating disorder patients, tracking outcomes through the National Death Index (Crow et al. 2008). Finally, the rationale for dietary restriction may lack temporal stability. Lee et al.'s (2001) retrospective study of 48 patients with AN demonstrated migration between fat-phobic and non-fat-phobic attributions in both directions.

FAMILY STUDIES

Robins and Guze's (1970) final criterion for diagnostic validity is familial coaggregation of the syndrome. Our literature review did not identify any studies examining the prevalence of NFP-AN in the first- or second-degree relatives of individuals with NFP-AN or any establishing NFP-AN concordance in monozygotic versus dizygotic twins. However, a small number of twin studies have evaluated the relative contribution of genetic versus environmental influences to related constructs in nonclinical samples. Although some twin studies have identified additive genetic effects for DT (Rutherford et al. 1993), feelings of fatness (Wade et al. 2003), and undue influence of weight and shape in self-evaluation (Wade and Bulik 2007), others have found shared or nonshared environmental influences to be more salient (Reichborn-Kjennerud et al. 2004; Wade et al. 1998).

Discussion

Available data on NFP-AN do not reach our standard for diagnostic validity. Clinical descriptions of NFP-AN arise in both Western and non-Western populations, psychological testing shows a consistent profile on measures of eating disorder psychopathology, and our meta-analytic findings suggest that NFP-AN can be differentiated from conventional AN by milder levels of eating pathology. However, follow-up studies have yielded inconsistent results, and studies of familial aggregation have been limited to analogous constructs studied in nonclinical samples.

First, with regard to clinical description, the specific literature on NFP-AN is modest, with relatively few papers published in the past 10 years—in fact, far fewer than the 50 papers Blashfield et al. (1990) suggested as a standard for adequate literature to establish a diagnosis. Lee and colleagues' studies dominate the literature on NFP-AN, notwithstanding their call for further investigation of this variant (Hsu and Lee 1993).

Second, available data support that NFP-AN is heterogeneous with diverse rationales for food refusal. Somatic complaints (abdominal discomfort, stomach bloating, lack of appetite, or lack of hunger) (Lee et al. 2001), religious motives, desire for control, and desire for familial impact are commonly endorsed. Absence of fat phobia has also been ascribed to fat phobia's lack of cultural salience as an idiom of distress, poor insight, and intentional nondisclosure of symptoms. Our meta-analytic findings of higher premorbid BMI in conventional AN than NFP-AN, coupled with the positive association between DT and BMI in previous work (Kok and Tian 1994; Striegel-Moore et al. 1995) suggest that the etiology of fat phobia may also be influenced by the local nutritional environment. The association between AN and a "culture of modernity," characterized by the high availability of food, has been asserted as an explanation for historical shifts in rationale for self-starvation (Bemporad 1996; Lee 1996).

Third, with regard to delimitation from other disorders, studies supporting culturally diverse rationales for self-starvation imply a conceptual congruence between NFP-AN and conventional AN. Moreover, crossover between rationale for food refusal indexing fat phobia or not (Lee et al. 2001), clinical observational data that endorsement of fat phobia can emerge with treatment (Soomro et al. 1995), and our own meta-analytic results highlighting comparable nutritional compromise (i.e., BMI) in AN versus NFP and low-DT-AN at presentation provide empirical support for these views. On the other hand, our meta-analytic results also indicate that NFP-AN exhibits less severe eating pathology than conventional AN, with effect sizes in the medium to large range. These quantitative findings provide some support for the conceptualization of NFP-AN as a distinct variant or disorder from conventional AN. Future studies utilizing taxometric analyses with multiple clinically relevant indicators would be necessary to determine whether these effects support categorical or dimensional differences between AN and NFP-AN.

Fourth, follow-up studies report inconsistent findings. Two of these suggest a more benign course (Lee et al. 2003; Strober et al. 1999), another one demonstrates similar response to treatment (Dalle Grave et al. 2008), and another demonstrates a higher mortality rate associated with low-DT-AN (Crow et al. 2008). Thus, existing data are insufficient to support the potential predictive validity of subtyping AN by presence or absence of fat phobia.

Fifth, there are no family or twin studies directly assessing the heritability of NFP-AN.

WHAT ARE THE OPTIONS FOR DSM-5 COVERAGE OF NON-FAT-PHOBIC ANOREXIA NERVOSA?

In 1993, Hsu and Lee called for careful assessment, treatment, and follow-up of NFP-AN patients, in part to characterize better their course, outcome, and overlap with AN. Subsequently, the National Institute of Mental Health–sponsored Culture and Diagnosis Committee recommended to the DSM-IV Task Force on Cultural Issues that a description of NFP-AN be included as an example of EDNOS (Weiss 1995). Fifteen years later, there are still insufficient data to clarify the relation between NFP-AN and AN. That said, extant data support heterogeneous presentations of AN that are geographically widespread and not associated with any one particular cultural context. Concerns remain, moreover, that lack of visibility for NFP-AN may undermine service delivery if clinicians are poorly equipped to recognize or evaluate these cases. On the basis of our review, we propose five possible coverage options for NFP-AN in DSM-5 (Table 20–3).

1. Modify or Eliminate Diagnostic Criterion B (i.e., the Requirement for Fear of Weight Gain or "Fat Phobia") for Anorexia Nervosa

One option would be to eliminate the requirement for "fat phobia" to meet diagnostic criteria for AN. Relatedly, Criterion B could be modified to allow more flexibility in rationale for food refusal or low weight. As Russell (1985) asserted, the centrality of body disturbance first emerged in Bruch's work in the 1960s and fear of fatness was not incorporated as a diagnostic criterion for AN until 1970. Bruch proposed a "pathoplastic" model in which fear of weight gain is (culturally) epiphenomenal to the core pathology of AN (Russell 1985). Lee et al. (1993) have been the most vociferous critics of the ethnocentrism of the current criteria and have proposed greater flexibility. Following these arguments, several investigators have proposed additional modifications for Criterion B. Alternate phrasings could include 1) a "phenomenologically pluralistic conceptualization of self-imposed emaciation" (Lee et al. 2001); 2) "ego-syntonic" weight loss (Rieger et al. 2001); 3) "no control phobia," referencing the negotiation of social (and often gendered) powerlessness (Katzman and Lee 1997); or 4) "overinvestment" in eating restraint (Palmer 1993).

The first advantage of rephrasing Criterion B in DSM-5 to encompass alternate rationales for food refusal is to avoid ethnocentrism that may be inherent in the fat phobia criterion. That is, a fat-phobic rationale for self-starvation depends upon a social context in which weight concerns are culturally salient. The second advantage would be to avoid the potential reification of the construct of eating pathology by diagnostic criteria based on, and measures initially developed for use in, Western populations. For example, the items composing the EDI Drive for Thinness scale may reference cultural norms that are not widely accessible or relevant to populations outside of North America (Garner et al. 1983). Indeed, norms for this construct appear to vary across even culturally similar populations (Kordy et al. 2001;

TABLE 20–3. Possible options for representing non-fat-phobic anorexia nervosa (NFP-AN) in DSM-5

	Pros	Cons
1. Modify or eliminate diagnostic Criterion B (i.e., the requirement for fear of weight gain or "fat phobia") for AN	• Would allow flexibility to encompass cultural variation in AN symptoms • Would promote the recognition of NFP-AN in clinical and community samples • Would reduce the proportion of individuals currently diagnosed with EDNOS	• NFP-AN appears to represent a milder variant of eating pathology than typical AN • Criterion B conceptually overlaps with Criterion C • Diagnostic specificity could be reduced
2. Subtype AN according to the presence or absence of fat phobia	• NFP-AN is associated with less severe eating pathology, which may indicate the presence of clinically meaningful subtypes	• NFP-AN may represent a heterogeneous group • Subtypes may be difficult to differentiate because of the diagnostic crossover between AN and NFP-AN and the dimensional nature of drive for thinness • Comparative outcomes for AN and NFP-AN remain unclear • Superimposition of a second AN subtyping scheme may reduce clinical utility

TABLE 20–3. Possible options for representing non-fat-phobic anorexia nervosa (NFP-AN) in DSM-5 *(continued)*

	Pros	Cons
3. Include NFP-AN as a provisional category nominated for further research	• May stimulate necessary research on NFP-AN (i.e., treatment outcome studies, longitudinal follow-up)	• May reify NFP-AN even if data are insufficient to support its clinical utility
4. Include NFP-AN as an example of EDNOS	• May promote clinical recognition of NFP-AN and may facilitate access to health care services • Inclusion of this variant allows flexibility for cultural diversity in eating disorders	• NFP-AN is already treated as an EDNOS variant in many research studies and has been identified in many clinical settings, so this relatively minor revision may not have much practical impact • It may be difficult to differentiate between AN and EDNOS given lack of consensus on operationalizing fat phobia
5. Do not include NFP-AN in DSM-5	• Conservative approach to inadequate data supporting the diagnostic validity of NFP-AN	• At least some data indicate that NFP-AN is associated with morbidity and mortality • Individuals with NFP-AN may have difficulty accessing appropriate health care services if clinicians are uninformed about this variant

Note. AN = anorexia nervosa; EDNOS = eating disorder not otherwise specified.

Schaeffer et al. 1998). In addition to the cultural relevance of specific item content, response style (Garner et al. 1983)—which can also be culturally driven—may have contributed to cross-population differences. A third advantage would be improved detection of NFP-AN in clinical and community settings by encouraging the use of screening instruments that do not require fat phobia for diagnosis. Crow et al.'s (2008) finding that the latent class most resembling NFP-AN exhibited greater mortality than the latent class most resembling conventional AN suggests that this group has significant pathology and risk that should not be overlooked. A fourth benefit would be the elimination of a substantial minority of cases from the heterogeneous EDNOS category. Individuals with NFP-AN present to eating disorder specialty clinics across the globe. Even in selected Western samples, approximately 17% (Ramacciotti et al. 2002) to 38% (Abbate-Daga et al. 2007) of consecutively referred patients with AN-like symptoms (i.e., low weight, amenorrhea) either do not meet the fat phobia criterion or present with low DT. However, these prevalence estimates have unknown generalizability to other clinical settings.

However, we also note several disadvantages associated with modifying the requirement for fat phobia. First, our meta-analytic findings indicate that both NFP-AN and low-DT-AN exhibit lower levels of eating pathology than conventional AN, even when utilizing conservative definitions of eating pathology, which exclude constructs with the potential for overlap with fat phobia. Second, the conceptual overlap between DSM-IV Criterion B ("intense fear of gaining weight or becoming fat, even though underweight") and Criterion C ("disturbance in the way in which one's body weight or shape is experienced") makes this approach problematic. How body image disturbance is manifested and assessed in the absence of weight concerns would require close examination (Hsu and Sobkiewicz 1991). Third, to date, NFP-AN has been studied mainly within the context of eating disorder specialty clinics where eating-related clinical impairment is a prerequisite for study inclusion. Thus, the sensitivity and specificity of the diagnosis in nonspecialty and community samples remain unknown, and without positive indicators of eating disorder psychopathology (i.e., Criteria B and C), it may be difficult to differentiate NFP-AN from low body weight because of 1) constitutional leanness, 2) co-occurring psychiatric illnesses associated with weight loss such as depression or conversion disorder (Garfinkel et al. 1983), 3) co-occurring physical illnesses associated with vomiting and weight loss such as achalasia (Marshall and Russell 1993), and 4) volitional restriction of caloric intake for potentially less pathological reasons (i.e., in hopes of achieving longer life, as in "caloric restriction for longevity" [Vitousek et al. 2004]).

2. Subtype Anorexia Nervosa According to the Presence or Absence of Fat Phobia

A second way to represent NFP-AN in DSM-5 would be to partition AN into fat-phobic versus non-fat-phobic subtypes. This option would feature the benefit of recognizing the similarities between NFP-AN and conventional AN while simultaneously reflecting research findings supporting their differential severity and course. However, there are insufficient data to support subtyping at this time. Observed differences in eating pathology in fat-phobic versus NFP-AN may reflect bias related to response style such as denial and minimization, which are common among individuals with AN (Couturier and Lock 2006; Vitousek et al. 1998). Individuals with AN who wish to provide a misleadingly positive account of their illness due to the ego-syntonic nature of low body weight or the demand for social desirability may score low on both attitudinal and behavioral measures of eating pathology (Ramacciotti et al. 2002). Moreover, findings of similar treatment outcomes for AN and low-DT-AN following inpatient cognitive-behavioral therapy (Dalle Grave et al. 2008) and the diagnostic crossover between NFP-AN and conventional AN in longitudinal studies (Lee et al. 2001) provide preliminary evidence that subtyping AN in this way may not be diagnostically valid. Finally, a reliable and clinically meaningful distinction between NFP-AN and AN may be problematic. Given the dimensional nature of DT and related constructs, the reliability and validity of a threshold distinguishing the two subtypes require further examination. Furthermore, the introduction of a secondary subtyping scheme—which would be superimposed on the extant "restricting" versus "binge eating/purging" subtyping scheme (American Psychiatric Association 2000)—may impose an unjustifiable burden of complexity on DSM readership.

3. Include Non-Fat-Phobic Anorexia Nervosa as a Provisional Category Nominated for Further Research

Including NFP-AN as a category for future research would feature many of the advantages of altering the fat phobia criterion or subtyping AN into fat-phobic versus non-fat-phobic (i.e., enhanced clinical recognition, stimulation of further research) but avoid some of the possible pitfalls (i.e., including non-eating-disordered individuals in the AN category) (Hsu and Lee 1993; Weiss 1995).

4. Include Non-Fat-Phobic Anorexia Nervosa as an Example of Eating Disorder Not Otherwise Specified

Another way to represent NFP-AN in DSM-5 is as an example of EDNOS. This would feature the advantage of enhanced clinical detection and stimulation of research without undermining the validity of the conventional AN diagnosis. On the other hand, NFP-AN may be overlooked in clinical and research settings if it is added to an already heterogeneous residual category. Another pitfall is the potentially arbitrary process of differentiating between AN and NFP-AN in clinical practice. The majority of NFP-AN studies have conferred diagnoses based on qualitative interviews, and although both EDI and EDE items have been utilized as proxies for fat phobia, there is no clearly accepted measure of this construct.

5. Do Not Include Non-Fat-Phobic Anorexia Nervosa in DSM-5

In our view, the least appealing option would be to continue to exclude NFP-AN from DSM-5. This option disregards data supporting both cultural diversity and heterogeneity of AN. Failure to address the variations of clinical presentation runs the risk of reifying the extant nosologic criteria presented in DSM through assessments that specifically capture relevant data but may miss cultural variants (Becker 2007; Cummins et al. 2005; Lee et al. 2002). Setting aside broader questions raised about increasing flexibility of diagnostic criteria across DSM-5, the literature on NFP-AN suggests that to accommodate cultural diversity, clinicians would benefit from an awareness of cultural patterning of the rationale for food refusal and alternate motivation for eating disorder symptoms. Unfortunate ethnic disparities in treatment access and outcomes persist for mental disorders in the United States. Sensitivity to cultural diversity in presentation will potentially enhance recognition and prompt treatment (Kam and Lee 1998; Ratan et al. 1998; Tareen et al. 2005).

Conclusion

Available data on NFP-AN are insufficient to meet our standard for diagnostic validity—either as a distinct diagnosis or as an AN subtype. Notwithstanding rich ethnographic and clinical details, the literature lacks a specific and consistent definition and operationalization of NFP-AN. Because the relation of NFP-AN and low-DT-AN remains unclear, findings from low-DT-AN studies cannot be extrapolated to apply to NFP-AN with confidence. Although our meta-analysis of published data suggests that NFP-AN may be a more clinically benign variant of AN or disorder, the small number of studies as well as some inconsistency in findings suggests that further studies are necessary.

The proposed revision of criterion B to encompass greater phenomenological diversity has great appeal on theoretical and practical grounds. However, we emphasize the inadequacy of existing data to support that NFP-AN and AN are variants of a single syndrome. On the other hand, NFP-AN has enduring and substantial presence in geographically and culturally diverse populations, and available data support its clinical significance. Raising its visibility by inclusion as an example of a common presentation of EDNOS will arguably enhance clinical detection. In turn, this will facilitate further research to describe NFP-AN and explore the critical role of social environment in shaping symptom phenomena and in modifying risk and course of AN.

References

Abbate-Daga G, Piero A, Gramaglia C, et al: An attempt to understand the paradox of anorexia nervosa without drive for thinness. Psychiatry Res 149:215–221, 2007

American Psychiatric Association: Diagnostic and Statistical Manual of Mental Disorders, 3rd Edition, Revised. Washington, DC, American Psychiatric Association, 1987

American Psychiatric Association: Diagnostic and Statistical Manual of Mental Disorders, 4th Edition. Washington, DC, American Psychiatric Association, 1994

American Psychiatric Association: Diagnostic and Statistical Manual of Mental Disorders, 4th Edition, Text Revision. Washington, DC, American Psychiatric Association, 2000

Banks CG: Culture in culture-bound syndromes: the case of anorexia nervosa. Soc Sci Med 34:867–884, 1992

Banks CG: There is no fat in heaven: religious asceticism and the meaning of anorexia nervosa. Ethos 24:107–135, 1996

Becker AE: Culture and eating disorders classification. Int J Eat Disord 40(suppl):S111–S116, 2007

Bemporad JR: Self-starvation through the ages: reflections on the pre-history of anorexia nervosa. Int J Eat Disord 19:217–237, 1996

Bennett D, Sharpe M, Freeman C, et al: Anorexia nervosa among female secondary school students in Ghana. Br J Psychiatry 185:312–317, 2004

Blashfield RK, Sprock J, Fuller AK: Suggested guidelines for including or excluding categories in the DSM-IV. Compr Psychiatry 31:15–19, 1990

Chan ZC, Ma JL: Family themes of food refusal: disciplining the body and punishing the family. Health Care Women Int 23:49–58, 2002

Couturier JL, Lock J: Denial and minimization in adolescents with anorexia nervosa. Int J Eat Disord 39:212–216, 2006

Crow S, Swanson S, Peterson C, et al: Mortality from eating disorders: association with latent class. Paper presented at the R-13 Meeting on Eating Disorders: Classification and Diagnosis, Washington, DC, September 2008

Cummins LH, Simmons AM, Zane WS: Eating disorders in Asian populations: a critique of current approaches to the study of culture, ethnicity, and eating disorders. Am J Orthopsychiatry 75:553–574, 2005

Dalle Grave R, Calugi S, Marchesini G: Underweight eating disorder without over-evaluation of shape and weight: atypical anorexia nervosa? Int J Eat Disord 41:705–712, 2008

Fairburn CG, Cooper Z, O'Connor ME: Eating Disorder Examination, in Cognitive Behavior Therapy and Eating Disorders, 16.0D Edition. Edited by Fairburn CG. New York, Guilford, 2008, pp 265–308

Garfinkel PE, Kaplan AS, Garner DM, et al: The differentiation of vomiting/weight loss as a conversion disorder from anorexia nervosa. Am J Psychiatry 140:1019–1022, 1983

Garner DM, Olmsted MP, Bohr Y, et al: The Eating Attitudes Test: psychometric features and clinical correlates. Psychol Med 12:871–878, 1982

Garner DM, Olmsted MP, Polivy J: Development and validation of a multidimensional eating disorder inventory for anorexia nervosa and bulimia. Int J Eat Disord 2:15–34, 1983

Goh SE, Ong SB, Subramaniam M: Eating disorders in Hong Kong (correspondence). Br J Psychiatry 162:276–277, 1993

Habermas T: In defense of weight phobia as the central organizing motive in anorexia nervosa: historical and cultural arguments for a culture-sensitive psychological conception. Int J Eat Disord 19:317–334, 1996

Hsu LK, Sobkiewicz TA: Body image disturbance: time to abandon the concept for eating disorders? Int J Eat Disord 10:15–30, 1991

Hsu LK, Lee S: Is weight phobia always necessary for a diagnosis of anorexia nervosa? Am J Psychiatry 150:1466–1471, 1993

Joughin N, Crisp AH, Halek C, et al: Religious belief and anorexia nervosa. Int J Eat Disord 12:397–406, 1992

Kam WK, Lee S: The variable manifestations and contextual meanings of anorexia nervosa: two case illustrations from Hong Kong. Int J Eat Disord 23:227–231, 1998

Katzman MA, Lee S: Beyond body image: the integration of feminist and transcultural theories in the understanding of self starvation. Int J Eat Disord 22:385–394, 1997

Khandelwal SK, Saxena S: Anorexia nervosa in people of Asian extraction. Br J Psychiatry 157:783–784, 1990

Kleinman A: Illness Narratives: Suffering, Healing and the Human Condition. New York, Basic Books, 1989

Kok LP, Tian CS: Susceptibility of Singapore Chinese schoolgirls to anorexia nervosa: part I (psychological factors). Singapore Med J 35:481–485, 1994

Kordy H, Percevic R, Martinovich Z: Norms, normality, and clinical significant change: implications for the evaluation of treatment outcomes for eating disorders. Int J Eat Disord 30:176–186, 2001

Lai KYC: Anorexia nervosa in Chinese adolescents—does culture make a difference? J Adolesc 23:561–568, 2000

Lau LLS, Lee S, Lee E, et al: Cross-cultural validity of the Eating Disorder Examination: a study of Chinese outpatients with eating disorders in Hong Kong. Hong Kong Journal of Psychiatry 16:132–136, 2006

Lee AM, Lee S: Disordered eating and its psychosocial correlates among Chinese adolescent females in Hong Kong. Int J Eat Disord 20:177–183, 1996

Lee HY, Lock J: Anorexia nervosa in Asian-American adolescents: do they differ from their non-Asian peers? Int J Eat Disord 40:227–231, 2007

Lee S: Anorexia nervosa in Hong Kong: a Chinese perspective. Psychol Med 21:703–711, 1991

Lee S: Self-starvation in context: towards a culturally sensitive understanding of anorexia nervosa. Soc Sci Med 41:25–36, 1995

Lee S: Reconsidering the status of anorexia nervosa as a Western culture-bound syndrome. Soc Sci Med 42:21–34, 1996

Lee S, Chiu HFK, Chen C: Anorexia nervosa in Hong Kong: why not more in Chinese? Br J Psychiatry 154:683–688, 1989

Lee S, Ho TP, Hsu LKG: Fat phobic and non-fat phobic anorexia nervosa: a comparative study of 70 Chinese patients in Hong Kong. Psychol Med 23:999–1017, 1993

Lee S, Lee AM, Leung T: Cross-cultural validity of the Eating Disorder Inventory: a study of Chinese patients with eating disorders in Hong Kong. Int J Eat Disord 23:177–188, 1998

Lee S, Lee AM, Ngai E, et al: Rationales for food refusal in Chinese patients with anorexia nervosa. Int J Eat Disord 29:224–229, 2001

Lee S, Kwok K, Liau C, et al: Screening Chinese patients with eating disorders using the Eating Attitudes Test in Hong Kong. Int J Eat Disord 32:91–97, 2002

Lee S, Chan YY, Hsu LK: The intermediate-term outcome of Chinese patients with anorexia nervosa in Hong Kong. Am J Psychiatry 160:967–972, 2003

Marshall JB, Russell JL: Achalasia mistakenly diagnosed as eating disorder and prompting prolonged psychiatric hospitalization. South Med J 86:1405–1407, 1993

Neumärker U, Dudeck U, Vollrath M, et al: Eating attitudes among adolescent anorexia nervosa patients and normal subjects in former West and East Berlin: a transcultural comparison. Int J Eat Disord 12:281–289, 1992

Ngai ES, Lee S, Lee AM: The variability of phenomenology in anorexia nervosa. Acta Psychiatr Scand 102:314–317, 2000

Noma S, Nakai Y, Hamagaki S, et al: Comparison between the SCOFF questionnaire and the Eating Attitudes Test in patients with eating disorders. Int J Psychiatry Clin Pract 10:27–32, 2006

Norvell N, Cooley E: Diagnostic issues in eating disorders: two cases of atypical eating disorder. Int J Psychiatry Med 16:317–323, 1986–1987

Ong YL, Tsoi WF, Cheah JS: A clinical and psychosocial study of seven cases of anorexia nervosa in Singapore. Singapore Med J 23:255–261, 1982

Palmer RL: Weight concern should not be a necessary criterion for the eating disorders: a polemic. Int J Eat Disord 14:459–465, 1993

Parry-Jones WLL: Archival exploration of anorexia nervosa. J Psychiatr Res 19:95–100, 1985

Pike KM, Mizushima H: The clinical presentation of Japanese women with anorexia nervosa and bulimia nervosa: a study of the Eating Disorder Inventory–2. Int J Eat Disord 37:26–31, 2005

Ramacciotti CE, Dell'Osso L, Paoli RA, et al: Characteristics of eating disorder patients without a drive for thinness. Int J Eat Disord 32:206–212, 2002

Ratan D, Gandhi D, Palmer R: Eating disorders in British Asians. Int J Eat Disord 24:101–105, 1998

Reichborn-Kjennerud T, Bulik CM, Kendler KS, et al: Undue influence of weight on self-evaluation: a population-based twin study of gender differences. Int J Eat Disord 35:123–132, 2004

Rieger E, Touyz SW, Swain T, et al: Cross-cultural research on anorexia nervosa: assumptions regarding the role of body weight. Int J Eat Disord 29:205–215, 2001

Robins E, Guze SB: Establishment of diagnostic validity in psychiatric illness: its application to schizophrenia. Am J Psychiatry 126:983–987, 1970

Russell GFM: The changing nature of anorexia nervosa: an introduction to the conference. J Psychiatr Res 19:101–109, 1985

Rutherford J, McGuffin P, Katz RJ, et al: Genetic influences on eating attitudes in a normal female twin population. Psychol Med 23:425–436, 1993

Schaeffer WK, Maclennan RN, Yaholnitsky-Smith S, et al: Psychometric evaluation of the Eating Disorder Inventory (EDI) in a clinical group. Psychol Health 13:873–881, 1998

Sjostedt JP, Schumaker JF, Nathawat SS: Eating disorders among Indian and Australian university students. J Soc Psychol 138:351–357, 1998

Soomro GM, Crisp AH, Lynch D, et al: Anorexia nervosa in 'non-white' populations. Br J Psychiatry 167:385–389, 1995

Steinhausen HC, Neumärker KJ, Vollrath M, et al: A transcultural comparison of the Eating Disorder Inventory in former East and West Berlin. Int J Eat Disord 12:407–416, 1992

Striegel-Moore RH, Schreiber GB, Pike KM, et al: Drive for thinness in black and white preadolescent girls. Int J Eat Disord 18:59–69, 1995

Strober M, Freeman R, Morrell W: Atypical anorexia nervosa: separation from typical cases in course and outcome in a long-term prospective study. Int J Eat Disord 25:135–142, 1999

Tareen A, Hodes M, Rangel L: Non-fat-phobic anorexia nervosa in British South Asian adolescents. Int J Eat Disord 37:161–165, 2005

Thomas JJ, Vartanian LR, Brownell KD: The relationship between eating disorder not otherwise specified and officially recognized eating disorders: meta-analysis and implications for DSM. Psychol Bull 135:407–433, 2009

Ung EK, Lee S, Kua EH: Anorexia nervosa and bulimia: a Singapore perspective. Singapore Med J 38:332–335, 1997

Vervaet M, van Heeringen C, Audenaert K: Is drive for thinness in anorectic patients associated with personality characteristics? Eur Eat Disord Rev 12:375–379, 2004

Vitousek K, Watson S, Wilson GT: Enhancing motivation to change in treatment-resistant eating disorders. Clin Psychol Rev 18:391–420, 1998

Vitousek KM, Manke FP, Gray JA, et al: Caloric restriction for longevity, II: the systematic neglect of behavioural and psychological outcomes in animal research. Eur Eat Disord Rev 12:338–360, 2004

Wade TD, Bulik CM: Shared genetic and environmental risk factors between undue influence of body shape and weight on self-evaluation and dimensions of perfectionism. Psychol Med 37:635–644, 2007

Wade T, Martin NG, Tiggemann M: Genetic and environmental risk factors for the weight and shape concerns characteristic of bulimia nervosa. Psychol Med 28:761–771, 1998

Wade TD, Wilkinson J, Ben-Tovim D: The genetic epidemiology of body attitudes, the attitudinal component of body image in women. Psychol Med 33:1395–1405, 2003

Weiss MG: Eating disorders and disordered eating in different cultures. Psychiatry Clin North Am 18:537–553, 1995

Willenberg H, Krauthauser H: "Weight phobia": a discussion of the problem of "atypical" and "not otherwise specified" eating and weight disorders [in German]. Psychother Psychosom Med Psychol 50:134–139, 2000

21

EATING DISORDERS IN JAPAN

Cultural Context, Clinical Features, and Future Directions

Kathleen M. Pike, Ph.D.

Yuko Yamamiya, Ph.D.

Haruka Konishi, B.A.

It is now widely recognized that eating disorders are not restricted to a single culture, socioeconomic class, or race (Becker 2004b; Becker et al. 2009; Soh et al. 2006). Early investigations conducted in Japan in the 1980s of clinical and nonclinical samples suggested that although eating disturbances existed, Japanese women were at reduced risk in comparison with women in the West (Huon and Brown 1984; Inaba and Takahashi 1989; Kiriike et al. 1988; Nishizono-Maher 1998; Suematsu et al. 1985). The difference in prevalence was often attributed to the protective factors of stable family systems, the traditional female role in society, healthy diet, and low rates of weight problems that characterized traditional Japanese culture.

In recent decades, Japan has witnessed an increase in the study of eating and weight disorders, and the data consistently document increases in both subclinical eating pathology and clinical cases of eating disorders (Nakai 2010; Nakamura et al. 1999). The expanding database and increased public awareness of eating disorders in Japan document a serious and growing psychiatric problem on the contemporary landscape. This chapter provides an overview of the cultural context and explores the clinical features of drive for thinness (DT) and weight and shape concerns in the exegesis of eating disorders. Recommendations for future studies highlight the need for rigorous and sophisticated research on risk factors for eating disorders in Japan.

Evidence of Increasing Eating Pathology in Japan

Epidemiological research based on representative samples utilizing rigorous diagnostic systems do not exist; however, a few large, nonclinical studies based on medical and educational records provide estimates of eating disturbances in Japan. Together with studies of clinical samples, the accumulating research from the second half of the twentieth century and beginning of the twenty-first century suggests that eating disorders have steadily increased during this period of time. These studies document a sixfold increase in eating disorders in Japan from the 1970s to the mid-1990s (Kiriike et al. 1998; Nadaoka et al. 1996; Suematsu et al. 1985; Takagi 1990). More recent survey studies among female university students estimated that 5.1%–7.5% had clinical levels of eating pathology (Makino et al. 2006; Yamatsuta and Nomura 2005). In studies of psychiatric samples, both the absolute number of eating disorders cases and the ratio to all psychiatric patients have increased during the past 25 years (Nadaoka et al. 1996; Nakai 2010).

Consistent with findings across the globe, adolescent and young adult women appear to be at greatest risk for eating disturbances in Japan; therefore, most studies focus on this segment of the population. In the late 1980s, school-based studies estimated that approximately 2% of high school girls (Takeda et al. 1993) and 2.9% of young women in college (Kiriike et al. 1988) met DSM criteria for bulimia nervosa (BN). Subclinical behavioral disturbances of binge eating were reported by approximately 1.3% of high school students and 4% of college students (Nogami et al. 1987). A large school-based study using growth charts from routine school health assessments reported a 2.3% cumulative incidence of probable anorexia nervosa (AN) for female students during their 6 years of junior high school and high school (Watanabe et al. 2003). Studies in recent decades document rates of extreme dysregulation of eating behaviors and weight control efforts that are comparable with those documented in the West (Koseisho 1993; Maruyama et al. 1993; Mukai et al. 1994; Nakamura et al. 1999; Pike and Mizushima 2005), with data estimating that the prevalence of AN is 0.4%; BN is 2.3%, and eating disorder not otherwise specified (EDNOS) is 12.5% among Japanese females (Nakai 2010).

Why Now and Why Women?

In framing the study of the development of eating disorders, Striegel-Moore et al. (1986) posed the questions "Why now?," "Why women?," and "Why some women and not others?" In Japan, particular changes in women's role in society as well as changes in population weight demographics are especially relevant for answering the questions of "Why women?" and "Why now?" We briefly describe these cultural changes to help elucidate the cultural context that serves as the backdrop for the rise of eating disorders in Japan.

GROWING UP FEMALE IN A RAPIDLY CHANGING SOCIETY

Profound economic, social, and political changes permeate every dimension of contemporary Japanese society, and nowhere is the change more apparent than in the revolution that has occurred in the lives of Japanese women (Pike and Borovoy 2004). Both international influences and domestic changes in legal and governmental institutions, demographics, industry, and labor have had a tremendous impact on transforming the role of Japanese women. In fact, during the past century, traditional Japanese society gave way to new social and political systems at an ever-increasing rate. As described by Iwao (1983), women born in the early twentieth century were raised by parents with prewar values who maintained that the model of the traditional woman is embodied in the expression *ryosai-kenbo* (the good wife and wise mother), whose primary responsibility is to maintain the *ie* (household). Women in the postwar generation were born into a society with a new constitution that affirmed gender equality, the establishment of coeducational institutions, and landmark changes in labor laws. Women in this generation came of age during a period when life expectancy increased dramatically and the birth rate decreased equally dramatically. Their prime adult years occurred during a period of great economic growth, societal fortitude, and pride in the modern Japanese institutions. Then the "bubble" burst. Since the latter part of the twentieth century, and extending into the beginning of the twenty-first century, Japan has faced a steady decline in economic standing at home and abroad. Japanese women coming of age today find that the twenty-first century is a radically different world from what women of previous generations knew, and although gender equality is constitutionally supported, Japanese society remains highly gender segregated; increased civil rights and education for women have not ipso facto resulted in greater autonomy and opportunity for women. Thus, the life choices for young Japanese women today are complex and dramatically different from those of their mothers or grandmothers, and few role models exist on how to navigate a different course.

As the study of eating disorders has expanded around the globe, the assumption is often made that Western influence and values are at the root of increasing rates of eating disorders in non-Western cultures. However, our view is that the concept of "westernization" is limited in its explanatory role of why eating disorders have increased in Japan during the latter part of the twentieth century and elsewhere in the newly industrialized areas of the world. As described by Gordon (2001) and Becker (2004a), the notion of "westernization" carries with it a certain geographic supremacy, when, in fact, societal factors that are often described as "Western" are more accurately understood as characteristics of modern, industrialized societies. It may be that the actual dynamic of social transformation—be it westernization, modernization, or industrialization—is what is especially relevant to increasing the risk for the development of eating disorders within a society (Katzman and Lee 1997). Miller (2006) has further argued that changes in body image and beauty ideals in Japan should be understood as a function of modernity and social change rather than simply as a function of emulating Western or foreign body styles, and thus as proposed by Nishizono-Maher (1998), perhaps it is more useful to describe eating disorders as "culture change syndromes."

Feminist scholarship analyzing the rise of eating disorders in the United States has emphasized the tension within American society because women are still expected to perform the traditional domestic care and nurturance of family and community while increasingly being expected to pursue gainful employment and public careers (Borovoy 2005; Gordon 2000; Hochschild and Machung 1989). In contrast, in Japan, expectations and meanings are such that independence and autonomy have historically been viewed as accessible within the structure of marriage and family, not outside them, and employment in the workforce has not been a path to self-sufficiency for Japanese women (Borovoy 2005; Pike and Borovoy 2004). Although the number of Japanese women entering the workforce has increased, the percentage of women employed in Japan is among the lowest of any industrialized nation (Gender Equality Bureau 2008), and men's and women's work remains dramatically polarized (Ono 2003). In fact, women earn only a little over 50% of what men earn on average, and in general, as women's income increases, their likelihood of marriage declines (Ono 2003). In contrast to the expansion of roles and opportunities that was central to the feminist movement in the United States, Japanese women still have few alternatives to the dominant cultural expectations associated with the role of housewife as the path to maturity, although the traditional social fabric has changed dramatically. The stage has been set for social conflict and dilemma whereby Japanese women are no longer satisfied with the traditional gender role expectations but have few alternative role models (Kelsky 2001). As a result, a quiet but profound protest is under way in Japan, where marriage and birth rates are among the lowest in the world (Ministry of Health, Labor, and Welfare 2009).

CHANGES IN WEIGHT DEMOGRAPHICS IN JAPAN

Changes in caloric consumption, food culture, and energy expenditure that come with the transformation to modern, industrialized society are well documented around the globe (Brownell 2010; Brownell et al. 2010). Most simply, such societal transformation is associated with dramatic increases in food supply, particularly high-calorie, prepared foods, coupled with more sedentary lifestyles. As a result, the twenty-first century is witnessing steady increases in population weight and overweight on a global scale. In the specific case of Japan, the rise of fast food and convenience stores and changes in nutrient intake over the past few decades clearly conform to patterns described in other parts of the world (Kageyama 2007). The number of convenience stores, where sales of fast foods and prepared foods account for approximately 75% of all sales, has exploded in Japan, and nutritional consumption has changed dramatically, with the consumption of grain dropping by half and consumption of meat and fats more than doubling in the past 20 years (Millstone and Lang 2008).

Although overweight and obesity remain uncommon in Japan compared with the United States, the overall trend for increasing population weight in Japan is clearly documented. According to Japanese Ministry of Health, Labor, and Welfare (2006) data, in 1980 Japan reported that 2% of its total population was obese (body mass index [BMI] > 30 kg/m^2). By 1990, the prevalence of obesity had increased to 2.3%, and by 2006 it had increased to 3.9%. Of course, these numbers are dwarfed by U.S. data indicating obesity prevalence estimates of 15%, 23.3%, and 34.3%, respectively; however, during this same period of time, overweight status (BMI > 25 kg/m^2) among Japanese men has climbed to 30.4%, a figure that is not far behind U.S. statistics.

As overall population weight increases, a finer analysis of the data reveals dramatically different trajectories for men and women at the low end of the weight continuum. Consistent with the overall population trend of increasing BMI, the likelihood that Japanese men fall within a low weight range has decreased steadily since 1980, with fewer than 5% of the adult male population reporting a BMI below 18.5 kg/m^2 (the body mass commonly used as a weight threshold for AN) as of 2004 (Ministry of Health, Labor, and Welfare 2006). In contrast, the number of Japanese women in this low weight category is steadily increasing. Between 1984 and 2004, the percentage of women whose BMI was less than 18.5 kg/m^2 increased from 15% to 22% for women in their twenties, from 9% to 15% for women in their thirties, and from 5% to 7% for women in their forties. Twenty-five years ago Japanese women under the age of 60 were twice as likely to be thin (BMI < 18.5 kg/m2) as overweight (BMI > 25 kg/m^2); now they are four times more likely to have a BMI less than 18.5 kg/m^2 as compared with 25 kg/m^2 or more (Ministry of Health, Labor, and Welfare 2006). Thus, although it is historically true that by international standards Japanese population weights are relatively low, these BMI data suggest a current trend among the adult female population that is not simply a reflection of a historical norm but rather a dramatic change in cultural ideals and behavioral practices around weight for women. The assumption that Japanese women are simply genetically predisposed to lower normative body mass is an oversimplification that fails to recognize that this subgroup's weight trajectory is the reverse of the majority of the population.

Dieting and Drive for Thinness in Japan

The weight loss and diet goods industry is expanding and lucrative in contemporary Japan. Despite the economic recession, "aesthetic salons" alone account for an annual $4 billion industry, and surveys indicate that weight loss is one of the top reasons for women's frequent visits (Miller 2006). As dieting increases in Japan, the number and variety of weight loss products have also exploded. Whereas a decade ago, terms such as "nonfat," "low calorie," and "sugar free" were virtually absent from Japanese vocabulary and grocery shelves, they are now pervasive. These products are typically marketed by touting their purifying effects, all-natural ingredients, and ancient Asian origins. These products are sold to assist individuals in combating the toxic, stressful demands of contemporary life that have contaminated an abstract, romanticized time when life was simple, pure, and authentically Japanese. These "functional foods," as they are often referenced, run the gamut from health teas to rice cookies, and they promise to protect individuals from the illnesses and weight gain that have been brought by modernity. In reality, many of these products are essentially laxatives that have been repositioned to create a commercial market that merges the traditional Japanese ideals of purity and simplicity and the modern ideals of beauty and thinness. Popular among Japanese women, more than 2,000 new products have been launched in the past 20 years, representing more than a $2 billion market in Japan (Miller 2006).

It would be impossible to survey popular media without taking note of the variety of diet fads that pervade women's magazines, daily publications, and visual advertising in public spaces in contemporary Japan. Some diets involve eating a single food item for every meal, such as pineapples, yogurt, bananas, or honey; in fact, the banana diet was such a rage that there were reported shortages in the supermarkets (Toyama 2008). Other dieting techniques run the gamut from the plausible (e.g., walking diet) to the outrageous (e.g., blood type diet, karaoke diet, and manicure diet). Scientific studies indicate that more than 50% of Japanese women report a history of dieting, and the majority of them start dieting during junior high or high school years (Nemoto and Shibata 2003). In a nonclinical study, more than 42% of normal-weight women reported significant dieting efforts to lose weight, 5.9% reported fasting to lose weight, 14.3% reported the misuse of diet pills, 10.3% reported the misuse of laxatives, and 3.7% reported the misuse of diuretics (Nakamura et al. 2000).

From elementary school through college, DT is increasingly documented in Japan. Kaneko et al. (1999) surveyed 280 girls in elementary schools and found that 22% of girls reported that they engaged in weight loss behaviors, 51% of them reported the desire to be thin, and 35% of them expressed the fear of weight gain, and these phenomena increased with age. Among junior high school girls, 48.4% reported dieting for the purpose of weight loss (Takeuchi et al. 1991), and even among preadolescent girls a significant percentage report dieting for the purpose of achieving a thin beauty ideal despite normal weight status (Kaneko et al. 1999; Matsumoto et al. 2001). Japanese high school girls and college-age women report DT that is comparable with similar groups in the West, with overall DT increasing with age (Nishizono et al. 2004). Widespread DT is further evident by the fact that Japanese college women have reported an average ideal body weight that is 5 kg less than actual weight (Nagatani et al. 2007).

Similar to historical trends described in the West, preoccupation with weight and shape and dieting has been of greater significance for women than men in Japan; however, increasingly the Japanese male physical ideal emphasizes thinness as well. Studies indicate higher social desirability for thinness over muscularity for men (Nemoto and Nagoya 2000; Nemoto and Shibata 2003), and popular male singers and actors are significantly more slender than in previous years (Fujino 2003). The importance of physical attractiveness in evaluating male partners has increased relative to educational background and professional status (Maruta 2004), and a number of documented cases of eating disorders among Japanese men have been described in the literature (Maruta 2004; Nagata 2000; Nemoto and Shibata 2003).

Weight and Shape Concerns and Eating Disorders in Japan

The popular press and scientific literature clearly document a thin beauty ideal and a pervasive practice of dieting in Japan. The question remains whether this preoccupation with thinness plays a central role in the etiology of eating disorders in Japan. The significance of dieting and weight and shape concerns in the clinical pathology of eating disorders has been intensely debated, and a thorough review has recently been conducted of the role of weight and shape concerns or fat phobia in AN (Becker et al. 2009). The actual data are complex and dynamic and vary across cultures within Asia. Moreover, as rates of eating disorders increase in Asian societies, and as public awareness of eating disorders increases, it appears that there is a concomitant evolution in ascribed meanings and etiological understandings such that what is true at one point in time may not hold true only a short time thereafter.

Consider, for example, pioneering research conducted by Sing Lee and colleagues in Hong Kong. In the original studies from the 1990s (Lee 1991; Lee et al. 1993), they described the eating pathology of individuals with AN in Hong Kong and reported that, contrary to the West, the majority of patients did not report fear of fat or weight and shape preoccupation as the rationale for food refusal. Instead, Lee and colleagues reported that patients with AN were likely to report physical problems such as stomach pains and loss of appetite as the rationale for food refusal, with 60% of the seventy anorexic patients reporting no conscious fear of becoming fat. Thus, Lee and colleagues advocated that the diagnostic criteria for AN be adapted to accommodate this variant form of AN, which they termed "non-fat-phobic AN." Fast-forward to the most recent studies of eating disorders in Hong Kong and mainland China, and a remarkable evolution has occurred in terms of clinical presentation. Whereas the majority of individuals with AN in the 1990s in Hong Kong reported no fat phobia, by 2007 fear of fat and weight and shape concerns had become the dominant rationale for food refusal among individuals with eating disorders (Lee et al. 2010). Similarly, a study conducted in mainland China reported a complete absence of cases of non-fat-phobic AN (Tong et al. 2010). In this study, results from interviews utilizing the Eating Disorder Examination (Fairburn and Cooper 1993), a highly regarded, standardized interview assessment of eating pathology, indicated that women with AN and BN from central China reported rates of weight and shape concerns comparable to those of similar groups in the West. Data from other parts of Asia also suggest that fear of fatness is not unique to Western settings and patients (Soh et al. 2006, 2008).

In the case of Japan, studies comparing Japanese groups with North American and European groups in terms of DT and body dissatisfaction have reported mixed findings. Whereas Kusano et al. (2000) found that Japanese females without eating disorders reported higher levels of DT than their German counterparts, Pike and Mizushima (2005) found that Japanese women without eating disorders reported lower levels of DT than the North American–referenced comparison. In comparisons of clinical samples, Japanese women with AN and BN report significantly higher rates of DT than non-eating-disordered individuals, documenting a role for fear of fat and weight and shape concerns in the exegesis of these eating disorders. However, compared with North American eating disorder groups, the Japanese AN and BN groups reported lower rates of DT, suggesting that although DT is significant in the pathology of eating disorders in Japan, it plays a moderating role compared with North American groups with the same disorders. In contrast, in terms of body dissatisfaction, Pike and Mizushima (2005) found that Japanese women with and without eating disorders reported rates of body dissatisfaction comparable with their respective reference groups in North America. Still other studies of nonclinical samples suggest that Japanese women experience higher rates of body dissatisfaction (despite lower BMI) than North American peers (Mukai et al. 1998; Nakai 1997; Yates et al. 2004).

Further studies are necessary to explore the meanings and relationship of DT and body dissatisfaction among Japanese women. Whereas weight dissatisfaction and body dissatisfaction are closely linked in the West, it appears that factors other than weight may play more salient roles in understanding body dissatisfaction among Japanese women. Given the fact that overweight and obesity are less common in Japan than North America, it may be that other dimensions of physical appearance carry more significance in understanding body dissatisfaction at this time for Japanese women. Dissatisfaction centered on other physical features, such as height, hair color, facial features, and curvaceous bodies, is often expressed in clinical case accounts of body dissatisfaction among Japanese women (Pike and Borovoy 2004).

Some of the complexity related to the role of weight concern and DT in the exegesis of eating disorders in Japan might be a function of evolving cultural meaning and attributions. It is noteworthy that although DT and weight and shape concerns are currently viewed as core diagnostic criteria in the DSM nosology, in the earliest writings on eating disorders such factors were not defining characteristics (Lee 1993, 2001). Hsu and Lee (1993) have proposed that fat phobia came to dominate the rationale for the disturbances in eating and weight regulation among individuals with eating disorders at least in part as a function of increasing tension that developed by the gap between the thin beauty ideal and the reality of increasing population weight. In the case of Japan, the cultural beauty ideal emphasizes thinness, but the actual rates of overweight and obesity are low. According to this line of reasoning, if Japanese population weight continues to climb, we should expect to see concomitant increases in DT and body dissatisfaction among individuals with eating disorders in Japan. Finally, it may be that cultural differences in DT and body dissatisfaction are more apparent in nonclinical samples, whereas cultural differences diminish in the case of clinical disorders in which severity of these symptoms comes to dominate the clinical picture across cultural groups as a function of the diagnostic systems employed to assess and treat such problems.

Risk Factors for Eating Disorders in Japan: Why Some Women and Not Others?

Clearly, eating disorders are multidetermined, and individual differences on multiple biological, psychological, and developmental factors will interact with and moderate the broad social context such that only some individuals actually develop eating disorders despite widespread exposure to certain environmental and cultural factors. The previous discussion on changes in women's social roles and population weight demographics in Japan highlights factors that are important in terms of general sociocultural conditions, and therefore they help answer the questions "Why now?" and "Why women?" The question "Why some women and not others?" requires a different level of analysis that focuses on the particular risk factors that distinguish among members of society by identifying the individual differences that are associated with increased risk.

The study of risk factors for eating disorders in Japan is in its infancy. To our knowledge, although a range of descriptive studies have been conducted in Japan to assess clinical features associated with eating pathology, prospective and interview-based studies of risk factors do not exist. Emotional neglect, problems in parent-child relationships, and familial discord have all been described as correlates of eating disorders in Japan (Nishizono-Maher 1998). Limited, retrospective data also suggest that trauma history, particularly in the form of physical and sexual abuse, may increase risk for the development of eating disorders in Japan (Nagata et al. 2001). However, the current knowledge base is limited to correlational studies that fail to establish time precedence of risk factors, and thus the degree to which these factors truly contribute to the etiological picture is unknown. Future studies that carefully establish time of exposure to putative risk factors and course of development of the eating pathology are necessary to establish risk factors for eating disorders in Japan. Case-control studies should inform prospective research that will ultimately identify those factors that put individuals at risk for eating disorders. This level of research is necessary to answer the third question posed by Striegel-Moore et al. (1986): Why some women and not others?

Considerations and Recommendations for the Study of Eating Disorders in Japan

This review of eating disorders in Japan focuses on a discussion of the cultural context and the role of DT and weight and shape concerns in the rise of eating pathology in Japan.

In terms of cultural context, there is incontrovertible evidence that Japanese society has been in a state of transformation, with ever-increasing momentum, for the past century. Societal change and evolution are as old as recorded history, but in the study of culture and eating disorders, it is essential to understand the particular changes that set the stage for the documented rise in eating and weight disturbances in modern Japan. Women have witnessed dramatic changes in terms of constitutional rights, education, and employment; however, societal expectations and pressures for women to conform to the traditional gender-defined pathways to maturity have created significant conflict and tension for women coming of age today. The reality is that in the private and public spheres, Japan remains highly gender defined and divided. Thus, women coming of age today are balking at the traditional roles of wife and mother but are still struggling to negotiate alternative pathways to maturity.

These broad social changes in gender development are coupled with particular changes in eating and weight patterns and disturbances in Japan. Research in this area documents a steady rise in overall population weight and a concomitant rise in the percentage of women falling into a very low weight range. Dieting and weight concerns have become normative among women in Japan, and concerns with weight loss, body dissatisfaction, and DT are increasingly extending to younger girls and to men. In addition to documented increases within the general population, the extant data suggest that clinical eating disorders are also increasing in Japan, and prevalence rates are comparable with those reported in the West.

Studies examining the role of DT and weight and shape concerns in the exegesis of eating disorders in Japan present a complex picture. Based on extant data, it appears that body dissatisfaction and DT are typical and pronounced among individuals with eating disorders in Japan, with symptom presentations on these dimensions conforming to the current nosology of eating disorders. However, the degree of DT and body dissatisfaction expressed by women with eating disorders in Japan compared with that in North America suggests that these factors may not dominate the clinical picture to the same extent. Further research is needed to examine the relatively complex and possibly changing role of body dissatisfaction and DT in understanding eating disorders among different cultures. Some data suggest that DT and body dissatisfaction will increase among the general population at least partially as a function of an increasing differential between real and ideal beauty standards, thereby creating a potentially more toxic environment for the risk of eating disorders.

Research on eating disorders in Japan requires more sophisticated methods to advance the field further. The extant database is limited, but it is sufficient to allow for more informed, hypothesis-driven research going forward. Epidemiological studies that are based on community samples and that utilize more rigorous diagnostic procedures would add substantially to incidence and prevalence data of eating disorders in Japan. These studies should be sufficiently broad in the assessment of eating and weight pathology that they allow for the identification and explication of eating disturbances that may be culture bound and unique to Japan. Clinical and nonclinical studies would also benefit from more rigorous, interview-based diagnostic procedures. Studies of clinical groups based on the dominant diagnostic nomenclature do not have the breadth of scope to shed light on "non-conforming" eating disturbances. More rigorous studies examining changing cultural values and population demographics related to gender roles and beauty ideals are necessary to advance the discourse on culture and eating disorders in Japan. Against this general backdrop of changes in social roles and changes in population weight, dieting, and shape concerns, it is essential to identify factors that can address the more specific question of why only some individuals develop clinical eating disorders within the population. Multilevel as well as multifactorial approaches will advance and enhance the knowledge base of etiological risk for eating disorders in Japan and thereby expand our understanding of eating disorders around the globe.

References

Becker AE: New global perspectives on eating disorders. Cult Med Psychiatry 28:433–437, 2004a

Becker AE: Television, disordered eating, and young women in Fiji: negotiating body image and identity during rapid social change. Cult Med Psychiatry 28:533–559, 2004b

Becker AE, Thomas JJ, Pike KM: Should non-fat phobic anorexia nervosa be included in DSM-V? Int J Eat Disord 42:620–635, 2009

Borovoy A: The Too-Good Wife: Alcoholism, Codependence, and the Politics of Nurturance in Postwar Japan. Berkeley, University of California, 2005

Brownell KD: In your face: how the food industry drives us to eat. Nutrition Action Healthletter 37:3–6, 2010

Brownell KD, Kersh R, Ludwig DS, et al: Personal responsibility and obesity: a constructive approach to a controversial issue. Health Aff 29:379–387, 2010

Fairburn CG, Cooper Z: The Eating Disorder Examination (12th edition), in Binge Eating: Nature, Assessment, and Treatment. Edited by Fairburn CG, Wilson GT. New York, Guilford, 1993, pp 317–360

Fujino K: The relationship between men with eating disorders and gender identity. Educ Clin Psychol Res 29:1–35, 2003

Gender Equality Bureau: White paper on gender equality 2008. Tokyo, Gender Equality Bureau, 2008

Gordon RA: Anorexia and Bulimia: Anatomy of a Social Epidemic, 2nd Edition. Oxford, United Kingdom, Blackwell, 2000

Gordon RA: Eating disorders East and West: a culture-bound syndrome unbound, in Eating Disorders and Cultures in Transition. Edited by Nasser M, Katzman MA, Gordon RA. New York, Taylor & Francis, 2001, pp 1–16

Hochschild A, Machung A: The Second Shift. New York, Viking, 1989

Hsu LKG, Lee S: Is weight phobia always necessary for a diagnosis of anorexia nervosa? Am J Psychiatry 150:1466–1471, 1993

Huon GF, Brown LB: Bulimia: the emergence of a syndrome. Aust N Z J Psychiatry 18:113–126, 1984

Inaba S, Takahashi T: Literature Review on Incidence and Prevalence of Anorexia Nervosa: Report on the Study of Anorexia Nervosa for the Fiscal Year. Tokyo, Ministry of Health, Labor, and Welfare, 1989

Iwao S: Japanese Woman: The Traditional Image and Changing Reality. Cambridge, MA, Harvard University Press, 1983

Kageyama Y: Fast-food binge continues to take Japan. Japan Times, April 6, 2007. Available at: http://search.japantimes.co.jp/print/nb20070406a1.html. Accessed November 29, 2010.

Kaneko K, Kiriike N, Ikenaga K, et al: Weight and shape concerns and dieting behaviors among pre-adolescents and adolescents in Japan. Psychiatry Clin Neurosci 53:365–371, 1999

Katzman MA, Lee S: Beyond body image: the integration of feminist and transcultural theories in the understanding of self-starvation. Int J Eat Disord 22:385–394, 1997

Kelsky K: Women on the Verge: Japanese Women, Western Dreams. Durham, NC, Duke University Press, 2001

Kiriike N, Nagata T, Tanaka M, et al: Prevalence of binge-eating and bulimia among adolescent women in Japan. Psychiatry Res 26:163–169, 1988

Kiriike N, Nagata T, Sirata K, et al: Are young women in Japan at high risk for eating disorders? Decreased BMI in young females from 1960 to 1995. Psychiatry Clin Neurosci 52:279–281, 1998

Koseisho: Shinkeisei syokuyoku fushin syo cyosa kenkyuhan heisei 4 nendo kenkyu houkokushyo 1993 [Government publication of annual report from Anorexia Nervosa Research Committee for 1993]. Tokyo, Koseisho, 1993

Kusano M, Ehara Y, Nakamura K, et al: Eating behavior research on a Japanese non-clinical group using the Eating Disorder Inventory–2: a cross-cultural validity study. Japanese Bulletin of Social Psychiatry 9:171–181, 2000

Lee S: Anorexia nervosa in Hong Kong: a Chinese perspective. Psychol Med 21:703–711, 1991

Lee S: How abnormal is the desire for slimness? A survey of eating attitudes and behaviour among Chinese undergraduates in Hong Kong. Psychol Med 23:437–451, 1993

Lee S: Fat phobia in anorexia nervosa: whose obsession is it? in Eating Disorders and Cultures in Transition. Edited by Nasser M, Katzman MA, Gordon RA. London, Brunner-Routledge, 2001, pp 40–54

Lee S, Ho TP, Hsu LKG: Fat phobic and non-fat phobic anorexia nervosa: a comparative study of 70 Chinese patients in Hong Kong. Psychol Med 23:999–1017, 1993

Lee S, Ng KL, Kwok K, et al: The changing profile of eating disorders at a tertiary psychiatric clinic in Hong Kong (1987–2007). Int J Eat Disord 43:307–314, 2010

Makino M, Hashizume M, Yasushi M, et al: Factors associated with abnormal eating attitudes among female college students in Japan. Arch Womens Ment Health 9:203–208, 2006

Maruta K: The main factors in male eating disorders. Okinawa University Department of Anthropology 5:55–64, 2004

Maruyama C, Ito K, Kimimoto R, et al: A first report of a study on eating disorders of school girls. Adolescentology 11:51–56, 1993

Matsumoto H, Takei N, Kawai M, et al: Differences of symptoms and standardized weight index between patients with early onset and late-onset anorexia nervosa. Acta Psychiatr Scand 104:6–71, 2001

Miller L: Beauty Up: Exploring Contemporary Japanese Body Aesthetics. Berkeley, University of California, 2006

Millstone E, Lang T: Risking regulatory capture at the UK's Food Standards Agency? Lancet 372:94–95, 2008

Ministry of Health, Labor, and Welfare: National Nutrition Survey. Tokyo, Ministry of Health, Labor, and Welfare, 2006

Ministry of Health, Labor, and Welfare: 2009 National Welfare Survey. Tokyo, Ministry of Health, Labor, and Welfare, 2009

Mukai T, Crago M, Shisslak CM: Eating attitudes and weight preoccupation among female high school students in Japan. J Child Psychol Psychiatry 35:677–688, 1994

Mukai T, Kambara A, Sasaki Y: Body dissatisfaction, need for approval, and eating disturbances among Japanese and American college women. Sex Roles 39:751–763, 1998

Nadaoka T, Oiji A, Takahashi S, et al: An epidemiological study of eating disorders in a northern area of Japan. Acta Psychiatr Scand 93:305–310, 1996

Nagata M: Men who binge and diet are in danger. Aera May 1–8:24–25, 2000

Nagata T, Kaye WH, Kiriike N, et al: Physical and sexual abuse histories in patients with eating disorders: a comparison of Japanese and American patients. Psychiatry Clin Neurosci 55:333–340, 2001

Nagatani T, Nagatani N, Inoue H, et al: A diet in youths with the possibility of the potential patient of an eating disorder: ideal weight of the youths in the questionnaire result. Journal of Shonan Tanki Daigaku 18:79–85, 2007

Nakai Y: Eating Disorder Inventory scores in eating disorders. Clin Psychiatry 39:47–50, 1997

Nakai Y: Change in prevalence of eating disorders and eating disorder symptoms. Seishin-igaku 32:379–383, 2010

Nakamura KY, Hoshino A, Watanabe K, et al: Eating problems and related weight control behavior in adult Japanese women. Psychother Psychosom 68:51–55, 1999

Nakamura K, Yamamoto M, Yamazaki O, et al: Prevalence of anorexia nervosa and bulimia nervosa in a geographically defined area in Japan. Int J Eat Disord 28:173–180, 2000

Nemoto K, Nagoya R: Female students' attitudes toward the shape of male body. Journal of Tokyo Kasei Gakuin University 40:9–16, 2000

Nemoto K, Shibata F: Body image, the desire to be thin, and eating disturbances. Journal of Tokyo Kasei Gakuin Daigaku 43:21–26, 2003

Nishizono A, Miyake Y, Nakane A: The prevalence of eating pathology and its relationship to knowledge of eating disorders among high school girls in Japan. Eur Eat Disord Rev 12:122–128, 2004

Nishizono-Maher A: Eating disorders in Japan: finding the right context. Psychiatry Clin Neurosci 52:230–232, 1998

Nogami Y, Kamata K, Momma K: Binge-eating among female students. Jpn J Psychiatry Neurol 41:151–152, 1987

Ono H: Women's economic resources, marriage, and cross-national contexts of gender. J Marriage Fam 65:275–290, 2003

Pike KM, Borovoy A: The rise of eating disorders in Japan: issues of culture and limitations of the model of westernization. Cult Med Psychiatry 28:493–531, 2004

Pike KM, Mizushima H: The clinical presentation of Japanese women with anorexia nervosa and bulimia nervosa: a study of the Eating Disorder Inventory–2. Int J Eat Disord 37:26–31, 2005

Soh NL, Touyz SW, Surgenor LJ: Eating and body image disturbances across cultures: a review. Eur Eat Disord Rev 14:54–65, 2006

Soh NLW, Touyz S, Dobbins T, et al: Body image disturbance in young North European and East Asian women with and without eating disorders in Australia and in Singapore. Eur Eat Disord Rev 16:287–296, 2008

Striegel-Moore RH, Silberstein LR, Rodin J: Toward an understanding of sociocultural risk factors for bulimia. Am Psychol 41:246–263, 1986

Suematsu H, Ishikawa H, Kuboki T, et al: Statistical studies on anorexia nervosa in Japan: detailed clinical data on 1011 patients. Psychother Psychosom 43:96–103, 1985

Takagi S: Recent trends of eating disorders in Keio University and Second Tokyo National Hospital. Japanese Journal of National Medical Services 44:153–158, 1990

Takeda A, Suzuki K, Matsushita Y: Prevalence of bulimia nervosa (DSM-III-R) among male and female high school students. Seishinigaku 35:1273–1278, 1993

Takeuchi S, Hayano J, Kamiya T, et al: Body image and self image in 712 junior high school students. Shinshin Igaku 31:367–373, 1991

Tong J, Shi J, Wang J, et al: Validity and reliability of the Chinese language version of the Eating Disorder Examination (CEDE) in mainland China: implications for the identity and nosology of the eating disorders. Int J Eat Disord January 12, 2010 [Epub ahead of print]

Toyama M: Japan goes bananas for a new diet. Time, October 17, 2008. Available at: http://www.time.com/time/world/article/0,8599,1850454,00.html. Accessed November 29, 2010.

Watanabe H, Tanaka T, Tokumura M, et al: A national epidemiological survey of anorexia nervosa and unhealthy thinness in junior and senior high school girls: an attempt for early detection of anorexia nervosa using growth charts based on regular school physical measurement data (in Japanese), in The Heisei 14 Report of the Health and Labor Science Research Grant (Research Project on the Comprehensive Research on Child and Family). Tokyo, Japanese Department of Health Labor and Science, 2003, 2003, pp 633–664

Yamatsuta K, Nomura S: Abnormal eating behavior among female university students: development, reliability and validity of a new body image dissatisfaction scale. Journal of Japanese Society of Psychosomatic Obstetrics and Gynecology 10:63–171, 2005

Yates A, Edman J, Aruguete M: Ethnic differences in BMI and body/self-dissatisfaction among whites, Asian subgroups, Pacific Islanders, and African-Americans. J Adolesc Health 34:300–307, 2004

22

COMPARISON OF FEMALE JAPANESE AND CANADIAN EATING DISORDER PATIENTS ON THE EATING DISORDER INVENTORY

Yoshikatsu Nakai, M.D., Ph.D.
Marion P. Olmsted, Ph.D., C.Psych.
Traci McFarlane, Ph.D., C.Psych.
Stephen A. Wonderlich, Ph.D.
Ross D. Crosby, Ph.D.

Japan differs from Western countries in customs in food, housing, education, religion, and family, including women's issues. However, during the past half-century, Japan has been rapidly developing, and this, along with a growing increase in Western culture, has brought many changes in the Japanese traditional lifestyle and cultural standards (Varadaman 2006). After the concept of anorexia nervosa (AN) was established firmly among Japanese doctors during the late 1950s, numerous reports of eating disorders in Japan were published, but most of them were written in Japanese (Nakai 1997; Shimosaka 1961). Moreover, cross-cultural studies assessing eating pathology between the Japanese and Western eating disorders are sparse (Pike and Mizushima 2005; Tachikawa et al. 2004).

The modern concept of AN has always contained the idea that concern about body weight, sometimes labeled *fear of fatness* or *drive for thinness* (DT), should be one of the defining and essential diagnostic criteria (American Psychiatric Association 1994). However, Lee et al. (1993) reported that 58.6% of 70 Chinese AN patients in Hong Kong did not exhibit any fear of fatness, although they were similar to Western AN patients in most other ways. This resulted in investigation of the symptom profiles of subjects with AN from different ethnic and social groups. Tareen et al. (2005) found that South Asian patients with AN presented less frequently with fat phobia compared with matched Caucasian English patients. These results suggest that morbid fear of fatness in AN may be culture bound and not necessarily universal among Asian culture. However, Strober et al. (1999) reported that 20.6% of 97 AN patients in the United States steadfastly denied fear of weight gain and showed a less malignant course and outcome compared with typical cases of AN.

The morbid fear of fatness is often measured by self-report as DT. The Eating Disorder Inventory (EDI; Garner et al. 1983) is the most widely used multidimensional instrument, consisting of 64 items that make up eight subscales: Drive for Thinness, Bulimia, Body Dissatisfaction, Ineffectiveness, Perfectionism, Interpersonal Distrust, Interoceptive Awareness, and Maturity Fears. The first three subscales assess attitude and/or behaviors related to eating disorders; the remaining five subscales assess psychopathology commonly associated with, but not unique to, eating disorders (Garner et al. 1983). The DT subscale measures preoccupation with body weight, a morbid fear of becoming fat, and excessive concern with dieting.

Lee et al. (1998) reported that in Hong Kong, non-fat-phobic AN patients ($n=11$) scored lower than fat-phobic AN patients ($n=12$) only on the DT subscale of the EDI. Shortly afterward, Ramacciotti et al. (2002) reported that 17% of 70 patients with eating disorders in Italy and 17% of 104 AN patients in Canada had low DT as measured by the EDI. The cutoff score of 7 was chosen to ensure low levels of DT in these patients relative to normal female college students. These atypical AN patients in Western countries scored lower than typical AN patients on most subscales of the EDI, reflecting less severe psychopathology. These results suggest that atypical AN patients with low DT in Western countries may be different from non-fat-phobic AN patients in Hong Kong. The percentage of AN patients with low DT is variable in Western countries, ranging from 17% to 38% (Abbate-Daga et al. 2007; Ramacciotti et al. 2002; Vervaet et al. 2004).

There were three papers using the EDI in Japanese clinical samples (Nakai 1997; Pike and Mizushima 2005; Tachikawa et al. 2004). In our previous study (Nakai 1997), the Japanese AN, restricting type (AN-R), AN, binge-purge type (AN-BP), and bulimia nervosa (BN) groups reported significantly less DT than the Canadian reference groups used in the development of the EDI. However, in the study of Pike and Mizushima (2005), the Japanese AN-BP group did not differ significantly from the corresponding Canadian reference group in terms of DT. Similarly, Tachikawa et al. (2004) reported that the Japanese AN-R and BN groups did not differ significantly from Canadian groups in terms of DT. Perhaps the sample sizes in these studies were too small to provide consistent results. Furthermore, to our knowledge there has been no report on atypical eating disorders with low DT in Japan.

The primary aim of this study was to assess whether cultural differences exist in eating disorder profiles between the Japanese and Western eating disorders. To test this idea, we compared the EDI between Japanese and Canadian eating disorder patients in a large sample. A secondary aim involved comparing Japanese and Canadian patients in terms of the frequency of an atypical form of AN, with low DT, and its associated clinical characteristics.

Methods

SUBJECTS

The Japanese sample consisted of 993 women with eating disorders who consulted the outpatient unit of Kyoto University Hospital. All patients met DSM-IV (American Psychiatric Association 1994) criteria for eating disorders and consisted of subtypes as follows: 247 (24.9%) AN-R; 137 (13.8%) AN-BP; 281 (28.3%) BN, purging type (BN-P); 72 (7.3%) BN, nonpurging type (BN-NP); and 256 (25.8%) eating disorder not otherwise specified (EDNOS). All patients were of Japanese ethnic descent.

The Canadian sample included 971 women with eating disorders from the Eating Disorder Program at Toronto General Hospital and consisted of subtypes as follows: 110 (11.3%) AN-R; 142 (14.6%) AN-BP; 319 (32.9%) BN-P; 51 (5.3%) BN-NP; and 349 (35.9%) EDNOS. Participants were selected from a larger sample of 1,196 based on age ($\leq$46 years) and body mass index (BMI$\leq$38 kg/m^2) to better match the characteristics of the Japanese sample.

ASSESSMENTS

In the Japanese sample, information was collected during the first consultation via semistructured interviews, including a history of illness, eating behaviors, and body perceptions. Objective weight and height were measured during the first consultation, and BMI was calculated. Patients completed a Japanese version of the EDI (Nakai 1997). The validity of the Japanese version of the EDI was described previously (Nakai 1997, 2007). Cronbach α coefficient for the Perfectionism subscale was 0.69, but for the remaining seven subscales α ranged from 0.80 to 0.84, reflecting adequate internal consistency (Nakai 2007).

In the Canadian sample, objective weight and height were measured at the pretreatment assessment. Patients completed the original English version of the EDI. The validity of the EDI has been previously described (Garner 1991; Garner et al. 1983).

STATISTICAL ANALYSIS

All data analysis was performed with PASW (formerly SPSS) Version 18.0.0. The Japanese and Canadian samples were compared on demographic and clinical characteristics at baseline using Fisher's exact tests for dichotomous variables, χ^2 for other categorical variables, and independent sample t tests for continuous measures. Japanese and Canadian samples within each diagnostic subgroup were compared on EDI scores using analysis of covariance controlling for age and BMI. Partial η^2 values were calculated to determine the proportion of unique variance in EDI scores accounted for by nationality. A small effect is reflected by a partial η^2 value of approximately 0.01, a medium effect is approximately 0.06, and a large effect is approximately 0.14 (Cohen 1988). Finally, we divided patients with AN into two groups based upon their DT score (Abbate-Daga et al. 2007; Ramacciotti et al. 2002; Vervaet et al. 2004): DT≤7 = atypical; DT>7 = typical. In the Japanese sample, the typical group consisted of 153 AN patients and the atypical group consisted of 231 patients; in the Canadian sample, the typical group consisted of 180 AN patients and the atypical group consisted of 67 patients. A two-way multivariate analysis of covariance was then performed comparing the remaining EDI subscale scores by sample (Japan vs. Canada), DT (atypical vs. typical), and the interaction, after controlling for age and BMI. A significance level of $P<0.05$ was used for all statistical tests.

Results

DEMOGRAPHIC AND CLINICAL CHARACTERISTICS

Demographic and clinical characteristics at intake for the Japanese and Canadian samples are presented in Table 22–1. In comparison to the Japanese sample, Canadian patients were significantly older, had a higher weight and BMI at intake, and were on average older at onset of the eating disorder. The distribution of eating disorder diagnoses was also significantly different between samples, with the Japanese sample having a higher proportion of AN-R patients and the Canadian sample having a higher proportion of EDNOS patients.

For both the Japanese and Canadian samples, the mean BMI (SD) for each diagnostic group was consistent with diagnosis:

- *Japanese sample:* AN-R, 14.5 kg/m² (1.5); AN-BP, 14.8 kg/m² (1.7); BN-P, 20.4 kg/m² (1.9); BN-NP, 21.2 kg/m² (2.8); EDNOS, 20.0 kg/m² (4.0)
- *Canadian sample:* AN-R, 16.3 kg/m² (1.4); AN-BP, 16.9 kg/m² (1.3); BN-P, 23.3 kg/m² (4.3); BN-NP, 24.8 kg/m² (4.8); EDNOS, 22.7 kg/m² (4.1)

TABLE 22–1. Demographic and clinical characteristics for the Japanese and Canadian samples

Intake characteristic	Sample		Significance
	Japanese ($n=993$)	Canadian ($n=971$)	
Female, n (%)	993 (100)	971 (100)	—
Age, years, mean (SD)	21.8 (5.0)	26.8 (7.0)	$t_{1962} = 18.12, P < 0.001$
Weight, kg, mean (SD)	45.6 (10.3)	57.9 (13.1)	$t_{1962} = 23.18, P < 0.001$
BMI, kg/m², mean (SD)	18.1 (3.8)	21.4 (4.7)	$t_{1962} = 17.42, P < 0.001$
Age at ED onset, years, mean (SD)	17.4 (4.1)	19.2 (6.3)	$t_{1791} = 7.04, P < 0.001$
DSM-IV eating disorder diagnosis			$\chi^2_4 = 72.71, P < 0.001$
AN-BP, n (%)	137 (13.8)	142 (14.6)	
AN-R, n (%)	247 (24.9)	110 (11.3)	
BN-NP, n (%)	72 (7.3)	51 (5.3)	
BN-P, n (%)	281 (28.3)	319 (32.9)	
EDNOS, n (%)	256 (25.8)	349 (35.9)	

Note. AN-BP = anorexia nervosa, binge-purge type; AN-R = anorexia nervosa, restricting type; BMI = body mass index; BN-NP = bulimia nervosa, nonpurging type; BN-P = Bulimia nervosa, purging type; ED = eating disorder; EDNOS = eating disorder not otherwise specified.

EATING DISORDER INVENTORY COMPARISON OF THE JAPANESE AND CANADIAN GROUPS

Comparisons of the Japanese and Canadian samples on EDI scores controlling for differences in age and BMI are presented separately by diagnostic group in Tables 22–2 through 22–6. Two notable patterns of differences between samples emerged. First, for the diagnoses of AN-BP (Table 22–2), AN-R (Table 22–3), and EDNOS (Table 22–6), the Canadian sample scored consistently and significantly higher on DT, Body Dissatisfaction, and Perfectionism. Second, except for the diagnosis of AN-R, the Japanese sample scored higher on Bulimia and Maturity Fears.

TABLE 22–2. Eating Disorder Inventory mean (SD) scores for anorexia nervosa, binge-purge subtype patients in the Japanese and Canadian samples

Intake characteristic	Sample		Significance[a]	Partial η^{2a}
	Japanese ($n=137$)	Canadian ($n=142$)		
Drive for Thinness	10.0 (6.2)	14.1 (6.3)	$F_{1,275} = 15.53; P < 0.001$	0.053
Bulimia	10.2 (6.6)	8.7 (6.4)	$F_{1,275} = 4.35; P = 0.038$	0.016
Body Dissatisfaction	12.6 (4.9)	17.2 (8.2)	$F_{1,275} = 11.30; P = 0.001$	0.039
Ineffectiveness	13.1 (6.8)	14.5 (8.2)	$F_{1,275} = 0.86; P = 0.354$	0.003
Perfectionism	6.6 (3.9)	9.7 (5.5)	$F_{1,274} = 19.49; P < 0.001$	0.066
Interpersonal Distrust	6.7 (6.6)	7.4 (5.1)	$F_{1,275} = 1.60; P = 0.207$	0.006
Interoceptive Awareness	12.4 (7.9)	14.6 (7.8)	$F_{1,274} = 2.99; P = 0.085$	0.011
Maturity Fears	9.4 (5.6)	6.1 (5.9)	$F_{1,273} = 8.14; P = 0.005$	0.029

[a]Controlling for age and body mass index.

TABLE 22–3. Eating Disorder Inventory mean (SD) scores for anorexia nervosa, restricting subtype patients in the Japanese and Canadian samples

Intake characteristic	Sample		Significance[a]	Partial η^{2a}
	Japanese ($n=247$)	Canadian ($n=110$)		
Drive for Thinness	5.2 (5.1)	11.8 (7.1)	$F_{1,353} = 53.28; P < 0.001$	0.131
Bulimia	2.0 (3.2)	1.5 (2.2)	$F_{1,352} = 0.24; P = 0.628$	0.001
Body Dissatisfaction	10.3 (4.0)	13.1 (8.1)	$F_{1,352} = 12.02; P = 0.001$	0.033
Ineffectiveness	8.0 (5.3)	11.7 (8.3)	$F_{1,353} = 9.24; P = 0.003$	0.026
Perfectionism	4.9 (4.0)	8.0 (5.1)	$F_{1,352} = 10.97; P = 0.001$	0.030
Interpersonal Distrust	4.4 (3.6)	6.3 (5.0)	$F_{1,353} = 2.69; P = 0.102$	0.008
Interoceptive Awareness	5.4 (6.1)	9.6 (7.1)	$F_{1,353} = 24.45; P < 0.001$	0.065
Maturity Fears	7.3 (4.6)	6.1 (6.1)	$F_{1,353} = 0.70; P = 0.405$	0.002

[a]Controlling for age and body mass index.

TABLE 22–4. Eating Disorder Inventory mean (SD) scores for bulimia nervosa, nonpurging subtype patients in the Japanese and Canadian samples

Intake characteristic	Sample		Significance[a]	Partial η^{2a}
	Japanese ($n=72$)	Canadian ($n=51$)		
Drive for Thinness	14.5 (5.1)	16.4 (4.0)	$F_{1,119} = 2.60$; $P = 0.109$	0.021
Bulimia	12.2 (5.3)	9.5 (5.0)	$F_{1,119} = 13.10$; $P < 0.001$	0.099
Body Dissatisfaction	18.0 (6.5)	20.1 (6.4)	$F_{1,119} = 0.00$; $P = 0.999$	0.000
Ineffectiveness	13.4 (6.3)	12.2 (7.4)	$F_{1,119} = 3.04$; $P = 0.084$	0.025
Perfectionism	7.2 (4.1)	9.0 (4.8)	$F_{1,119} = 3.31$; $P = 0.071$	0.027
Interpersonal Distrust	6.4 (4.3)	5.4 (4.2)	$F_{1,119} = 1.78$; $P = 0.185$	0.015
Interoceptive Awareness	12.6 (6.0)	12.2 (6.9)	$F_{1,118} = 0.42$; $P = 0.517$	0.004
Maturity Fears	7.9 (5.0)	5.2 (5.1)	$F_{1,119} = 6.14$; $P = 0.015$	0.049

[a]Controlling for age and body mass index.

TABLE 22–5. Eating Disorder Inventory mean (SD) scores for bulimia nervosa, purging subtype patients in the Japanese and Canadian samples

Intake characteristic	Sample		Significance[a]	Partial η[2a]
	Japanese (*n*=281)	Canadian (*n*=319)		
Drive for Thinness	13.5 (5.7)	15.8 (4.6)	$F_{1,596} = 19.92; P < 0.001$	0.032
Bulimia	14.2 (5.3)	12.5 (5.0)	$F_{1,594} = 22.12; P < 0.001$	0.036
Body Dissatisfaction	18.1 (6.7)	19.7 (7.3)	$F_{1,596} = 0.02; P = 0.885$	0.000
Ineffectiveness	14.2 (6.2)	13.8 (7.4)	$F_{1,596} = 0.28; P = 0.595$	0.000
Perfectionism	7.5 (4.3)	8.3 (5.0)	$F_{1,595} = 2.66; P = 0.104$	0.004
Interpersonal Distrust	6.6 (4.2)	6.6 (4.6)	$F_{1,595} = 0.07; P = 0.794$	0.000
Interoceptive Awareness	13.7 (7.5)	14.0 (7.3)	$F_{1,596} = 0.42; P = 0.518$	0.001
Maturity Fears	8.9 (5.7)	5.2 (5.2)	$F_{1,596} = 31.01; P < 0.001$	0.041

[a]Controlling for age and body mass index.

TABLE 22–6. Eating Disorder Inventory mean (SD) scores for eating disorder not otherwise specified patients in the Japanese and Canadian samples

	Sample		
Intake characteristic	Japanese (n=256)	Canadian (n=346)	Significance[a]	Partial η_1^{2a}
Drive for Thinness	10.2 (6.5)	14.5 (5.9)	$F_{1,598} = 68.44; P < 0.001$	0.103
Bulimia	7.9 (6.4)	6.1 (5.5)	$F_{1,597} = 24.03; P < 0.001$	0.039
Body Dissatisfaction	15.0 (7.8)	19.2 (7.8)	$F_{1,601} = 21.75; P < 0.001$	0.035
Ineffectiveness	11.8 (6.7)	12.9 (8.2)	$F_{1,601} = 3.38; P = 0.067$	0.006
Perfectionism	6.3 (4.2)	8.6 (5.3)	$F_{1,600} = 26.71; P < 0.001$	0.043
Interpersonal Distrust	6.2 (4.2)	6.1 (4.9)	$F_{1,601} = 0.39; P = 0.531$	0.001
Interoceptive Awareness	10.2 (8.4)	11.7 (7.7)	$F_{1,601} = 10.13; P = 0.002$	0.017
Maturity Fears	8.0 (5.3)	5.1 (5.0)	$F_{1,597} = 25.70; P < 0.001$	0.041

[a]Controlling for age and body mass index.

COMPARISON OF TYPICAL AND ATYPICAL ANOREXIA NERVOSA PATIENTS ON EATING DISORDER INVENTORY SCORES

The atypical (low DT) AN group included 58.6% of AN patients in the Japanese sample but only 27.1% of AN patients in the Canadian sample. Multivariate comparisons revealed significant main effects for sample and DT as well as the interaction (all P values < 0.001). Information on the univariate tests is provided in Table 22–7. Significant differences were found between the Japanese and Canadian AN samples on five of the EDI scales, with the Canadian sample scoring higher on Body Dissatisfaction, Perfectionism, and Interoceptive Awareness, whereas the Japanese sample scored higher on Bulimia and Maturity Fears. However, the magnitude of the differences between the Japanese and Canadian samples based upon partial η^2 were quite small (0.001–0.026) compared with those for DT comparisons (0.055–0.229), where the typical DT group scored significantly higher than the atypical DT group on all EDI scales. The sample-by-DT interaction was significant for the Bulimia scale (partial $\eta^2 = 0.007$), for which the Japanese sample with typical DT showed the highest scores, and for the Body Dissatisfaction scale (partial $\eta^2 = 0.096$), for which the Canadian sample with typical DT was much more elevated than other groups.

Discussion

We compared large samples of Japanese and Canadian eating disorder patients on the EDI subscales. In the present study there were differences between samples in the subscales related to core eating disorder symptoms (DT, Bulimia, Body Dissatisfaction). Across most diagnostic subgroups the Japanese sample scored significantly higher on the Bulimia subscale and lower on the DT and Body Dissatisfaction subscales than their Canadian counterparts. It is not clear whether this pattern of differences reflects differences in the frequency or severity of behavioral symptoms or reflects a difference in the way the illness is experienced or reported across cultures.

To further study the cultural difference on the DT subscale, we divided the AN sample into two groups based on DT scores consistent with previous studies (Abbate-Daga et al. 2007; Ramacciotti et al. 2002; Vervaet et al. 2004). More than half of the Japanese sample (58.6%) had low DT, compared with just over one-quarter (27.1%) of the Canadian sample. Atypical AN patients (i.e., low DT) scored lower on almost all the EDI subscales compared with typical AN patients, both in the Japanese sample and in the Canadian sample, reflecting less severe psychopathology across both cultures. Our test of the idea that the characteristics of atypical AN would differ between cultures was largely unsupported, except for the findings that Japanese patients showed greater typical versus atypical differences

TABLE 22–7. Eating Disorder Inventory subscale mean (SD) scores for typical and atypical anorexia nervosa in Japanese and Canadian samples

Subscale	Japan		Canada		Significance (partial η^2)[a]		
	Atypical DT (n=231)	Typical DT (n=153)	Atypical DT (n=67)	Typical DT (n=180)	Japan vs. Canada	Atypical vs. typical DT	Interaction
Bulimia	2.4 (4.2)	8.6 (6.8)	2.6 (4.2)	6.7 (6.5)	0.001 (0.017)	< 0.001 (0.141)	0.034 (0.007)
Body Dissatisfaction	10.6 (3.8)	12.0 (5.2)	8.2 (5.0)	18.0 (7.9)	0.033 (0.007)	< 0.001 (0.158)	< 0.001 (0.096)
Ineffectiveness	7.6 (5.1)	13.3 (6.6)	8.6 (6.9)	15.1 (8.2)	0.530 (0.001)	< 0.001 (0.150)	0.293 (0.002)
Perfectionism	4.5 (3.7)	7.0 (4.2)	7.2 (4.8)	9.7 (5.4)	< 0.001 (0.025)	< 0.001 (0.060)	0.689 (0.000)
Interpersonal Distrust	4.3 (5.3)	6.7 (4.1)	4.9 (4.9)	7.7 (5.0)	0.455 (0.001)	< 0.001 (0.055)	0.579 (0.000)
Interoceptive Awareness	4.0 (5.5)	13.1 (7.3)	7.0 (6.0)	14.4 (7.6)	0.042 (0.007)	< 0.001 (0.229)	0.306 (0.002)
Maturity Fears	6.9 (4.7)	9.8 (5.2)	4.1 (4.6)	6.9 (6.2)	< 0.001 (0.026)	< 0.001 (0.059)	0.988 (0.000)

Note. DT = drive for thinness.
[a]Controlling for age and body mass index.

on the EDI Bulimia scale than did Canadian patients. Also, Canadian patients displayed greater typical versus atypical differences on the EDI Body Dissatisfaction scale than did Japanese patients. Overall, there was little evidence to suggest that the typical versus atypical comparison differed across cultures.

There were also significant differences between Japanese and Canadian patients across several other subscales of the EDI. For example, the Japanese eating disorder patients scored significantly higher on Maturity Fears than the Canadian counterparts across all groups except AN-R, although the effect sizes were not large. Lee et al. (1993) reported similar findings and hypothesized that a high score may reflect a strong parent-child relationship in China. Characteristics of Japanese culture, especially for the family environment, may resemble Chinese culture. However, high Maturity Fears scores were also seen in some European countries, including Sweden (Norring and Sohlberg 1988), Germany (Kordy et al. 2001), Bulgaria (Boyadjieva and Steinhausen 1996), and Hungary (Rathner et al. 1995). Therefore, this subscale may reflect social structure rather than Asian culture itself.

Relative to their respective Canadian groups, the Japanese AN-R, AN-BP, and EDNOS groups scored significantly lower on the Perfectionism subscale. This is consistent with previous studies (Nakai 1997; Pike and Mizushima 2005; Tachikawa et al. 2004). Yet we should be cautious in the interpretation of these results, because Cronbach α was 0.65 in the study by Tachikawa et al. (2004) and 0.67 in the present study, indicating that this measure taps into a less homogeneous construct in Japanese samples than in Canadian samples.

In summary, a low-DT form of AN was more common in Japan (59% of AN) than in Canada (27% of AN) and was accompanied by lower scores on all other subscales of the EDI both in Japan and in Canada. This finding is in keeping with the recent review paper by Becker et al. (2009), who concluded that low-DT AN patients are characterized by lesser eating pathology but similar nutritional compromise to typical AN patients. In addition, some cultural differences were identified. Japanese patients had higher maturity fears and bulimic tendencies and lower DT and body dissatisfaction than the Canadian patients. These results indicate that there may be both cultural and social differences in eating disorders and that we need further transcultural study related to the experience, diagnosis, and classification of eating disorders on non-Western countries.

References

Abbate-Daga G, Pierò A, Gramaglia C, et al: An attempt to understand the paradox of anorexia nervosa without drive for thinness. Psychiatry Res 149:215–221, 2007

American Psychiatric Association: Diagnostic and Statistical Manual of Mental Disorders, 4th Edition. Washington, DC, American Psychiatric Association, 1994

Becker AE, Thomas JJ, Pike KM: Should non-fat phobic anorexia nervosa be included in DSM-V? Int J Eat Disord 42:620–635, 2009

Boyadjieva S, Steinhausen HC: The Eating Attitudes Test and the Eating Disorders Inventory in four Bulgarian clinical and nonclinical samples. Int J Eat Disord 19:93–98, 1996

Cohen J: Statistical Power Analysis for the Social and Behavioral Sciences, 2nd Edition. Hillsdale, NJ, Lawrence Erlbaum, 1988

Garner DM: Eating Disorder Inventory–2: Professional Manual. Odessa, FL, Psychological Assessment Resources, 1991

Garner DM, Olmsted MP, Polivy J: Development and validation of a multidimensional eating disorder inventory for anorexia nervosa and bulimia. Int J Eat Disord 2:15–34, 1983

Kordy H, Percevic R, Martinovich A: Norms, normality, and clinical significant change: implications for the evaluation of treatment outcomes for eating disorders. Int J Eat Disord 30:176–186, 2001

Lee S, Ho TP, Hsu LKG: Fat phobic and non-fat phobic anorexia nervosa: a comparative study of 70 Chinese patients in Hong Kong. Psychol Med 23:999–1017, 1993

Lee S, Lee AM, Leung T: Cross-cultural validity of the Eating Disorder Inventory: a study of Chinese patients with eating disorders in Hong Kong. Int J Eat Disord 23:177–188, 1998

Nakai Y: Eating Disorder Inventory scores in eating disorders. Clinical Psychiatry (Tokyo) 39:47–50, 1997

Nakai Y: The Eating Disorder Inventory in Japanese clinical and nonclinical samples, presented at the 10th general meeting of the ECED, Porto, 2007

Norring C, Sohlberg S: Eating Disorder Inventory in Sweden: description, cross-cultural comparison and clinical utility. Acta Psychiatr Scand 78:567–575, 1988

Pike KM, Mizushima H: The clinical presentation of Japanese women with anorexia nervosa and bulimia nervosa: a study of the Eating Disorder Inventory–2. Int J Eat Disord 37:26–31, 2005

Ramacciotti CE, Dell'Osso L, Paoli RA, et al: Characteristics of eating disorder patients without a drive for thinness. Int J Eat Disord 32:206–212, 2002

Rathner G, Túry F, Szabó P, et al: Prevalence of eating disorders and minor psychiatric morbidity in central Europe before the political changes in 1989: a cross-cultural study. Psychol Med 25:1027–1035, 1995

Shimosaka K: Psychiatrische Studien über pubertätsmagersucht [in Japanese with German abstract]. Psychiatria et Neurologia Japonica 63:1042–1082, 1961 (in Japanese with German abstract).

Strober M, Freeman R, Morrell W: Atypical anorexia nervosa: separation from typical cases in course and outcome in a long-term prospective study. Int J Eat Disord 25:135–142, 1999

Tachikawa H, Yamaguchi N, Hatanaka K, et al: The Eating Disorder Inventory–2 in Japanese clinical and non-clinical samples: psychometric properties and cross-cultural implications. Eat Weight Disord 9:107–113, 2004

Tareen A, Hodes M, Rangel L: Non-fat-phobic anorexia nervosa in British South Asian adolescents. Int J Eat Disord 37:161–165, 2005

Varadaman JM: Contemporary Japanese History: Since 1945. Tokyo, IBC Publishing, 2006

Vervaet M, van Heeringen C, Audenaert K: Is drive for thinness in anorectic patients associated with personality characteristics? Eur Eat Disord Rev 12:375–379, 2004

23

A LATENT PROFILE ANALYSIS OF THE TYPOLOGY OF BULIMIC SYMPTOMS IN AN INDIGENOUS PACIFIC POPULATION

Evidence of Cross-Cultural Variation in Phenomenology

Jennifer J. Thomas, Ph.D.

Ross D. Crosby, Ph.D.

Stephen A. Wonderlich, Ph.D.

Ruth H. Striegel-Moore, Ph.D.

Anne E. Becker, M.D., Ph.D., Sc.M.

Portions of this paper were presented at the National Institute of Mental Health (NIMH)–sponsored R-13 meeting on Eating Disorder Classification in Arlington, Virginia, on March 16, 2009; and the American Psychological Association Convention in Toronto, Canada, on August 6, 2009. The full manuscript was previously published in *Psychological Medicine* (41:195–206, 2010), which provided permission for reprinting in this monograph.

This project was funded by NIMH K23 MH 068575 (A.E.B.), a Harvard Research Enabling Grant (A.E.B.), and a Klarman Foundation Post-Doctoral Fellowship (J.J.T.). The authors report no competing financial interests.

We gratefully acknowledge the assistance of Dr. Lepani Waqatakirewa, CEO, Fiji Ministry of Health, and his team; the Fiji Ministry of Education; Joana Rokomatu, the late *Tui Sigatoka;* Dr. Jan Pryor, Chair of the FN-RERC; Dr. Tevita Qorimasi; Professor Bill Aalbersberg; A. Nisha Khan; Asenaca Bainivualiku; Professor Jane Murphy; Lauren Richards; Aliyah Shivji; Amy Heberle; Kesaia Navara; and members of the Senior Advisory Group for the HEALTHY Fiji Study. Finally, we thank all the Fiji-based principals and teachers who facilitated this study.

The clinical utility of the DSM-IV (American Psychiatric Association 1994, 2000) eating disorder classification system has been critiqued because the residual category, eating disorder not otherwise specified (EDNOS), is the most common eating disorder diagnosis in clinical settings. In contrast to the diagnostic categories of anorexia nervosa (AN) and bulimia nervosa (BN), EDNOS is phenomenologically heterogeneous (Thomas et al. 2009), and few clinical trials support relevant treatment strategies. As a result, the upcoming publication of DSM-5 has inspired a wave of research on empirical approaches to reconsider optimal eating disorder nosology. To date, 10 published studies (Bulik et al. 2000; Duncan et al. 2007; Eddy et al. 2009; Keel et al. 2004; Mitchell et al. 2007; Pinheiro et al. 2008; Striegel-Moore et al. 2005, 2008; Sullivan et al. 1998; Wade et al. 2006) have used latent class analysis (LCA) or latent profile analysis (LPA) to derive eating disorder subtypes empirically based on the co-occurrence of attitudes and behaviors in symptomatic samples. These analyses have proved invaluable in highlighting the strengths and weaknesses of DSM-IV diagnoses. For example, whereas several LCA and LPA studies have confirmed the existence of latent classes resembling AN (Bulik et al. 2000; Keel et al. 2004) and BN (Bulik et al. 2000; Eddy et al. 2009; Keel et al. 2004; Pinheiro et al. 2008; Striegel-Moore et al. 2005; Sullivan et al. 1998), others have identified subgroups not yet recognized as formal diagnostic categories in DSM-IV, including binge eating disorder (Bulik et al. 2000; Eddy et al. 2009; Mitchell et al. 2007; Pinheiro et al. 2008; Striegel-Moore et al. 2005), purging disorder (Mitchell et al. 2007; Pinheiro et al. 2008; Striegel-Moore et al. 2005), and night eating syndrome (Striegel-Moore et al. 2008).

The generalizability of previous LCA and LPA findings to populations underrepresented in mental health research may be limited, however, by the demographic homogeneity of study samples. Specifically, only three studies have included participants from outside the United States, including Canada (Keel et al. 2004), Europe (Keel et al. 2004; Pinheiro et al. 2008), and Australia (Wade et al. 2006), and only one study has included a large proportion of non-Caucasian participants (Striegel-Moore et al. 2005). To date, no LCA or LPA studies have investigated the latent structure of eating pathology among participants outside high-income countries. This lack of broad ethnic, social, and cultural representation is consistent with meta-trends in the broader psychiatric literature, in which just 6% of articles published in the field's top journals originate from the global regions outside of Western Europe, North America, Australia, or New Zealand that represent more than 90% of the world's population (Patel and Sumathipala 2001).

Designated a priority area for adolescent mental health by the World Health Organization (2003), eating disorders have global distribution and public health significance. Because eating pathology may present differently outside of North America and Europe, empirical typologies derived from previous eating disorder LCA and LPA studies may not capture the full range of possible presentations. For example, epidemiological and case-finding investigations have found AN to be rare among majority blacks in Curaçao (Hoek et al. 2005), Kenya (Njenga and Kangethe 2004), and Ghana (Bennett et al. 2004). However, a non-fat-phobic variant of AN has been identified in Hong Kong (Lee et al. 2001), Singapore (Ong et al. 1982), and Ghana (Bennett et al. 2004). Interestingly, although two LCA studies (Bulik et al. 2000; Keel et al. 2004) have identified latent classes resembling AN, and five LCA and LPA studies have identified subgroups of low- to normal-weight participants exhibiting moderate weight concerns (Bulik et al. 2000; Eddy et al. 2009; Keel et al. 2004; Mitchell et al. 2007; Wade et al. 2006), none has identified a class clearly resembling non-fat-phobic AN. This pattern of findings is consistent with etiological theories that link the core psychopathology of eating disorders—i.e., weight and shape concerns—to specific cultural and historical contexts (Becker et al. 2009; Lee et al. 2001).

The purpose of the present study was to conduct an LPA of eating disorder phenotypes in an ethnic Fijian study sample to examine potential ethnic and cultural variation in optimal categorization. Ethnic Fijians, a small-scale indigenous Pacific Islander population, are ethnically and culturally distinct from Western populations utilized in previous LCA studies. Although there is no indigenous Fijian nosologic category for eating disorders, weight management strategies are common among Fijian youth (McCabe et al. 2009), and ethnic Fijian cultural traditions support attention to appetite, eating, and weight (Becker 1995; Mavoa and McCabe 2008). However, in the setting of globalizing economic and cultural influences on the nutritional environment (Hughes and Lawrence 2005), urban migration, and social norms for appearance, eating pathology (Becker et al. 2002) and obesity (Becker et al. 2005; Mavoa and McCabe 2008) have become more common in ethnic Fijian females. Weight management strategies include use of an extensive traditional herbal pharmacopoeia *(dranu)* both to prevent weight loss (Becker 1995) and to prevent weight gain (Becker et al. 2010b) and suggest the potential for cross-cultural plasticity in eating disorder presentation.

Therefore, our primary hypothesis was that an LPA utilizing both conventional DSM-IV and uniquely Fijian eating disorder symptoms as indicators would identify novel and culture-specific subgroups with possibly greater local relevance than those identified in previous eating disorder LCAs and LPAs. Our secondary hypothesis was that symptomatic latent classes would differ from asymptomatic classes on external validators, including eating pathology, clinical impairment, and general psychopathology. Finally, a post hoc aim was to explore whether symptomatic latent classes were associated with differential social and cultural characteristics.

Methods

SAMPLE CHARACTERISTICS

Ethnic Fijian schoolgirls ($N=523$) enrolled in 12 secondary schools registered within one sector of the Fiji Ministry of Education participated in this study, which was part of a larger investigation on social transition and psychopathology risk. Girls aged 15–20 years were eligible for inclusion. All of the invited schools agreed to participate, and 71% of eligible students enrolled in the study. Participants' mean age was 16.67 (SD = 1.09) years, and mean body mass index (BMI) was 23.96 (SD = 3.35) kg/m^2. Participants were evenly divided between rural (50%, n = 262) and peri-urban (50%, n = 261) locations. Fewer than half (41%, n = 216) lived in relative material affluence (i.e., operationalized as having household access to electricity, a gas stove, a refrigerator, and running water); the majority (59%, n = 307) lived in relative material poverty (i.e., lacking one or more of these goods or services). Furthermore, 41% (n = 216) reported having sometimes gone hungry in the past month due to insufficient food in the home.

PROCEDURE

The study used data originally collected as part of a two-stage design described previously (Becker et al. 2010b, 2010c). Briefly, all participants completed a self-report battery at Stage 1. Assessments were offered in either English (the language of formal instruction) or the vernacular (Fijian) language. For LPA indicators, we drew from Stage 1 self-report and anthropometric data available for the full sample (N = 523). Stage 2 interview data were available for a subsample (n = 215) selected by eligibility criteria specified in a related study identifying symptomatic (n = 178) and asymptomatic (n = 37) groups (described in Becker et al. 2010b and 2010c). The Partners Human Research Committee, Harvard Medical School Human Subjects Committee, and Fiji National Research Ethical Review Committee approved the data collection. The Partners Human Research Committee approved the secondary data analyses.

MEASURES

Eating Pathology

We assessed eating pathology with the Eating Disorder Examination Questionnaire (EDE-Q) Version 5.2, adapted to include an item assessing herbal purgative use. The EDE-Q is a self-report measure evaluating the domains of Restraint, Eating Concern, Shape Concern, and Weight Concern (Fairburn and Beglin 1994). All participants rated the frequency of eating disorder symptoms over the past 28 days on a Likert scale ranging from "no days" to "every day." Internal consistency, retest reliability, and construct validity were adequate in our sample (Becker et al. 2010c).

Herbal Purgative Use

We evaluated herbal purgative use as a potential LPA indicator with the following item incorporated into the EDE-Q: "Over the past 28 days, how many times have you taken traditional Fijian *dranu* to cause diarrhea, clean out your stomach, or suppress your appetite as a means of controlling your shape or weight?" We previously reported that self-reported herbal purgative use was prevalent in our sample and significantly associated with both eating pathology (Becker et al. 2010c) and eating-related clinical impairment (Becker et al. 2010b).

Evaluation of Herbal Purgative Use to Qualify It as a Potential Indicator of Eating Pathology

Because the phrasing of this single assessment item could conceivably encompass nonpathological (i.e., culturally sanctioned medicinal) use of *dranu,* we sought to ascertain that herbal purgative use was rationalized as a mode of weight management by at least some participants, in order to justify its inclusion as an LPA indicator. In order to interrogate the rationales for herbal purgative use and confirm its local cultural relevance as a potential sign of eating pathology, we examined portions of Stage 2 interview transcripts from a convenience sample of 19 respondents who had endorsed this behavior on the EDE-Q. Transcripts were from a semi-structured interview based on the Eating Disorder Examination Version 16.0 (Fairburn and Beglin 1994) and adapted for this population by adding culturally and developmentally appropriate probe questions addressing the presence, motivation, and context of herbal purgative use. Of the 19, 74% ($n=14$) confirmed using herbal purgatives specifically in order to influence their shape or weight, whereas 26% ($n=5$), exclusively provided rationales less clearly linked to—or even independent of—eating pathology, such as the alleviation of postprandial discomfort after overeating ($n=1$), the prevention of appetite loss ($n=2$), or the treatment of physical illness ($n=2$). Table 23–1 displays interview transcript excerpts from six participants who affirmed that their herbal purgative use was linked to weight management and purging, although some excerpts illustrate plural rationales. Indeed, herbal purgative use was compensatory for specific overeating episodes (e.g., cases 2, 3, 4), as well as non-compensatory, but still motivated by weight management goals (e.g., cases 1, 5, 6). Notably, we found evidence that family members sometimes encouraged or enabled herbal purgative use (e.g., cases 1, 3, 4, 6). Consistent with our study aim to encompass a broad range of behaviors that might reflect culture-specific variation in eating pathology, we conceptualized herbal purgative use as a possible eating disorder symptom and utilized it as an indicator variable in our LPA.

Body Mass Index

BMI was calculated as weight in kilograms divided by height in meters squared, using height and weight estimates generated from measured values at Stage 1. We measured weight with an electronic scale to the nearest 0.2 kg and height with a portable stadiometer to the nearest millimeter with subjects in light clothing without shoes. Weight estimates were corrected for clothing by subtracting 0.5 kg, and height estimates were rounded to the nearest centimeter.

TABLE 23–1. Excerpted Eating Disorder Examination (EDE) interview transcript data illustrating a rationale for herbal purgative use to compensate for episodes of overeating and/or control shape or weight among six study participants who self-reported herbal purgative use in the past 28 days

Case number	Frequency of herbal purgative use in past 28 days[a]	Peri-urban school	Age	BMI	EDE-Q Global Score	Excerpts from participant responses to the initial EDE probe item: "Over the past 4 weeks, have you taken *dranu* as a means of controlling your shape or weight?"
1	1	No	18	24.14	2.48	"Yes, madam. [INT] [...] It's [called] *kura*. [INT] [...] [It causes] vomiting [INT] [...] and sometimes I get diarrhea. [INT] [...] It's, uh, Fijian medicine [...] [My parents] think that, uh, inside their body can come out and have the body to lose weight. [INT: And they want you to lose weight?] Yes, ma'am."
2	1	Yes	18	28.12	4.19	"Yes, I tried to vomit. [INT] I drank to my mom's, like, herbal medicine I don't know for a cough, and I just tried it to take care of things, and I just drank it and then I started feeling sick and started vomiting. [INT: Did you do it because you wanted to get rid of the food?] Yes. [...] [INT: Did you do it after you felt like you had eaten too much, or did you just do it?] No, after I ate too much."
3	2	Yes	16	23.93	3.08	"Yes, ma'am. [INT] [...] Fijian *dranu*. [INT] [...] My mother gave it to me [INT] [...] so it, um, because my stomach, to clean it out. [INT: Why did you feel like you needed to clean your stomach?] Because I had a lot to, I ate a lot. [INT: So you ate a lot?] Yes, ma'am. [INT: And you wanted to get rid of it? But not to change your shape or weight?] Yes. [INT: Or to stay the same?] Yes, ma'am. [INT: Was it to stay the same shape and weight?] Yes, ma'am."

TABLE 23–1. Excerpted Eating Disorder Examination (EDE) interview transcript data illustrating a rationale for herbal purgative use to compensate for episodes of overeating and/or control shape or weight among six study participants who self-reported herbal purgative use in the past 28 days *(continued)*

Case number	Frequency of herbal purgative use in past 28 days[a]	Peri-urban school	Age	BMI	EDE-Q Global Score	Excerpts from participant responses to the initial EDE probe item: "Over the past 4 weeks, have you taken *dranu* as a means of controlling your shape or weight?"
4	5	Yes	17	22.11	3.36	"Yes. [INT] A Fijian one. [INT] It was in liquid form [INT] from a plant. [INT] We usually drink it as a whole family [INT] […] to cut down on my eating habits and to lose weight. [INT] […] It cleans out my stomach and makes me go to the loo most of the time. [INT: Did you do this after you felt you had eaten too much, like those times we talked about, or did you do it when you weren't eating too much?] When I was eating too much [INT] […] so that all the unwanted stuff could come out and that you could lose weight, be fit and all."
5	5	No	17	22.77	2.28	"Yeah. [INT] It was, uh, it was before, when my father told me that I was like overweight. […] I was, like, um, very, um, not satisfied with my weight, so I tried Fijian medicine [INT] […] I took it and I tried to like make me sick so that I could, uh, vomit and like […] [have] diarrhea […] so that it could wash out. […] [INT: This was to control your shape and weight?] Shape and weight. [INT: Because your father told you that you were too big?] Yeah, that's why I took it."

TABLE 23–1. Excerpted Eating Disorder Examination (EDE) interview transcript data illustrating a rationale for herbal purgative use to compensate for episodes of overeating and/or control shape or weight among six study participants who self-reported herbal purgative use in the past 28 days *(continued)*

Case number	Frequency of herbal purgative use in past 28 days[a]	Peri-urban school	Age	BMI	EDE-Q Global Score	Excerpts from participant responses to the initial EDE probe item: "Over the past 4 weeks, have you taken *dranu* as a means of controlling your shape or weight?"
6	28	Yes	18	24.82	3.24	"Yes. [INT] [...] It was a liquid. [INT] [INT] My mother [gave it to me]. [INT] Um, she says it's for girls [INT] to clean the stomach from, uh, everything. [INT] [...] It helps. [INT] It makes me go to the, use the toilet. [INT: And did you do this to lose weight, too? Did you use it to control your weight?] Yes. [INT] Sometimes I take it, like, every day. [INT] [...] Just for keeping safe and, uh, control something, control anything that can happen. [...] [INT: Do you also do it to lose weight?] Yes. [INT: To be slim?] Uh-hmm."

Note. BMI = body mass index; *dranu* = a generic term for indigenous Fijian medicinal herbal preparations; EDE-Q = Eating Disorder Examination Questionnaire; [INT] = interviewer question omitted; *kura* = a specific Fijian herbal preparation. [...] = participant comment omitted.
[a]Reported on the EDE-Q.

Impairment and Comorbid Psychopathology

The Clinical Impairment Assessment (Bohn et al. 2008) evaluates the extent to which eating disorder symptoms negatively impact mood, cognitive functioning, and relationships, with four-point response options ranging from "not at all" to "a lot." It was adapted and administered to Stage 2 participants (*n*=215) as a structured interview. Internal consistency was adequate in our sample (Becker et al. 2010b). The Center for Epidemiologic Studies Depression Scale is a self-report measure of depressive symptoms (e.g., low mood, hopelessness) over the past 7 days (Radloff 1977) and was used to measure psychopathology that is often comorbid with disordered eating. The items, which are scored on a four-point Likert scale ranging from less than 1 day to 5 or more days, have been used successfully in non-Western adolescent populations (Ghubash et al. 2000; Yang et al. 2004). For this study, participants received scores as long as they responded to at least 90% of the scale items.

Cultural Orientation

We assessed cultural orientation with composite measures derived from Likert items relating multiple dimensions of both Western/global and ethnic Fijian cultural orientation. Development, translation, and psychometric evaluation of these measures are described elsewhere (Becker et al. 2010a). For this study, participants received scores as long as they answered at least 80% of scale items.

Indigenous Practices: *Kava* and *Dranu* Use

As an additional proxy for traditional Fijian orientation, we queried the use of indigenous health and social practices. We evaluated use of *kava* (a ceremonial and social traditional beverage prepared from dried *Piper methysticum* root) in the past 30 days on a Likert scale ranging from 0 (no days) to 5 (every day). We also assessed whether participants had used traditional herbal medicine to prevent and/or treat an indigenous illness, *macake* (characterized by loss of appetite; see Becker 1995), in the past month.

Peer Eating Pathology

We evaluated the perceived prevalence of peer eating pathology in participants' social networks by asking them to estimate the proportion of "your five or so closest friends" who had engaged in dieting, fasting, and vomiting/laxative abuse in the past 30 days on a four-point Likert scale ranging from "none of them" to "all of them." These items exhibited "moderate" test-retest reliability ($\kappa=0.41$ for dieting; $\kappa=0.48$ for fasting: $\kappa=0.53$ for vomiting/laxative use) (Landis and Koch 1977).

LATENT PROFILE ANALYSIS

LPA is a technique that utilizes maximum likelihood estimation to assign participants to mutually exclusive populations called latent classes. Classes are latent because membership is not directly observable but instead can be inferred by evaluating the pattern of inter-correlations among indicator variables. The purpose of LPA is to identify the smallest number of classes that could account for these inter-correlations, thus minimizing the associations among indicator variables within each latent class and achieving a state of conditional independence. In contrast to LCA, which accepts only dichotomous indicator variables, LPA utilizes nominal, ordinal, or continuous indicators.

Consistent with previous LCA and LPA studies utilizing community samples (Bulik et al. 2000; Striegel-Moore et al. 2005; Sullivan et al. 1998), we included only symptomatic participants in our LPA in order to enhance statistical power to identify multiple pathological groups. Because the base rate of AN symptoms was quite low in our sample (i.e., only 1% had a BMI less than 17.5 kg/m^2 and 4% endorsed amenorrhea), we restricted our LPA to symptoms characterizing a diagnosis of BN. Therefore, we included only those participants who self-reported vomiting or herbal purgative use in the past 28 days via the EDE-Q ($n=222$). LPA indicator variables reflected the frequency of EDE-Q bulimic symptoms, with the addition of herbal purgative use. Because both symptom frequencies and Likert endorsement of our indicator variables were positively skewed, we transformed indicators into dichotomies or ordered categories based on natural breaks in the distributions. Our LPA indicator variables were as follows: 1) overvaluation of weight and shape ("not at all" [mean of EDE-Q overvaluation items <1], "slightly" [mean of EDE-Q overvaluation items ≥1, <3], "moderately" to "markedly" [mean of EDE-Q overvaluation items ≥3]); 2) binge eating (0, 1–3, 4 or more episodes); 3) vomiting (0 vs. ≥1 episode); 4) laxative use (0 vs. ≥1 episode); 5) fasting (0 vs. ≥1 episode); 6) driven exercise (0, 1–4, 5 or more episodes); and 7) herbal purgative use (0 vs. ≥1 episode).

We conducted our LPA using Latent GOLD 4.5 (Vermunt and Magidson 2005). We evaluated conditional independence by identifying the class solution associated with the lowest values of the Bayesian information criterion and the consistent Akaike information criterion as well as the minimization of cross-classification probabilities. We examined bivariate residuals (indices of the remaining correlations among indicator variables within latent classes) to ensure that none was greater than 5. Because no more than 2% of participants had missing values on any indicator variable, all 222 participants who endorsed self-induced vomiting or herbal purgative use in the past 28 days were submitted to LCA, and the remaining 301 participants served as a nonpurging control group in subsequent validation analyses.

VALIDATION ANALYSES

We hypothesized that if purging is a valid marker of psychopathology among ethnic Fijian girls, then the latent classes would score significantly higher than nonpurging participants with regard to 1) eating pathology (EDE-Q), 2) clinical impairment associated with disordered eating symptoms (Clinical Impairment Assessment), and 3) depressive symptoms (Center for Epidemiologic Studies Depression Scale). Furthermore, given the potential confounding effect of impoverished food environment on the cross-cultural assessment of eating pathology (le Grange et al. 2004), we wanted to ensure that the classes did not differ from one another or from the nonpurging group on the 1-month prevalence of hunger due to lack of food in the home. To evaluate these hypotheses, we conducted a series of analyses of variance and χ^2 tests. To reduce type I error, we set α to 0.01 for each omnibus test. To follow up statistically significant F tests, we utilized Fisher's least significant difference post hoc comparisons. To follow up statistically significant omnibus χ^2 tests, we utilized a Bonferroni correction by dividing $\alpha = 0.05$ by the number of unique pairwise comparisons. We conducted our validation analyses on SPSS Version 16.0 (SPSS 2007).

POST HOC CLASS COMPARISONS OF POTENTIAL ETIOLOGICAL VARIABLES

A third aim of the study was to generate hypotheses about the social and cultural characteristics that could provide insights into the potentially distinct etiologies of symptomatic latent classes. Therefore, we used t tests and χ^2 analyses to compare levels of cultural orientation, indigenous health practices, and peer eating pathology across classes. We again set α to 0.01 to reduce type I error and conducted these post hoc analyses on SPSS Version 16.0.

Results

LATENT PROFILE ANALYSIS

We evaluated models with one to five classes (model fit indices available upon request from the first author).[1] In order to meet the assumptions of the LPA model, we allowed for the conditional dependence of three pairwise correlations of indicators in which bivariate residuals were greater than 5: 1) herbal purgative use/laxative use, 2) driven exercise/overvaluation, and 3) laxative use/overvaluation.

---

[1]Because of our recruitment strategy, participants could be considered nested within school. Class membership was associated with school ($\chi^2_{22} = 34.92$, $P = 0.04$), but the effect size was small (Cramer's $V = 0.18$). We therefore re-ran our LPA with school as a covariate. Results were similar with regard to number of classes, proportion of participants in each class, and characteristics of each class, so we chose to present the final results of our LPA without controlling for school.

Bayesian information criterion and consistent Akaike information criterion were lowest for the two-class model with 21 parameters. Table 23–2 displays the relative endorsement of each indicator variable in the two latent classes, and Figure 23–1 provides a graphical depiction of these data.

The first class comprised 39% ($n = 86$) of the purging sample and was characterized primarily by high prevalence of self-induced vomiting (100%) and binge eating (90%). Members of this "BN-like class" also had moderate prevalence of herbal purgative use (58%) and laxative use (39%). In addition, the majority endorsed exercise for weight control (87%). More than half endorsed fasting (56%), and approximately one-third affirmed that weight and shape figured "moderately" to "markedly" into their self-evaluation (35%).

The second class comprised 61% of the purging sample ($n = 136$). All members of this "herbal purgative class" endorsed herbal purgative use. Other forms of purging, such as vomiting (11%) and laxative use (10%), were infrequently endorsed. Participants defined by this class also endorsed binge eating (58%) and exercise for weight control (60%) less frequently than members of the BN-like class. However, the prevalences of fasting (47%) and "moderate" to "marked" overvaluation of shape and weight (43%) were comparable with those observed in the BN-like class. Notably, had we not added this culturally relevant item to the EDE-Q, 71% of participants in the herbal purgative class would have been classified as nonpurging because of their negative responses to the items probing self-induced vomiting and laxative use.

VALIDATION ANALYSES

Results of the validation analyses are presented in Table 23–3; the P values presented represent Fisher's least significant difference post hoc pairwise comparisons, which we conducted to follow up omnibus tests that already met our $\alpha = 0.01$ criterion for statistical significance.

Eating Pathology

Participants in the BN-like and herbal purgative classes endorsed similar levels of eating pathology on the EDE-Q. As hypothesized, the BN-like and herbal purgative classes both endorsed significantly greater EDE-Q Global, Restraint, Eating Concern, Shape Concern, and Weight Concern scale scores than the nonpurging group (all P values < 0.05). The BN-like class, however, endorsed significantly greater eating concern than the herbal purgative class ($P = 0.03$).

Impairment and Comorbid Psychopathology

Contrary to our expectations, the herbal purgative class endorsed significantly greater clinical impairment related to disordered eating than the BN-like class ($P = 0.03$), and the BN-like class did not differ from the nonpurging group with re-

TABLE 23–2. Prevalence of eating disorder symptom endorsement in the latent profile analysis–derived bulimia nervosa (BN)-like class and herbal purgative class

	BN-like (*n*=86) *n* (%)	Herbal purgative (*n*=136) *n* (%)
Overvaluation of weight and shape		
0 ("Not at all"/mean of EDE-Q overvaluation items < 1)	8 (9)	21 (15)
1 ("Slightly"/Mean of EDE-Q overvaluation items ≥1, <3)	**48 (56)**	57 (42)
2 ("Moderately" to "markedly"/mean of EDE-Q overvaluation items ≥3)	30 (35)	**58 (43)**
Binge eating		
0 (None)	9 (10)	57 (42)
1 (1–3 episodes)	**60 (70)**	**62 (46)**
2 (≥4 episodes)	17 (20)	16 (12)
Self-induced vomiting		
0 (None)	0 (0)	**119 (89)**
1 (≥1 episode)	**86 (100)**	15 (11)
Laxative use		
0 (None)	**51 (61)**	**121 (90)**
1 (≥1 episode)	33 (39)	13 (10)
Fasting		
0 (None)	38 (44)	**72 (53)**
1 (≥1 episode)	**48 (56)**	64 (47)
Driven exercise		
0 (None)	11 (13)	**53 (40)**
1 (1–4 episodes)	**51 (59)**	51 (39)
2 (≥5 episodes)	24 (28)	28 (21)
Herbal purgative use		
0 (None)	36 (42)	0 (0)
1 (≥1 episode)	**50 (58)**	**136 (100)**

Note. Within each cell, the bolded percentage indicates the modal response for that variable within that latent class. Numbers in some cells do not add up to the total number of participants in that latent class due to missing data on that variable.
EDE-Q=Eating Disorder Examination Questionnaire.

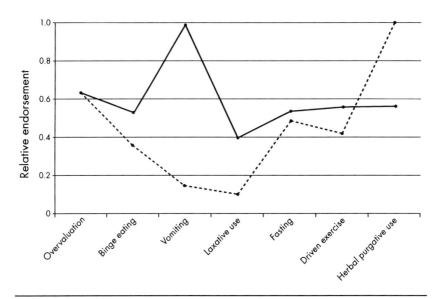

FIGURE 23–1. Relative endorsement of eating disorder symptom indicators in the bulimia nervosa–like class (represented by the *solid line*) and herbal purgative class (represented by the *dashed line*).

For dichotomous variables (vomiting, laxative use, fasting, and herbal purgative use), relative endorsement is plotted as the percentage of participants in each class who endorsed that symptom. For ordinal variables (overvaluation, binge eating, and driven exercise), relative endorsement is plotted as the mean of the three ordered categories (assigned point values of 0, 1, and 2 for increasingly greater frequencies) divided by two, so as to fit on a 0–1 scale.

gard to clinical impairment. In line with predictions, the herbal purgative class endorsed greater clinical impairment than the nonpurging group ($P<0.001$). As expected, both the BN-like ($P=0.005$) and herbal purgative ($P=0.01$) classes reported higher levels of comorbid depressive symptoms than the nonpurging group.

Demographics

The two classes did not differ from one another or from the nonpurging group on demographic characteristics, including age, BMI, peri-urban school location, relative material poverty, and hunger.

POST HOC CLASS COMPARISONS OF POTENTIAL ETIOLOGICAL VARIABLES

No significant sociodemographic or cultural differences were identified between BN-like and herbal purgative classes, including cultural orientation, indigenous practices, and peer eating pathology (Table 23–4).

TABLE 23–3. Comparison of external validators in the latent profile analysis–derived bulimia nervosa (BN)–like and herbal purgative classes versus the nonpurging group

	Mean (SD) or n (%)			F_{df} or χ^2_{df}	P	Effect size
	BN-like (n=86)	Herbal purgative (n=136)	Nonpurging (n=301)			
Eating pathology						
EDE-Q Global	2.08 (0.93)[a]	1.90 (1.11)[a]	1.49 (1.05)[b]	$F_{2,519} = 13.60$	< 0.001	$\eta^2_p = 0.050$
EDE-Q Restraint	1.28 (1.09)[a]	1.20 (1.24)[a]	0.71 (0.88)[b]	$F_{2,519} = 16.39$	< 0.001	$\eta^2_p = 0.059$
EDE-Q Eating Concern	1.84 (1.01)[a]	1.51 (1.20)[b]	1.28 (1.09)[c]	$F_{2,519} = 9.14$	< 0.001	$\eta^2_p = 0.034$
EDE-Q Shape Concern	2.62 (1.28)[a]	2.50 (1.45)[a]	2.09 (1.47)[b]	$F_{2,520} = 6.77$	0.001	$\eta^2_p = 0.025$
EDE-Q Weight Concern	2.55 (1.33)[a]	2.39 (1.39)[a]	1.90 (1.42)[b]	$F_{2,520} = 10.18$	< 0.001	$\eta^2_p = 0.038$
Impairment and comorbid psychopathology						
Clinical Impairment Assessment[†]	11.47 (10.43)[a]	15.39 (11.57)[b]	8.69 (10.15)[a]	$F_{2,212} = 6.34$	0.002	$\eta^2_p = 0.056$
CES-D	21.48 (7.14)[a]	20.85 (8.41)[a]	18.85 (7.25)[b]	$F_{2,514} = 5.76$	0.003	$\eta^2_p = 0.022$
Demographics						
Age (years)	16.70 (1.14)	16.74 (1.14)	16.65 (1.06)	$F_{2,520} = 0.33$	n.s.	$\eta^2_p = 0.001$
Body mass index	24.03 (3.12)	24.11 (3.29)	23.88 (3.45)	$F_{2,520} = 0.23$	n.s.	$\eta^2_p = 0.001$
Peri-urban school location	38 (44)	62 (46)	161 (54)	$\chi^2_2 = 3.69$	n.s.	$V = 0.08$
Relative material poverty	54 (63)	79 (58)	174 (58)	$\chi^2_2 = 0.71$	n.s.	$V = 0.04$
Hunger due to insufficient food (past 30 days)	41 (48)	55 (41)	120 (40)	$\chi^2_2 = 1.71$	n.s.	$V = 0.06$

Note. Within each row, means and percentages with different superscripts (a, b, c) differ significantly from one another (utilizing Fisher's least significant difference post hoc comparisons to follow up significant omnibus F tests, and Bonferroni corrections to follow up significant omnibus χ^2 tests). CES-D = Center for Epidemiologic Studies Depression Scale; df = degrees of freedom; EDE-Q = Eating Disorder Examination Questionnaire; n.s. = nonsignificant; η^2_p = partial eta squared; SD = standard deviation; V = Cramer's V. [†] Data available for Stage 2 participants only (n=215).

Discussion

To our knowledge, this study is the first LCA or LPA of eating disorder symptoms in a small-scale indigenous population and outside a high-income country. Our LPA of ethnic Fijian schoolgirls identified two latent classes associated with comparable levels of eating and general psychopathology, which we have characterized as "BN-like" and "herbal purgative" classes, respectively. The BN-like class, with its high rates of binge eating and vomiting, is phenomenologically similar to the BN classes described in previous North American and European LCAs and LPAs (Bulik et al. 2000; Eddy et al. 2009; Keel et al. 2004; Pinheiro et al. 2008; Striegel-Moore et al. 2005; Sullivan et al. 1998). In contrast, the herbal purgative class, which was characterized primarily by the use of indigenous herbal purgatives, has not been observed in previous LCAs and LPAs, nor is it represented as a distinct subtype in DSM-IV. Although the two classes were distinguished by self-reported purging modalities, they appeared to share core pathology by exhibiting remarkably similar profiles of eating and general psychopathology. Our results highlight the importance of including as LPA indicators locally meaningful behaviors that might be culture specific, such as herbal purgative use, in order to enhance the generalizability of empirically derived nosologic schemes.

Contrary to expectations, our post hoc analyses of social and cultural characteristics did not find evidence that the herbal purgative class differed from the BN-like class on either Fijian or Western/global cultural orientation or perceived disordered eating among peers. However, our study was only sufficiently powered to detect medium to large effects. Moreover, the multiple dimensions of acculturation likely have heterogeneous impacts on health outcomes (Becker et al., in press; Guarnaccia et al. 2007), and the two classes may differ on a facet of cultural orientation that we did not assess. An alternative interpretation is that ethnic Fijian girls view the two types of purging as interchangeable. Indeed, given that herbal purgatives are used to induce vomiting or diarrhea, it is conceivable that there is more overlap in purging modality than the self-report responses suggest, reflecting a response bias related to the perception that herbal purgative use is more socially acceptable than other modes of purging. Relatedly, it is possible that within-class variation with respect to purging confounds the relation between sociocultural variables and class membership. For example, the BN-like class contains respondents who also use herbal purgatives, and the herbal purgative class may include respondents who do not explicitly link their herbal purgative use to weight management or who espouse plural rationales for herbal purgative use. Moreover, the herbal purgative class we identified may not be culturally unique; surveys of North American eating disorder patients indicate that 13% (Trigazis et al. 2004) to 64% (Steffen et al. 2006) have used herbal products to induce weight loss or vomiting. Of these products, the ingestion of ipecac syrup to induce emesis in Western populations (Silber 2005) bears the greatest phenomenological similarity to the herbal

TABLE 23–4. Class comparisons of selected potential etiological variables in the latent profile analysis–derived bulimia nervosa (BN)–like and herbal purgative classes

	Mean (SD) or n (%)				
	BN-like ($n=86$)	Herbal purgative ($n=136$)	t_{df} or χ^2_{df}	P	Effect size
Cultural orientation					
Global/Western Orientation Scale	4.54 (0.90)	4.44 (0.78)	$t_{220} = 0.88$	n.s.	$d = 0.12$
Ethnic Fijian Orientation Scale	4.99 (1.48)	4.74 (1.58)	$t_{220} = 1.04$	n.s.	$d = 0.16$
Indigenous health practices					
Kava use (Likert frequency in past month)	1.30 (0.51)	1.45 (0.62)	$t_{220} = 1.91$	n.s.	$d = 0.25$
Indigenous herbal medicine use to prevent *macake*[a] (yes in past month)	44 (56)	73 (60)	$\chi^2_1 = 0.34$	n.s.	$V = 0.04$
Peer eating pathology: close friends					
Dieting	1.99 (0.75)	1.93 (0.85)	$t_{219} = 0.49$	n.s.	$d = 0.07$
Fasting	1.74 (0.83)	1.63 (0.77)	$t_{219} = 1.05$	n.s.	$d = 0.15$
Vomiting/laxative use	1.48 (0.71)	1.32 (0.62)	$t_{219} = 1.69$	n.s.	$d = 0.24$

Note. $d=$Cohen's d; df=degrees of freedom; n.s. =nonsignificant; $V=$Cramer's V.

[a]*Macake* is an indigenous illness characterized by appetite loss.

purgative use observed in Fiji. Indeed, because no previous eating disorder LCA or LPA has used ipecac or herbal product use as an indicator variable, we cannot be certain whether the emergence of an herbal purgative class in our ethnic Fijian sample reflects actual culture-specific phenomenological heterogeneity or our more inclusive operational definition of disordered eating behaviors.

The substantial prevalence of herbal purgative use in our sample suggests local vulnerability to disordered eating that could benefit from additional research attention and clinical resources. However, there are several additional implications of our findings, beyond their immediate public health relevance for the local populace. First, these results suggest that the application of a "universal" criteria set for eating disorders developed from a largely Euro-American evidence base may be insufficient to characterize the full range of phenomenological heterogeneity across populations outside of these regions; indeed, a broader—and more culturally informed—scope of symptom phenomena should be considered (Kleinman 1977). Second, indigenous nosologic categories may not identify all symptom profiles as culturally salient, even if they are associated with distress and impairment. Third, "unsupervised learning techniques" such as LCA (Magidson and Vermunt 2002, p. 38), in which group size and composition are not known a priori, may mitigate some of the limitations inherent to the application of solely etic or emic perspectives in cross-cultural evaluation by identifying novel symptom patterns. Fourth, this study provides further evidence that social environment may promote unique symptom presentations. It would be misleading, however, to interpret these results to mean that cultural context results only in superficial epiphenomenal variants on universal core pathology. Additional data are necessary to establish whether the herbal purgative class represents a clinical phenomenon with a course and outcome similar to or distinct from eating disorders described in high-income countries. For example, our preliminary qualitative data analysis suggests that characteristics of Fijian girls' herbal purgative use—insofar as it is sometimes abetted by parents or temporally unrelated to overeating—may be distinctive from purging typical of BN.

Also of note, the BN-like class in our study endorsed EDE-Q scores substantially lower than those reported for BN-like classes identified in an American LPA (Eddy et al. 2009) and European LCA (Pinheiro et al. 2008) but comparable with the population median for American female undergraduates (Luce et al. 2008). Notably, more than half of participants in both classes endorsed the use of traditional herbal therapy to prevent an indigenous illness, *macake,* which is characterized by poor appetite. The juxtaposition of a weight loss prevention strategy with purgative use suggests that weight and shape concerns may not be central to all eating disorder presentations in Fiji. Eating disorders resembling AN but presenting in the absence of weight concerns have been also been described in non-Western populations (Bennett et al. 2004; Lee et al. 2001; Ong et al. 1982). Taken together, this cultural variation in the presentation of eating pathology supports the possibility that cultural context may attenuate or exacerbate the cognitive symptoms associated with disordered eating.

Our findings should be interpreted in light of design strengths and limitations. With regard to strengths, first, we developed and adapted assessments to be culturally appropriate and in the local vernacular language, drawing from foundational ethnographic data and expert local knowledge. Second, we considered and excluded potential confounding by impoverished food environment (le Grange et al. 2004). Third, the mean Clinical Impairment Assessment score for the herbal purgative class approached the clinical cutoff of 16 that separated eating disorder cases from noncases in the original validation sample (Bohn et al. 2008), which supports our interpretation of herbal purgative use as an eating disorder symptom.

A limitation is the use of primarily self-report data to identify and validate the latent classes. Moreover, our characterization of the heterogeneity and complexity of rationales for herbal purgative use in this sample is preliminary and incomplete. Indeed, in our evaluation of herbal purgative use via narrative data, a sizeable minority of respondents did not explicitly attribute their herbal purgative use to shape and weight. Therefore, it is likely that at least some of the herbal purgative use observed in the present study may have been motivated by alternative socially sanctioned indications (e.g., medicinal usage). On the other hand, it is also conceivable that individuals may not formulate herbal purgative use as motivated by weight concerns if they do not regard weight control as a socially legitimate pursuit. Relatedly, other investigators have commented on the validity of evaluating eating pathology with self-report versus interview assessment, highlighting the potentially greater candor evidenced in self-reports of socially stigmatized behaviors (Keel et al. 2002; Mond et al. 2007). A second limitation is that our selection of LPA indicators and validators—although informed by extensive ethnographic work with this population—necessarily reflects our Western conceptual models of disordered eating and related distress. A third limitation is that because we did not observe the two respective classes longitudinally, we could not evaluate crossover between classes or the directionality of the relation between class membership and external validators. Lastly, LPA cannot distinguish differences in kind versus differences in degree. Indeed, there were more similarities than differences between the BN-like and herbal purgative classes, and future taxometric work is needed to ascertain the nature of the boundary between groups.

This study augments empirical support for cultural variation in patterning of eating disorder symptom presentation (Franko et al. 2007; Lee et al. 2001) and also has implications for clinical practice. For example, without appropriate breadth to identify clinically relevant variation, clinical and research assessment of eating pathology can result in misclassification of true cases as noncases (Bennett et al. 2004; Lee et al. 2001) and noncases as cases (le Grange et al. 2004). Indeed, the majority of participants in the herbal purgative class would have been classified as nonpurging by the EDE-Q had we not included an item referencing a culture-specific means of purging. In summary, the inclusion of populations with culturally distinctive traditions and symptoms in latent structure modeling may enhance the clinical utility of statistically derived nosological schemes in both diverse social contexts and multicultural populations.

References

American Psychiatric Association: Diagnostic and Statistical Manual of Mental Disorders, 4th Edition. Washington, DC, American Psychiatric Association, 1994

American Psychiatric Association: Diagnostic and Statistical Manual of Mental Disorders, 4th Edition, Text Revision. Washington, DC, American Psychiatric Association, 2000

Becker AE: Body, Self, and Society: The View From Fiji. Philadelphia, University of Pennsylvania Press, 1995

Becker AE, Burwell RA, Gilman SE, et al: Eating behaviours and attitudes following prolonged exposure to television among ethnic Fijian adolescent girls. Br J Psychiatry 180:509–514, 2002

Becker AE, Gilman SE, Burwell RA: Changes in prevalence of overweight and in body image among Fijian women between 1989 and 1998. Obes Res 13:110–117, 2005

Becker AE, Thomas JJ, Pike KM: Should non-fat-phobic anorexia nervosa be included in DSM-V? Int J Eat Disord 42:620–635, 2009

Becker AE, Fay K, Agnew-Blais J, et al: Development of a measure of 'acculturation' for ethnic Fijians: methodologic and conceptual considerations for application to eating disorders research. Transcult Psychiatry 47:754–788, 2010a

Becker AE, Thomas JJ, Bainivualiku A, et al: Adaptation and evaluation of the Clinical Impairment Assessment to assess disordered eating related distress in an adolescent female ethnic Fijian population. Int J Eat Disord 43:179–186, 2010b

Becker AE, Thomas JJ, Bainivualiku A, et al: Validity and reliability of a Fijian translation and adaptation of the Eating Disorder Examination Questionnaire. Int J Eat Disord 43:171–178, 2010c

Bennett D, Sharpe M, Freeman C, et al: Anorexia nervosa among female secondary school students in Ghana. Br J Psychiatry 185:312–317, 2004

Bohn K, Doll HA, Cooper Z, et al: The measurement of impairment due to eating disorder psychopathology. Behav Res Ther 46:1105–1110, 2008

Bulik CM, Sullivan PF, Kendler KS: An empirical study of the classification of eating disorders. Am J Psychiatry 157:886–895, 2000

Duncan AE, Bucholz KK, Neuman RJ, et al: Clustering of eating disorder symptoms in a general population twin sample: a latent class analysis. Psychol Med 37:1097–1107, 2007

Eddy KT, Crosby RD, Keel PK, et al: Empirical identification and validation of eating disorder phenotypes in a multisite clinical sample. J Nerv Ment Dis 197:41–49, 2009

Fairburn CG, Beglin SJ: The assessment of eating disorders: interview or self-report questionnaire? Int J Eat Disord 16:363–370, 1994

Franko DL, Becker AE, Thomas JJ, et al: Cross-ethnic differences in eating disorder symptoms and related distress. Int J Eat Disord 40:156–164, 2007

Ghubash R, Daradkeh TK, Al Naseri KS, et al: The performance of the Center for Epidemiologic Study Depression Scale (CES-D) in an Arab female community. Int J Soc Psychiatry 46:241–249, 2000

Guarnaccia PJ, Pincay IM, Alegria M, et al: Assessing diversity among Latinos: results from the NLAAS. Hisp J Behav Sci 29:510–534, 2007

Hoek HW, van Harten PN, Hermans KME, et al: The incidence of anorexia nervosa on Curaçao. Am J Psychiatry 162:748–752, 2005

Hughes RG, Lawrence MA: Globalisation, food and health in Pacific Island countries. Asia Pac J Clin Nutr 14:298–306, 2005

Keel PK, Crow S, Davis TL, et al: Assessment of eating disorders: comparison of interview and questionnaire data from a long-term follow-up study of bulimia nervosa. J Psychosom Res 53:1043–1047, 2002

Keel PK, Fichter M, Quadflieg N, et al: Application of a latent class analysis to empirically define eating disorder phenotypes. Arch Gen Psychiatry 61:192–200, 2004

Kleinman AM: Depression, somatization, and the "new cross-cultural psychiatry." Soc Sci Med 11:3–10, 1977

Landis J, Koch G: The measurement of observer agreement for categorical data. Biometrics 33:159–174, 1977

Lee S, Lee AM, Ngai E, et al: Rationales for food refusal in Chinese patients with anorexia nervosa. Int J Eat Disord 29:224–229, 2001

le Grange D, Louw J, Breen A, et al: The meaning of 'self-starvation' in impoverished black adolescents in South Africa. Cult Med Psychiatry 28:439–461, 2004

Luce KH, Crowther JH, Pole M: Eating Disorder Examination Questionnaire (EDE-Q) norms for undergraduate women. Int J Eat Disord 41:273–276, 2008

Magidson J, Vermunt JK: Latent class models for clustering: a comparison with K-means. Canadian Journal of Marketing Research 20:37–44, 2002

Mavoa HM, McCabe M: Sociocultural factors relating to Tongans' and indigenous Fijians' patterns of eating, physical activity and body size. Asia Pac J Clin Nutr 17:375–384, 2008

McCabe MP, Ricciardelli L, Waqa G, et al: Body image and body change strategies among adolescent males and females from Fiji, Tonga and Australia. Body Image 6:299–303, 2009

Mitchell JE, Crosby RD, Wonderlich SA, et al: Latent profile analysis of a cohort of patients with eating disorders not otherwise specified. Int J Eat Disord 40:S95–S98, 2007

Mond JM, Hay PJ, Rodgers B, et al: Self-report versus interview assessment of purging in a community sample of women. Eur Eat Disord Rev 15:403–409, 2007

Njenga FG, Kangethe RN: Anorexia nervosa in Kenya. East Afr Med J 81:188–193, 2004

Ong YL, Tsoi WF, Chea JS: A clinical and psychosocial study of seven cases of anorexia nervosa in Singapore. Singapore Med J 23:255–261, 1982

Patel V, Sumathipala A: International representation in psychiatric literature: survey of six leading journals. Br J Psychiatry 178:406–409, 2001

Pinheiro AP, Bulik CM, Sullivan PF, et al: An empirical study of the typology of bulimic symptoms in young Portuguese women. Int J Eat Disord 41:251–258, 2008

Radloff LS: The CES-D scale: a self-report depression scale for research in the general population. Appl Psychol Meas 1:385–401, 1977

Silber TJ: Ipecac syrup abuse, morbidity, and mortality: isn't it time to repeal its over-the-counter status? J Adolesc Health 37:256–260, 2005

SPSS: Statistical Package for the Social Sciences, 16.0 for Macintosh. Chicago, IL, SPSS, 2007

Steffen KJ, Roerig JL, Mitchell JE, et al: A survey of herbal and alternative medication use among participants with eating disorder symptoms. Int J Eat Disord 39:741–746, 2006

Striegel-Moore RH, Franko DL, Thompson D, et al: An empirical study of the typology of bulimia nervosa and its spectrum variants. Psychol Med 35:1563–1572, 2005

Striegel-Moore RH, Franko DL, Thompson D, et al: Exploring the typology of night eating syndrome. Int J Eat Disord 41:411–418, 2008

Sullivan PF, Bulik CM, Kendler KS: The epidemiology and classification of bulimia nervosa. Psychol Med 28:599–610, 1998

Thomas JJ, Vartanian LR, Brownell KD: The relationship between eating disorder not otherwise specified (EDNOS) and officially recognized eating disorders: meta-analysis and implications for DSM. Psychol Bull 135:407–433, 2009

Trigazis L, Tennankore D, Vohra S, et al: The use of herbal remedies by adolescents with eating disorders. Int J Eat Disord 35:223–228, 2004

Vermunt JK, Magidson J: Latent GOLD 4.5. Belmont, MA, Statistical Innovations Inc, 2005

Wade TD, Crosby RD, Martin NG: Use of latent profile analysis to identify eating disorder phenotypes in an adult Australian twin cohort. Arch Gen Psychiatry 63:1377–1384, 2006

World Health Organization: Caring for Children and Adolescents With Mental Disorders: Setting WHO Directions. Geneva, Switzerland, World Health Organization, 2003

Yang H-J, Soong W-T, Kuo P-H, et al: Using the CES-D in a two-phase survey for depressive disorders among nonreferred adolescents in Taipei: a stratum-specific likelihood ratio analysis. J Affect Disord 82:419–430, 2004

INDEX

Page numbers printed in **boldface** *type refer to tables or figures.*